Urban Mental Health

Urban Mental Health

Edited by

Dinesh Bhugra
Emeritus Professor of Mental Health and Cultural Diversity,
Centre for Affective Disorders, Institute of Psychiatry,
King's College London, UK

Antonio Ventriglio
Psychiatrist, Department of Mental Health, and Department
of Clinical and Experimental Medicine, University of Foggia,
Foggia, Italy

João Castaldelli-Maia
University of São Paulo Medical School, São Paulo, Brazil

Layla McCay
Director, Centre for Urban Design and Mental Health,
London, UK

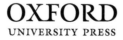

OXFORD
UNIVERSITY PRESS

OXFORD

UNIVERSITY PRESS

Great Clarendon Street, Oxford, OX2 6DP,
United Kingdom

Oxford University Press is a department of the University of Oxford.
It furthers the University's objective of excellence in research, scholarship,
and education by publishing worldwide. Oxford is a registered trade mark of
Oxford University Press in the UK and in certain other countries

© Oxford University Press 2019

The moral rights of the authors have been asserted

First Edition published in 2019

Impression: 1

Published in the United States of America by Oxford University Press
198 Madison Avenue, New York, NY 10016, United States of America

British Library Cataloguing in Publication Data

Data available

Library of Congress Control Number: 2018966914

ISBN 978–0–19–880494–9

Printed and bound by
CPI Group (UK) Ltd, Croydon, CR0 4YY

Preface

The overall proportion of people living in urban areas has been increasing rapidly, and the speed and extent of urbanization has been astonishing. The concept of cities has given way to urban areas, sprawls, or urban conurbations. The worldwide urbanization has been caused by a number of factors, of which globalization and industrialization are only two of the factors. These have certainly contributed to the speed of urbanization.

Why should living in cities be bad for one's mental health? It is not an idealized perception that the rural idyll is better. Epidemiological findings from a number of countries and settings confirm higher rates of psychiatric disorders, including alcohol and substance use in urban areas, although many authors have challenged this view and findings. Often, healthcare facilities are more likely to be situated in urban areas—whether these meet the demand or are due to ease of urban comfort is debatable.

Architecture, structures, urban spaces, and processes all play a role in the mental health of individuals is debatable. Culture embedded in urban spaces and areas is also important in moulding mental health and help seeking. Youth culture has its own needs and is influenced by urban spaces. Social determinants affect mental health and well-being, and these include urban poverty, lack of green spaces, unemployment, overcrowding, lack of proper public transport, and other factors. Aspiration and discrepancy with achievement can add to poor mental health. Migrants, even when they are from the country, do carry with them stressors related to life events and lost support and values, which can precipitate or contribute to poor mental health.

In this volume we bring together experts in the field of urban studies and mental health. We have been fortunate in our authors, who have delivered their chapters in spite of their busy schedules. We are grateful for their enthusiasm and their contributions.

Our thanks are also due to Pete Stevenson, Senior Commissioning Editor at Oxford University Press, and to his team, especially Lauren Tiley and Rachel Goldsworthy, for their unstinting support.

Dinesh Bhugra
Antonio Ventriglio
João Castaldelli-Maia
Layla McCay

Contents

Section 2 **Mental ill health in cities**

Section 3 **Challenges in urban settings**

Contributors

Suraj Beloskar, Medical Officer, Ganesh Darshan Co-op Society, Mumbai, India

Vishal Bhavsar, Department of Psychosis Studies, Institute of Psychiatry, London, UK

Dinesh Bhugra, Emeritus Professor of Mental Health and Cultural Diversity, Centre for Affective Disorders, Institute of Psychiatry, King's College London, London, UK

Jed Boardman, Consultant Psychiatrist and Senior Lecturer in Social Psychiatry, Institute of Psychiatry, Psychology & Neuroscience King's College London, London, UK

Richard Bradlow, Psychiatric Registrar, Hornsby Hospital, Sydney, NSW, Australia

Jorge Javier Caraveo-Anduaga, Senior Researcher, National Institute of Psychiatry 'Dr. Ramón de la Fuente Muñiz', Mexico City, Mexico

Mauro G. Carta, Department of Social Sciences and Public Health, University of Cagliari, Cagliari, Italy

João Castaldelli-Maia, University of São Paulo Medical School, São Paulo, Brazil

Anna Chang, Southern California Institute of Architecture, Los Angeles, CA, USA

Santosh K. Chaturvedi, Professor of Psychiatry & Dean Behavioural Sciences, National Institute of Mental Health and Neuro Sciences, Bangalore, India

Fiona Choi, Research Associate, Institute of Mental Health, Department of Psychiatry, The University of British Columbia, Vancouver, Canada

Tom K.J. Craig, Professor of Social Psychiatry, Institute of Psychiatry, Psychology & Neuroscience King's College London, London, UK

Debby Darmansjah, Resident Medical Officer, Latrobe Regional Hospital, Traralgon, Victoria, Australia

Diego de Leo, Emeritus Professor of Psychiatry, Australian Institute for Suicide Research and Prevention, Griffith University, Brisbane, Australia

Jan Golembiewski, Psychological Design, Sydney, Australia

Kerry L. Jang, Professor, University of British Columbia, Vancouver, Canada

Gurvinder Kalra, Psychiatrist, Flynn Adult Inpatient Psychiatric Unit, Latrobe Regional Hospital Mental Health Services, Victoria, Australia

James B. Kirkbride, PsyLife Group, Division of Psychiatry, University College London, London, UK

Kairi Kõlves, Principal Research Fellow and Course Convener at the Australian Institute for Suicide Research and Prevention, Griffith University, Brisbane, Australia

Michael Krausz, UBC-Providence Leadership Chair for Addiction Research, Department of Psychiatry, University of British Columbia, Vancouver, Canada

Todd Litman, Victoria Transport Policy Institute, Victoria, Canada

Shubhada Maitra, Professor, Centre for Health and Mental Health, Project Director, Tarasha and Muskaan School of Social Work, Tata Institute of Social Sciences, Mumbai, India

Narayana Manjunatha, Assistant Professor of Psychiatry, National Institute of Mental Health and Neuro Sciences, Bangalore, India

Layla McCay, Director, Centre for Urban Design and Mental Health

Anthony M. Orum, Professor Emeritus, Department of Sociology, University of Illinois at Chicago, IL, USA

José Erazo Pérez, Research Assistant, Autonomous Metropolitan University, Mexico City, Mexico

Alice Roe, Programme Manager, Health Influencing, Age UK, UK

Jenny Roe, DeShong Professor in Design and Health and Director, Center for Design and Health, School of Architecture, University of Virginia, Charlottesville, VA, USA

Victoria Ross, Research Fellow, Australian Institute for Suicide Research and Prevention, Griffith University, Mt Gravatt Campus, Brisbane, Australia

Peter Schofield, MRC Fellow and Wolfson Lecturer in Population Health, School of Population Health Sciences, King's College London, London, UK

Neha Singh, Medical Officer, Kalamboli, Mumbai, India

Francesca Solmi, PsyLife Group, Division of Psychiatry, University College London, London, UK

Michael Jae Song, Researcher, Department of Psychiatry, University of British Columbia, Canada

Verena Strehlau, Scientist at the Centre of Health Evaluation and Outcome Sciences (CHEOS), Vancouver, Canada

Emily Suzuki, Tokyo Medical and Dental University, Tokyo, Japan

Nora Angélica Martínez Vélez, Researcher, National Institute of Psychiatry 'Dr. Ramón de la Fuente Muñiz', Mexico City, Mexico

Antonio Ventriglio, Psychiatrist, Department of Mental Health, and Department of Clinical and Experimental Medicine, University of Foggia, Foggia, Italy

Shuo Zhang, Health Service and Population Research, Institute of Psychiatry, London, UK

Abbreviations

ACC	anterior caudal cortex	ICD-10	10th Revision of the International Classification of Diseases
ACT	assertive community treatment		
ADHD	attention deficit–hyperactivity disorder	ICM	intensive case management
		IOM	International Organization for Migration
ÆSOP	Aetiology and Ethnicity in Schizophrenia and Other Psychoses		
		IPS	Individual Placement and Support
aHR	adjusted hazard ratio	LAMI	low-and-middle-income
AOT	Assertive Outreach Team	LGBTQI	lesbian, gay, bisexual, transgender, queer, and intersex
AR	augmented reality		
ASD	autism spectrum disorder		
BIS	Brief Impairment Scale	LIT	Lost in Transition
BMI	body mass index	NCD	non-communicable disease
CAC	community amenity contribution	NIMBY	Not in My Back Yard
		NYC	New York City
CBTD	Brief Screening and Diagnostic Questionnaire	pACC	perigenual anterior caudal cortex
CES-D	Center for Epidemiologic Studies Depression Scale	PAN	permanent account number
		rDLPFC	right dorsolateral prefrontal cortex
CI	confidence interval		
CMD	common mental disorders	RE	restorative environment
DCC	day-care centre	RN	restorative niche
DHS	Directorate of Health Services	SCARF	Schizophrenia Research Foundation
DOHMH	Department of Health and Mental Health Hygiene		
		SMHC	School Mental Health Consultants
DSM-IV	Diagnostic and Statistical Manual of Mental Disorders, 4th Edition		
		TMG	Tokyo Metropolitan Government
DUP	duration of untreated psychosis	UNCRPD	United Nations Convention on Rights of Persons with Psychosocial Disabilities
ELSA Brazil	Brazilian Longitudinal Study of Adult Health		
FEP	first-episode psychosis	URC	Urgent Response Center
GAPS	Green, Active, Pro-social and Safe Places	VPD	Vancouver Police Department
		WHO	World Health Organization
GSM	gender and sexual minority		
ICD	International Classification of Diseases		

Section 1

Urbanization and processes

Chapter 1

Introduction

Dinesh Bhugra, Antonio Ventriglio,
João Castaldelli-Maia, and Layla McCay

The rapid increase in the number of people living in urban areas raises a number of health-related issues. These include both physical and mental ill health. However, by and large, healthcare providers with the latest diagnostic tools and facilities (including machines) are much more likely to be based in urban sprawls and urban conurbations. The real two-tier health care—one level for urban areas and another, perhaps more low-key, in rural areas—is much more striking in low- and middle-income countries. Even in countries as rich as the USA, the health care provided comes from very many centres of excellence, most likely to be based in urban areas. In the UK, even with its National Health Service (NHS), most of the regional specialist facilities are in urban areas. This interaction between high demand and high supply does create a differential healthcare system. There is no doubt that many healthcare issues in urban areas are also related to social determinants such as unemployment, poverty, overcrowding, lack of green spaces, and so on. Furthermore, these social determinants are strongly influenced by geopolitical determinants, which lead to migration and migrants often settle in urban areas and conurbations. That is not to say that these factors do not occur in rural areas, which are sometimes described as idyllic. That view of idyllic rural life remains a fantasy in many settings and countries.

Urban spaces also raise specific issues in the setting of people and their activities. Within urban areas are special spaces for individuals, community, work, and sex.

Prakash [1] reminds us that nearly as old as the modern city is the critical attention given to it by writers and commentators. He argues that the concept of a city (which was seen as a clearly defined unit) has been replaced by the amorphous and expanding spaces of modern networks. Hence, the notion of the urban sprawl or conurbation starts to emerge. These may be linked by public transport systems or by geographical accessibility, but with the advent of social media, contact between individuals, whether they are family members or strangers, has become much more rapid and often demands instant gratification. The urban or city centre and peripheral sprawls have not only superseded the city, but also the ideas related to living in such spaces [2]. A further complicating dimension attached to all this is the culture of the groups, communities, and individuals who live in these geographical areas, thereby contributing to the culture of the place. Big cities do not have a homogenous culture; it is groups that give the city its cultural patina.

Over the last 100 years, the pace of change in generating a bustling metropolis with millions of people living cheek by jowl has been truly impressive. The rate of development and progress of large urban areas has moved from North America and Europe to Asia and Africa. There is no doubt that Mexico City, São Paulo, and Mumbai, along with many other cities around the globe, are all experiencing massive growth and expansion in terms of geographical spread and, as a result, of movement of people. Migration is often of the within-country variety and largely rural to urban, although people from smaller cities are equally likely to move into metropolitan cities. In China, this has resulted from rapid expansion of manufacturing and rapid economic growth. Regional urban constellations have started emerging in China.

There is no doubt that historical aspects of the building of cities and their spaces are likely to affect an individual's health and consequent functioning. Prakash [1] suggests that historical processes in the urban form itself (not only the form and the structure of the city, but also the architecture of the urban life and representations) lead to the formation of society, the economy, culture, and politics. All these are of relevance to people's mental health.

Prakash [1] goes on to highlight that, as a result of globalization, different legal regimes have started to emerge. The original capitalist interpretations and impact of urbanization is giving way to informational networks and 'private modernity', which have marginalized old urban solidarities [3]. Virlio [4] predicted the dissolution of the city by media and communication, but it can also be argued that there are different levels and types of communication and networks; therefore, the impact will also be variable. There is the physical architectural network of the city. This is accompanied by the physical–emotional network of the people living in a communal or in a community space. Then there is the physical–emotional space, which could thrive on social media and its links. Finally, it could be argued that there exists a cognitive network between individuals, which will influence their 'self' and self-esteem. From the central space in urban areas or what were described and known as urban centres or city centres, these centres have now moved to the periphery and cities may now contain

multiple centres. Koolhas [5] described these as occurring as a result of spontaneous fragmentation also related to a massive increase in consumption. From
the perspective of the study of mental health, such fragmentation also leads to
fragmentation in whatever networks the individuals (or city dwellers) have. In
addition, social support starts to appear at a distance. In the past, such support
may well have contributed to resilience, but in the urban sprawl and with the social media, the degree and the quality of the support is likely to change dramatically. The changes in family networks and the shift from kinship-based settings
in many low- and middle-income countries to more individualistic settings has
meant that an additional dimension must be taken into account while trying to
develop healthcare delivery. The multiple public spaces in urban areas, such as
shopping malls, cineplexes, railway stations, airports, sports complexes, public
parks, and other spaces, are both general and individual in that their meanings
to urban dwellers may be both general and individual. Living in crowded spaces
the individual dweller may see the public green space as both personal, providing respite, and general, where individuals can meet others, as seen in Hong
Kong, where, on Sunday afternoons, domestic employees congregate according
to their country of origin and spend the afternoon talking to each other, sharing
food and space. These 'formally informal' networks allow individuals to share
their concerns and support each other. Cities also raise aspirations among those
who migrate to the cities, but the discrepancy between aspiration and achievement may contribute to mental ill health.

Prakash [1] points out that Lefebvre [2] writes of urban space as occupation
(by the individuals and the community). Urban spaces mould political concerns as political concerns are a projection of urban spaces so, in turn, they influence public spaces. Urban spaces can generate political concerns, which may
further contribute to mental ill health. The portrayal of urban spaces in cinema
(which is viewed in an urban space) highlights the role cities play in the lives
of individuals and their families, as well as employers. An additional factor that
needs detailed examination in the city is youth culture—gangs, games, entertainment venues, and access to alcohol and other substances affect youth culture and youth mental health. The cultural forms and cultural norms both very
strongly influence mental health and urbanicity. Embedded within the urban
values is also the concept of traditionalism or modernity. Small towns that have
grown into big urban sprawls can carry within their spaces traditional small
businesses and traditional values living in parallel with modern values and expectations. Recent developments in many cities around the world where high-
street shops are closing down and/or being taken over by cafes and meeting
places, thereby changing the function of the previously well-recognized shopping areas. Thus, dystopian perspectives attributed to modernity—especially

in cultures-in-transition—may impact upon traditional attitudes and values, thereby affecting an individual's self and self-esteem.

This volume discusses a number of issues, from the impact of globalization to urban mental health to the impact of architecture on the epidemiology of mental illness.

Layla McCay, in her chapter on urban design (Chapter 3), argues that any associations between the urban living environment and mental health are becoming increasingly apparent. People who live in a city often have increased pre-existing risk factors for mental illness. However, it is entirely possible that the intrinsic features of the city's built environment further exacerbate people's risk. Cities can expose vulnerable people to further socio-economic disparities and discrimination, deliver sensory input overload, and further erode many of the protective factors that are associated with maintaining good mental health. McCay suggests that one way forward will be to work with urban planners and designers in promoting and supporting public mental health. Urban mental health may be improved by designing cities to provide residents with regular access to green space, integrating physical activity opportunities, facilitating positive, natural social interactions, and fostering feelings of safety further public mental health education, which may facilitate better mental health and well-being.

Anthony Orum, in Chapter 2, sets the scene for sociology of urban studies and mental health, and emphasizes that not only cities, but also urban places are a fascinating focus of study. He points out that when studying not only physical urban spaces, but also processes that happen in urban spaces, sociology can provide a helpful insight. Historically, various schools of study of sociology have highlighted various aspects of urban places and areas. For several decades the Chicago School of Sociology shaped urban sociology as a whole by seeing and recognizing the city as a place consisting of different concentric zones. These zones will include a manufacturing zone, for example, as well as a red light district, as well as particular ethnic settlements. However, as manufacturing has moved out of many cities, these derelict zones have developed further areas of concerns, although in many settings artists and others have moved into such urban spaces, creating new settings. There is no doubt that each of these zones carries with it various issues related to mental health, well-being, and levels of mental illness. Some of the earliest studies in urban mental health originated from Chicago, recognizing the impact of urbanicity on people's well-being. Several chapters in this volume remind us of the concept of public space and its functioning, which, in turn, are likely to create a number of issues that need exploration. On the one hand, these urban spaces allow, and indeed encourage, people to get together and, on the other, it has been argued that the reality of the world today has eliminated the notion of public space. This chapter explores these issues within the broader context of globalization. Kalra et al. link globalization with urbanization and argue that the processes related to globalization, and indeed globalization itself, affect health directly and indirectly in a number of ways. One aspect of globalization is an increase in the movement of people and resources both within the country and across countries, which create problems of its own. The variations reported in rates of various psychiatric and physical illnesses are often ignored and the focus is often on similarities across cultures, thereby creating a homogeneous global culture with an emphasis on the premise to universalize the provision of health treatment for all people in a Westernized allopathic care ignoring local models of care. It is important to bear this in mind because with urbanization as a direct correlate of globalization and resulting industrialization, social, economic, and political transitions are taking place, which at one level are not only increasing economic growth, but also discrepancies, but on another level changing expectations of the individual patients and their families. It is worth recognizing that politically and in civic terms globalization has become an oft-used and abused term to describe a collection of processes all involving social economic and cultural *exchanges*. The abuse of the term is related to its negative aspects and political interpretations, leading to xenophobia and nationalism. However, the term retains a wide currency and usage, which focuses on debates about economics, development, international relations, and, increasingly, health. Furthermore, the processes related to globalization have influenced health care, resources, policy making, and provision in global circles of influence for much of the past 30 years. Developing the same theme further, Shuo Zhang, Vishal Bhavsar and Dinesh Bhugra focus in Chapter 12 on the prevalence and incidence of schizophrenia, which is shown to have a higher urban incidence. The approach in social psychiatry so far has been to concentrate on the impact of the urban environment on psychosis and to associate, correlate, and classify factors of interest. The individual's experience of and in the city can be conceptualized in terms of cross-cultural contact across constructed boundaries of identity, ethnicity, and class. Acculturation is a useful beginning in thinking about how the modern city causes illness. However, Francesca Solmi and James B. Kirkbride confirm that rates of many psychiatric disorders in cities over the last seven decades or so are high, starting from Chicago studies, especially those of schizophrenia, other psychoses, mood disorders, and non-affective psychoses (Chapter 10). Reasons for the variation are many. Initially, it was hypothesized that people migrate into urban areas because of their illness, but it has also been considered whether the urban environment is the cause. This significant change thus reduced the likelihood that exposure status was a consequence of the prodromal phase of disorder, a form of reverse leading to social drift where individuals with early signs and symptoms of psychotic disorder move into more deprived, fragmented, or marginal areas. Whether this is also due to a decline in socio-economic status or desire for anonymity (a perverse feature of modern, densely populated environments) deserves further exploration. In his chapter on research, Todd Litman (Chapter 12) highlights that although studies proclaim that urban living increases mental illness and unhappiness, it is his view that a critical evaluation of the research evidence indicates that much of this research is incomplete and biased. There is little doubt that the issues are complex, often involving trade-offs between the impact of and our understanding of risk factors. The factors impacting on city living may increase some forms of psychosis and mood disorders, drug addiction, and some people's unhappiness, but may well reduce rates of dementia, alcohol abuse, and suicide. Litman reminds us that from the perspective of mental well-being, many people are happier in cities than they would be in smaller communities.

Jenny and Alice Roe, in Chapter 13, suggest that the number of young people living in cities has increased and it is inevitable that they face unprecedented social, cultural, and economic challenges as a result of globalization and rapid urbanization complicated by the fact that many cultures around the globe are in transition between traditional and modern values, with a degree of tension. Additional factors that influence the individual development of adolescents and their brains go on to affect their relationships and further social functioning. Thus, understanding the dynamic brain development that is strongly influenced by the social environment is critical as it then goes on to shape the capabilities an individual takes forward into adult life. In addition, promoting positive well-being in adolescence and self-esteem can help lay the foundations for positive well-being in adult life. Investing in young people can bring a triple dividend of benefits now, into adult life and for the next generation. We know that nearly half of psychiatric disorders in adulthood start before the age of 15; therefore, the importance of mental health promotion and prevention of mental ill health has not only to be included at a number of levels in childhood and adolescence, but also in the context of learning about parenting, addictions, and other strategies. In Chapter 14, Jorge J. Caraveo-Andaga et al. confirm some of these observations. They argue that among Mexican children there appears to be an urgent need to not only understand the needs of young people in rapidly developing urban spaces, but also to develop interventions at individual and population levels. They argue that prospective long-term studies are needed that can enable researchers and clinicians to look at aetiological factors affecting both physical and psychological development. In this chapter they present reported changes in the behavioural symptoms and syndromes in

Mexican children living in different geographical locations within Mexico City. They report that across all age groups, nervousness, restlessness, inattentiveness, irritability, and explosiveness have shown significant increases over the years. They emphasize that any relationship between the environment and psychological symptoms is of great interest, especially in preschool-age children who are likely to be irritable, which will affect their functioning at a number of levels, including scholastic achievements. They note that depressive syndrome with both irritable and depressed mood as core symptoms shows an increasing prevalence from preschool age to late childhood, while depressive syndrome with only one core symptom (predominantly irritable mood) shows a consistent increase across all age groups. Interestingly, explosiveness possibly associated with brain damage shows a significant increase, most notably for older school-age children. This raises significant questions about the environment within which children live, play, and grow up. Furthermore, if confirmed elsewhere, these findings help us set up public mental health programmes for mental health promotion and prevention of mental illness.

Todd Litman, in Chapter 21, reminds us that mental health is strongly influenced by a number of factors that affect individuals' mental health and happiness, and recommends various ways to use this information to create cities he calls saner and happier. Litman also notes specific mechanisms through which urban living can affect mental health and happiness, and identifies practical strategies that communities and individuals can use to increase urban mental health and happiness. A considerable amount of research has focused its attention on the risk factors associated with living in the cities. Although many of these studies have found associations of both social and environmental determinants to living in cities and a high rate of schizophrenia and other mental disorders given the hectic, haphazard, and rapid processes of global urbanization, robust research mixing qualitative and quantitative data and prospective approaches are needed to explore and clarify the causal links of the associations so far highlighted and the interactions between environmental and genetic factors. Studies on positive adaptation factors to the city are not yet sufficient. There is little doubt that like all living environments humans are strongly influenced by their functioning, and in examining how urban living affects residents' mental health and happiness, Litman suggests ways to use this information to create saner and happier cities. In exploring how urban living can affect mental health and happiness it should be possible to change the urban environment.

Jan Golembewski, in Chapter 9, argues that the actual perception of the physical environment by the brain is critically important for a number of reasons. Such an understanding of the relationship between built environment and the brain is crucial not only to the successful functioning of human beings, but also inevitably for the upbringing and functioning of future generations, too. The way the brain processes perceptions of the physical environment is of interest in understanding the aetiology, as well as epidemiology, of mental and physical health. Recent findings that the city—the locus of human endeavours—is one of the most predictable factors of the development of some disorders are of interest for a number of reasons, from understanding causality but perhaps more importantly helping develop interventions and strategies for mental health promotion, arguing that different approaches may be needed in cities than in rural areas. Golembewski points out that the ecological model of perception is an excellent model for enabling us to understand the relationship between the mental health and the physical environment, as well as their interrelationship. The observation that visual perception does not commence a cognitive process but is part of the way the brain reacts to the demands for action that are intrinsic to objects and forms within the environment is an important one. Golembewski goes on to trace key neural differences between urban and rural populations to explain this ecological perception phenomena, in what has been called the Ecological Hypothesis for Schizophrenia: how it is that the perceptions afforded by life (particularly urban life) become directly symptomatic. This chapter raises important issues related to the built environment and those who are responsible for these, for example town planners, architects, designers, urban designers, artists, and other city builders. Inevitably, it is in the interest of clinicians to work together with city planners to provide a better understanding of various issues, which, in the long run, will help to not only reduce rates of mental illness, but also likely improve therapeutic adherence.

While Jang et al. (Chapter 19) also remind us that urbanization and mental health are inter-linked, they urge that as there appears to be an increasing pressure on healthcare services as expectations of patients and their carers and families are changing along with changes in family structures, especially in urban areas, it is vital that services fit in with the needs of patients. They argue that provision of healthcare services can inevitably be constrained as a result of financial and human resource problems. Discussing Vancouver and New York, they compare service provision in these two cities and point out that the two approaches, falling on a continuum, raise specific issues for the development and delivery of mental health services. It is well recognized that in most countries there exist three levels of government: the national or federal, state or provincial assemblies, and city or municipal councils. In theory, each order is relatively independent, with its own taxation powers, policy jurisdictions, and responsibilities, but there also appears to be a tremendous amount of inter-dependency and in many settings federal government controls local funding. Local or municipal governments typically derive their powers from state or provincial law in the form of a municipal act, which inevitably places clear statutory limitations on what cities are responsible for, as well as restrictions on how, and where, the municipality may raise and spend monies. The primary responsibility of municipal governments lies in land use, which is relevant for urban spaces. In the UK, for example, many sites cannot be developed as a result of such policies. Some raise local taxes, but healthcare policies may be developed at federal or national levels, and, paradoxically, their delivery is expected at local levels raising specific issues and expectations along with pressures on local authorities who are often in the line of attack and expectations. Layla McCay et al., in Chapter 20, use Tokyo as an example. Tokyo is one of the most populous urban areas in the world, with a city population of over 13 million people and a metropolitan area extending to 36 million people. Not surprisingly, urban planning in Tokyo has not traditionally focused on mental health. A policy review along with interviews with urban practitioners examined how Tokyo applies the key principles of urban planning and design for the population's mental health. Various observations were made, which showed that Tokyo is well placed to leverage the urban environment and can improve mental health through increasing awareness among architects and planners. In addition, by introducing simple measures such as facilitating bicycle lanes and rides, developing waterways and green space, which will improve and increase physical activity along with positive social interactions, can help optimize the workplace for mental health. There is no doubt that many other cities could learn from Tokyo's empowering residents to green their neighbourhoods, and pedestrianized areas that prioritize greenery, walkability, bikeability, and other social activities. Interior place-making in shopping malls and offices can also help improve health, including mental well-being. These authors suggest that for women urban spaces are important at a number of levels and in a variety of ways. Reintegration of women with mental disorders is a long and arduous effort. Shubhda Maitra, in Chapter 22, illustrates this from the point of view of India, where women living with mental disorders experience long-term institutionalization and often abandonment by their families. These women may be admitted to hospital in their late twenties or early thirties and may find it difficult to get out of the institutions, in spite of being asymptomatic, owing to a lack of community-based accommodation. Maitra describes a community-based project working with women surviving mental disorders. The project links shelter, livelihoods, and psycho-social issues to facilitate women's recovery and reintegration by negotiating urban spaces in order to reduce stigma and discrimination.

In Chapter 8, Michael Krausz et al. present a research overview of vulnerable urban individuals and suggest that as mental illness and substance use disorders are risk factors for social marginalization, homelessness, and poverty, policymakers need to take this into account. They point out that a majority of homeless individuals report having experienced early childhood trauma, maltreatment, foster care, and family dysfunction, all of which contribute to their vulnerability. This is further complicated by limited access to physical and mental healthcare continuity, especially in urban areas, which further marginalizes those who are already vulnerable and creates social exclusion. The general migration of people towards big metropolitan areas also increases pressure on infrastructure and health care in urban centres. This movement constitutes a significant public health threat and heralds the need to reposition the healthcare system, including mental health services.

Describing sex in the city, Dinesh Bhugra and Antonio Ventriglio emphasize that sexual acts are at the basis of human life and necessary for procreation, although cultural differences may exist. The numbers of male and female sex workers are often significant in urban areas and their mental health needs are different. Sex trafficking adds another dimension of stress and illness for children and women. They argue that the risks of resulting sexually transmitted diseases are higher and, consequently, physical and psychiatric comorbidity may be higher. The theory of sex markets focuses on sexual partnering and describes it as a fundamentally local process, meaning that the two people must live within reasonable geographical proximity to initiate and develop a physical sexual relationship. However, in recent times, things have changed and through Tindr and Grindr, and other apps, as well as through cybersex, ideas of pleasure are changing. Often people do indulge in cybersex for which adequate electronic and Wi-Fi facilities have to be available, which are more likely in urban areas rather than rural areas. Economic aspects and perspectives may play a major role in transient sexual partnering. In Chapter 18, Bradlow et al. relate gender and sexual minority groups with their living environments and their mental health. It can be argued that urban settings are a hot spot of sociocultural evolutions that attract individuals from gender and sexual minority (GSM) groups. Inevitably, this can not only increase rural-to-urban area migration, but also those from other countries who are looking for safe spaces. As in other types of migration, various push-and-pull factors in both the rural and urban areas play a role in facilitating migration. These authors recognize that while rural areas present with challenges such as social isolation within a homophobic/transphobic environment, urban areas also have their own unique set of challenges for the GSM population, especially when they develop mental illness and are seeking help.

In Chapter 7, M.G. Carta and Dinesh Bhugra describe that rapid growth of the urban population worldwide is one of the current critical challenges for public mental health as urban living exposes populations to several risk factors that may cause mental ill health risks. These risks of various types and can be classified into macro-social; relational/support; macro-environment; and evolutive/(eu) genetic. Of course, these are inter-linked at different levels and their impact may well be cumulative. In this chapter they present a synthesis of some of the research findings related to urbanization and increased psychopathological risks. They argue that it is inevitable that there is an urgent need to study urban rehabilitation interventions in the context of whole-population models. They recommend that such approaches should take a multidisciplinary collaborative approach involving skills and knowledge ranging from architecture to urban planning to anthropology and to human wellness and mental health.

Ventriglio and Bhugra recognize that the recent spate of migration across the globe for geo-political reasons hides the fact that migration of humans has been constant over several millennia (Chapter 5). Perhaps in recent times, the immediacy of social media has led to acute awareness of the impact of immigration on social, political, and economic aspects of the new country, thereby creating tensions and leading to xenophobia and nationalistic attitudes. Surprisingly, the contributions that migrants make to these spheres are often ignored or even forgotten. There is little doubt that in order to survive arduous journeys migrants, by and large, are psychologically and physically resilient, but the acculturation processes may not always go smoothly, thereby leading to increasing stigma and discrimination against migrants. There is no getting away from the fact that some migrant groups do show higher rates of psychiatric disorders, but these have to be seen in the context of discrimination in policies of employment, housing, eand so on. In addition, other factors such as poverty and overcrowding may play a role. Other political, social, and economic factors may lead to depression among migrants to urban areas. There may be specific social factors that influence the individual's functioning soon after arrival, but other factors may emerge after moving into the city. Studying refugee populations in urban areas, Peter Schofield (Chapter 6) notes that these groups are also at an increased risk of mental disorders, including psychosis and post-traumatic stress disorder. This may well be attributable to the post-migration context in which they live, typically socio-economically deprived urban areas. Factors related to the neighbourhoods where refugees live are relevant and important to mental health outcomes. Although not a consistent finding, neighbourhood ethnic density is related to the incidence of psychosis and other mental disorders for members of ethnic minority groups. One consequence of dispersal policies of refugees, where they are placed in urban areas far from others from their country of origin, may cause isolation and may impact on their mental health. It is entirely possible that refugees may be more exposed to other neighbourhood factors, such as high levels of social deprivation and low levels of social cohesion, which may affect their mental well-being. These are, however, potentially modifiable risk factors.

Santosh Chaturvedi and Narayana Manjunatha, in Chapter 15, note that the common mental disorder are the commonest psychiatric disorders in the general population, as well as at primary care, and include a triad of illnesses—depression, anxiety disorders, and somatoform disorders. It is possible that various factors in urban areas, such as poverty, overcrowding, and unemployment, contribute to these high rates in spite of cities providing various opportunities for economic growth and comparatively better healthcare facilities. The models of explaining mental illnesses are critical in our understanding and developing interventions. However, while looking at rates of suicide in urban areas, Kairi Kõlves et al. (Chapter 16) recognize that urban living is linked to increased stress and illness, confirming higher levels of mental health disorders, such as depression, anxiety, and schizophrenia, and altered human brain responses, resulting in higher sensitivity to social stressors. They argue that given the stressful effects of urbanicity on brain function and mental health, a complex relationship exists between city life and suicide. Historically, suicide rates have been higher in urban areas, but a general trend of decline in urban suicide rates and an increase in rural trends has been observed. It is entirely possible that social integration plays a role in influencing the rates of suicide. They argue that some researchers blame this variation on rural areas becoming more socially isolated and have lower levels of social integration. Other factors, such as social fragmentation, social deprivation, social marginalization, and poverty, also play a role. The method of suicide also depends upon ease of availability. For example, in highly urbanized cities such as Singapore and Hong Kong, where most of the population live in multi-storey buildings, jumping from a height is the most common suicide method. Similarly, using metros, subways, or underground trains is not an uncommon method of suicide in many cities. Prevention of access to means, such as physical barriers at popular jumping sites, and suicide pits, platform screen doors, and blue lights in subways, has been shown to be effective in preventing urban suicides. These authors go on to recommend that a combination of the most appropriate strategies should be tailored to the city or suburb context, depending on the socio-economic background, level of deprivation, and demographic composition.

Jed Boardman and Tom Craig, in Chapter 23, describe the relationship between unemployment and mental disorders, which, although complex, has a bidirectional causality. There is a recognized causal impact of losing employment on mental health, as illustrated by studies looking at unemployment rates due to economic recession and mental ill health. However, mental ill health problems can also lead to unemployment and, once unemployed, it may well be impossible to find and sustain suitable employment. These authors note that whereas it was previously taken for granted that people with disabilities associated with enduring mental health problem required a lengthy period of re-training before job seeking, such an approach has been turned on its head, starting first with job placement and following this with ongoing support to both employee and employer. Such an approach has been shown to be a more effective approach across several countries albeit tempered by structural factors such as the state of the wider economy and availability of state welfare support.

Rapid urbanization and further fragmentation within urban sprawls have a major impact on an individual's social functioning and their interactions with others. Human beings are social animals and require support networks in a number of ways. The needs of urban settlers also require an understanding of the careful impact of gender, age, socio-economic and educational status, as well as other factors. Common to these living factors are cultural factors, which are changing and in transition at varying speeds. Clinicians and urban planners and architects need to work together to create safe spaces and green spaces with opportunities for physical activities, as well as interaction with others.

Urbanization and mental health require a deeper understanding of the causal pathways. It is entirely possible that multiple other factors contribute to a web of causation that may interact with resilience and other mitigating factors and influence the individual's mental health. Supporting factors such as social capital, family support, and physical environments may be protective. However, poverty, overcrowding, and unemployment can contribute to vulnerability to mental illness. The focus in this book is on urban design and somewhat different ways of looking at urbanicity and mental health.

References

1. **Prakash G.** Introduction. In: G Prakash, KM Kruse (eds) *The Spaces of the Modern City: Imaginaries, Politics and Everyday Life*. Princeton, NJ: Princeton University Press, 2008, 1–18.
2. **Lefebvre H.** *The Production of Space* (translated by David Nicholson Smith). Oxford: Blackwell, 1991.
3. **Appadurai A, Holson J.** Introduction: cities and citizenship. In: J Holston (ed.) *Cities and Citizenship*. Durham,NC: Duke University Press, 1999, pp 1–20.
4. **Virlio P.** *The Lost Dimension* (translated by Daniel Moshenberg). Paris: Seiotexte, 1991.
5. **Koolhas R.** Postscript: introduction for new research 'Contemporary City'. In: *Architecture and Urbanism*. Reprinted in K. Nesbitt (ed.) *Theorizing a New Agenda for Architecture*. New York: Princeton Architectural Press, 1988, p. 217.

Chapter 2

Sociology and the study of cities

Anthony M. Orum

Introduction

The study of cities has a long and rich history in the field of sociology. The great historian Max Weber was among the first scholars to offer a number of insights into cities, chief among them his claim that the market, or as we would now say, the economy, furnished the foundations for the origins of cities [1]. But the major theoretical effort began with Georg Simmel. Simmel wrote a famous essay on the metropolis in which he argued that the emerging metropolis in the nineteenth century represented an entirely new social form, one in which elements of the past were upended [2]. The manner of thinking in the metropolis, he suggested, was entirely different than that in previous societies. People in this new age were compelled to think quickly and rationally, to make assessments about others not based on their personal qualities, but rather on the manner in which they transacted with one another. Indeed, transactions became the signal quality of this new social form, replacing the interpersonal ties and qualities of the past. Simmel's essay represented an imaginative view of the new world, one that represented the key foundation for the growing sociological interest in cities.

The Chicago School of Sociology

The sociological interest in cities really took off a few years later. A new Department of Sociology had been established at the University of Chicago. Here some key players came on the scene. They included Robert Park, who had received some training in ecology in Germany; Louis Wirth who would write a seminal essay on the metropolis, one that drew in part on the ideas of Simmel; and Ernest Burgess, who would come to help develop a research project on the city of Chicago that would guide generations of sociologists, as well as geographers, interested in cities [3]. Park relied on analogies between the worlds studied by ecologists and the world of interest to sociologists [4]. Thus, he wrote about the dynamics of populations, for example, as well as the conflicts and struggles within cities. The evidence for his claims came directly from the world emerging around him in Chicago. By the late nineteenth century the city of Chicago was becoming home to tens of thousands of new immigrants from abroad. They came from countries like Italy and Poland, as well as Ireland. Driven out for various reasons from their European homes, they made new lives in Chicago, creating new urban settlements and recreating the cultures of their European homes. They thus remade the city of Chicago; but their struggles to create settlements, as well as the replacement of one ethnic group by another in specific sites, came to furnish the basis for Park's new urban ecology, as well as for Burgess' map of the city of Chicago as a city of concentric zones (Figure 2.1) [5]. There were other important voices as well, including those of Jane Addams, the founder of Hull House on Chicago's West Side, as well as

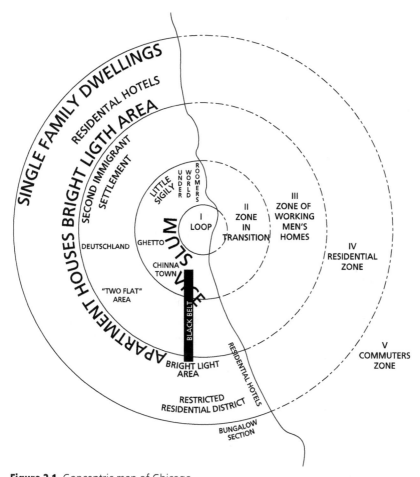

Figure 2.1 Concentric map of Chicago.

Reproduced from *Contained in the City: Suggestions for Investigation of Human Behavior in the Urban Environment*, Robert Ezra Park and Ernest Watson Burgess. With permission from University of Chicago Press, 1925 and 1967.

that of W.E.B. DuBois, America's first African American sociologist, whose pioneering studies of Philadelphia helped to give rise to a number of important ideas, including that of the 'double-consciousness' of African Americans [6, 7].

For several decades, then, the Chicago School of Sociology shaped urban sociology as a whole. Urban sociologists, whether at Chicago or elsewhere, now came to think of the city as a place consisting of different concentric zones—a zone of manufacturing, for example, as well as a red light district, and particular ethnic settlements.

Moreover, following the work of Wirth, sociologists also thought of the city as a place where people were anonymous and unknown to one another [8]. This image replaced the earlier sociological image of the town wherein people shared close ties with one another and knew each other intimately. Impersonality reigned in the vision of Wirth as it had earlier in the imagery of Georg Simmel. Sociologists now did empirical studies of populations of people, how they settled, and how they moved from one part of the city to another. An important line of work also developed whereby sociologists studied the under-represented and mistreated groups in the city—figures like thieves and prostitutes. Life histories became a new method to gain insight into the lives of such people and how cities shaped those lives. Life histories became a popular method among the sociologists of the city who wished to do qualitative rather than quantitative research. Both population studies and life histories furnished evidence about the emerging character of life in cities. They thus helped to create the field of urban sociology. There are countless works that originated in the writings of the Chicago School scholars, as well as those who followed in their footsteps.

The neo-Marxist critique

The Chicago School and its various theoretical ideas remained popular among urban scholars until the 1970s. Then a whole new set of ideas burst on the scene. They were inspired, in part, by two European scholars, Manuel Castells and David Harvey. Castells essentially insisted that the population dynamics of the city found in the writings of Park and his followers completely misunderstood the nature of the city. It was not the conflicts between population segments like ethnic groups that gave rise to urban conflicts, but rather the underlying economic elements and dynamics of cities [9]. Cities, Castells insisted, were economic formations that resulted from the growth and development of modern capitalism. Thus, issues of conflict and struggle represented forms of class conflict, of the struggle of the poor against the rich: the economy lay the basis for the modern city and thus its developments shaped the ways of urban life. Castells also maintained that cities were changing from sites of production to sites of consumption, and that the city should therefore be seen as the site where struggles over consumption took place. In this sense he updated the ideas of Karl Marx. Likewise, David Harvey produced a fundamental reorientation of how geographers, as well as sociologists, should approach the study of cities [10]. Instead of dwelling on population dynamics as though they were ecological in nature, he argued that cities are socially constructed through the developments of modern capitalism. As such, the periodic crises of capitalism were manifest in urban life, forcing a reinvestment of capital from business firms into real estate ventures. At the same time, just as Marx had written of the fundamental flaws of capitalism, Harvey pointed to the ways in which injustice was revealed in urban life, especially in the ways in which capital incessantly sought profits by remaking urban areas. This became part of the story of the continuing uneven development of cities, and the growing gap between the older parts of cities that became less valuable and the newer outlying sections where land development brought in higher profits [11].

Marxist interpretations thus replaced the ecological interpretations of the Chicago School of Sociology by the late 1970s. A very popular interpretation of urban growth along the same lines emerged in the writing of Harvey Molotch, and his colleague, John Logan [12]. In a seminal paper published in 1976 Molotch argued that the city should be seen as like a 'growth machine' [13]. Cities necessarily sought to grow, he argued, and to do so they mobilized various urban forces to make such growth happen. Thus, he argued, local government officials value growth because it increases their own power, as well as revenues for the city. Likewise, real-estate developers value growth because it generates profits for them. And even the local media come to adopt growth as a slogan because it enhances their circulation plus their visibility in the world of media. Ultimately, out of these and other factions, a pro-growth coalition arises that pushes relentlessly for the growth of the city. But, once unleashed, growth has a host of unfortunate consequences, less for the growth coalition and more directly for local residents. Neighbourhoods are uprooted as new zoning laws are passed that serve the interests of the growth coalition. Economic growth and development, which seem to enhance the fortunes of cities, like those of the growth coalition, often result in disrupting the lives of countless residents.

The neo-Marxist writings about cities have retained much of their popularity over the past several decades, especially as the welfare state has declined and the forces of neo-liberalism—i.e. the state aiding capitalist development—have been unleashed. A great deal of writing today about urban development emphasizes the economy and the ways in which the upper classes are doing much better than the middle and working classes. *Gentrification*, or the remaking of older urban areas into wealthy, high-end neighbourhoods represents part of this new emphasis [14, 15]. Many sociologists, but a number of other kinds of scholars as well, write of urban development today as a process whereby the residents of poor areas are forced to move out because of the rising costs of housing and local goods. This transformation of the city has taken place across the globe, but especially in urban areas in the West. Moreover, it is in the West that a narrative has emerged about urban decline, a decline that set in with the deindustrialization of cities. Such occurrences took place in Europe, as well as in the United States. And the resulting social consequences—the loss of jobs, the growing poverty of people of colour, the growth in crime and homelessness—became the standard portrait of many urban areas after the 1970s [16].

The global city and the creative class

But there were new twists on these arguments as well, especially from those who sought to explain not the decline of the industrial city, but the rise of the new post-industrial city. Two arguments came to dominate much of this post-industrial literature. One argument is that of Saskia Sassen. Sassen argues that a new kind of city has emerged since the 1980s, the global city [17]. Taking as her examples the cases of London, New York City, and Tokyo, she insists that such cities now act as the control centres for capitalist development in the world. They house the emerging and dominant forms of capitalism—in particular, finance, insurance, and real estate. These corporations, she found, exercised a tremendous amount of control over how monies accumulate and flow between cities: and they have been the centres for the accumulation of capital. Among other consequences, she suggests, is that such cities have bypassed states as the leading centres of power in the world. Her view was immensely popular until recently, when the major sovereign powers began to realign themselves. Obviously, Brexit in the United Kingdom will fundamentally shift the fortunes of bankers and their allies in London. But also the growing number of conflicts and schisms in different parts of the world will have serious consequences for development, and for urban residents, everywhere but especially in countries like Syria.

The second argument regarding the development of cities in the post-industrial era is that of Richard Florida. Florida insisted that in the post-industrial era economic growth was being driven by the efforts of a 'creative class' of people [18]. These were people especially in the area of high technology and its allied enterprises. They were the new entrepreneurs of the post-industrial age, people like Steve Jobs and Bill Gates, figures who were sparkling with lots of new ideas and ways to deploy technology. Moreover, he argued, in the process of creating new industries and jobs they also fostered a new kind of social atmosphere to cities. Such cities showed a higher rate of tolerance, Florida discovered, and therefore they made life better for everyone. Cities like Austin, Texas; San Jose, California; and Seattle, Washington exemplified the attributes of the creative class and the creative city. But Florida's ideas, while immensely popular with political officials who wished to see their cities grow, inspired a host of legitimate criticisms. One of the main criticisms is that the new wealth created in such cities failed to raise people out of poverty or solve the racial tensions existing in so many cities.

Culture and the city

Besides these views there are others that consider the nature of the culture of cities today. The writings of the sociologist Sharon Zukin focuses on cities and the cultures of such cities [19, 20]. She argues, like Manuel Castells before her, that cities today are more focused on consumption than on production. Further consumption has taken on a life all its own. The cultures of cities have flourished in the post-industrial era. Art and architecture have blossomed, evident in the construction of new museums, as well as public art. But, in addition, cities have become enlivened by the variety of new cultural and ethnic groupings that have opened up a variety of new shops and restaurants, all of which make the city a far more interesting, even spectacular, place than the older industrial cities. (But note that Zukin's emphasis on culture can be read as the other side of gentrification: gentrification itself produces new art and lively new urban spaces but at the expense of displacing many older and poorer urban residents.)

Emerging ideas and views

New ideas continue to emerge about cities today. One of the most important is the idea that the cities of the Global North differ from those of the Global South. This is a very important argument, one that is gaining increasing attention. Cities of the Global North, for example, were those created by the Industrial Revolution [21, 22]. They included cities like Manchester, England, and Milwaukee, Wisconsin. They are cities that were bifurcated between the very wealthy and the very poor, and they are cities that today are experiencing not only deindustrialization, but also the lingering effects of deep ethnic and racial tensions. Cities of the Global South are set along an entirely different path. Not only are they configured in spatially different ways, but their social groups and even their growth is far different. Places like Shanghai, China; or Mumbai, India; or Johannesburg, South Africa, all are growing more rapidly, developing into megacities and thus outpacing the growth of the older cities of the Global

North. But more than that they also face far different challenges and offer far different prospects for the future.

Reimagining power, space, and justice: new directions for urban and spatial research

We now want to move beyond the conventional wisdom about cities and to suggest some new directions for sociological and spatial research. In particular we want to focus primarily on two concepts: power and space. Power as a concept has actually disappeared from virtually all urban research, thereby making such research far less realistic than it should be. Here, we shall argue that power and space are concepts that are deeply intertwined and inextricably connected with one another. We do so with one ambition in mind. Having shown that power and space are intertwined with one another we want to create a perspective of the world that allows us to gain greater insight, to assemble empirical data, and eventually to insist on a way that political efforts can and should be mobilized to address the ways that the powerful shape the lives of the powerless. In the end our main purpose is political: to expose the ways that power and space are intertwined in our world today, and therefore the ways they must be disentangled to help those people and groups that are powerless. It is our contention that unless we realize the ways that power and space are intertwined we will never be able to effectively address and to overcome the elements of injustice.

Space

Space is various and rich, and capable of being produced and reproduced in many ways, following the character of society and social developments themselves. But there is one critical distinction to which we want to draw attention here: the distinction between private and public space. Let us begin with some preliminary observations on both kinds of spaces.

Public space is that social space where people come together and meet. It is the space where people in effect get outside themselves and where they engage in a variety of ways with other people [23–25]. It may be the public space in the home, such as a living room, where different people gather; it may be the public spaces of a community of people where the various and different parties gather; it may be sidewalks; it may also may be the quarters where the political work of a city is done. The essential element is that those people who compose a household or a community or a city or a neighbourhood have equal access to and equal interest in gathering in the public spaces. Such spaces are where the very elements of a family or a community or a neighbourhood are constituted. They are where the objective character of the entity is transformed into something that is subjective—that links the fates and fortunes of the diverse members of the group together. It is, to use a Hegelian expression, where the thing in itself becomes transformed to a thing for itself, a concept, of course, that played a major role in Marx's thinking about social classes.

In an absolutely perfect and imagined world the public space of a place would be open to all people and to all varieties of activity. The quintessential form is that of a gathering place, whether a park or an actual assembly hall, to which all people are equally welcome. There they can engage with one another in activities that they normally might do on their own, if at all. The typical image of such space is that of a town hall, or even a political forum, where people gather and engage in issues of common concern. The nature of such public space is such that various and diverse groups of people gather there freely and engage with one another freely. It represents the essence of a democratic space, like an open forum, where issues can be raised and examined, where people can voice their opinions, and where differences among them may be considered and addressed. Moreover, in an ideal world a wide variety of activities can take place in public spaces, not just talk. Indeed, a rich conception of human activity would suggest that people would be free in public spaces to do all sorts of public things, or things together: dance, sing, chat, and other such human activities. In other words, various publics can emerge and develop in public spaces themselves.

Of course, apart from works of fiction or of fictionalized history, we know very little of such actual public spaces. The real world, the one in which we live, is, in fact, very different from this idealized version. (Nevertheless, of course, it is the task of political philosophers to construct such images of an ideal world in order to assess how far any real world may be from this ideal.) Critical social theory, such as the form we have in mind here, addresses how and why the real, the actual, world is different from this idealized form. Marxist writings, as well as that of the neo-Marxist writers today, dig deeply and widely to show how much the idealized world of public space, where democracies can bloom, is different from the actual world. Regarding urban and metropolitan spaces, writers like David Harvey and Henri Lefebvre point to the many ways in which the institutions of modern capitalism carve their ways through public spaces, effectively diminishing the abilities of people to freely and openly enjoy the opportunities to engage with one another in such spaces—and to air and examine and consider their differences, and how they might be resolved [26].

But one need not be a Marxist, or attentive to the real and growing inequalities of modern capitalism, to provide a critical view of how public spaces seem to bring out the worst rather than the best in people (today). The elements of power, and the workings of social exclusion, in fact, are to be found diminishing the potentials of public spaces everywhere today. Where power exists, where the institutions of a particular place create advantages for one group to exercise its power over another, then public spaces themselves will reveal such power and how it operates. This is how space, public space, and power come together: some groups, the outsiders, simply do not enjoy the advantages, the privileges, the rights enjoyed by other groups in public spaces. They may be women who fear the violence of men in such public spaces; they may be African Americans who fear the police in such spaces; or they may be simply people who are disabled and who, because of the lack of facilities for them, find it difficult, if not impossible, to negotiate the distances across public spaces, like sidewalks, or even public transportation.

Public spaces, to repeat, should, in principle, be open to all people so regardless of who you are or what you do you may enjoy such spaces. In a home such spaces may be the living rooms, or family rooms, that offer the opportunity for all the members of the family to gather there, to enjoy one another's company, to constitute themselves as a family. In a public park, the various and diverse groups of people also should, in principle, be able to do what they wish in such a park—dance, sing, chat, run, play soccer. That is the very character of public spaces in principle: to allow different publics to emerge, to effectively exclude no one nor any form of activity in which members of the public engage.

But, of course, such public spaces often, if not always, are restricted spaces. For example, such spaces like public parks may be restricted to only the residents of a particular city. Thus, the residential status of people determine who can occupy such parks and who cannot [27]. Often, public spaces like parks have restrictions that prevent 'vagrants' from staying or 'loitering' in the parks. Or there may be public spaces like the meeting rooms of local councils that are only open to those people who are actual residents of a place. Thus, although it is claimed that such assemblies are open to the ideas and exchanges of everyone concerning a specific issue, they are, in fact, not: they may only be open to those residents who are property owners.

On and on such restrictions can pile atop one another until it becomes clear in many, if not most, instances that most public spaces are heavily restricted: they only permit certain kinds of people to enter and to engage with one another in such spaces. And this, of course, takes us to the next critical element about public spaces: who administers them and who decides who can enter? Here is where power, and those who deploy it, show their brutal face. Power, in particular, power of one group over another emerges in the exercise of control over entry into public spaces. Typically, there are guards, or police, who determine who may enter and who may not. Such figures make critical everyday decisions, for example, who is to be identified as a vagrant and who is not; or who is a resident and who is not. (The prison is the quintessential form of this kind of public space.) But even other people who occupy public spaces, like parks or neighbourhood sidewalks, may act to exercise such control. Surveillance and control, like social exclusion itself, are present everywhere and among everyone. And the insiders always seem to have the inside track.

The other kind of space that exists is that of *private space*. It is the space that defines the life of an individual, in effect, apart from the issue of public concerns. Typically, such space has been conceived as the space of the home and of the family. These are private matters, of course, presumably not subject to public discussion or interference by public forces. Yet, as many feminist theorists point out, this distinction between the home/family and the public/community often results in demeaning the role and significance of women in the public sphere. Theories developed by men and under the rule of patriarchies establish the public realm as that of men, and the private realm as that of women. Here we wish to move beyond those categories and to consider for the purposes of public space, as well as public discussion, the role of women, as well as the ways in which they are typically excluded. That must also be a central presupposition here: that exclusion by gender is as demeaning as exclusion, say, by race or poverty, and must be addressed in the same way we address any other forms of domination and power in a city, community, or society.

Moreover, as Crawford and others point out, the distinction between those spaces that are public and those that are private have become blurred in recent times [28]. Take the case of the homeless. They exist everywhere today, and seem to be growing in number. Often they have no place to turn for shelter and are compelled to build their own homes on the streets and sidewalks, even under bridges and overpasses—the public spaces. They are people whose lives have been torn asunder by the pace and development of modern cities, and thus they become multiple victims of social exclusion: not only their minds, but also their bodies and self-respect endure constant assaults. They have no private place to turn, to seek to meet their needs at local social agencies across urban areas, and thus they are exposed relentlessly by the daily routines of cities and their occupants.

Conceptualizing two ways to think about space and power

A little reflection on the preliminary discussion above suggests that there exists a genuine intellectual division and tension between those who insist that public space permits people to gather and to express themselves freely and those who insist that the reality of the world today is such that there is no such thing as public space that is truly open, accessible, and free. There are, in fact, intelligent observers on both sides of a kind of divide regarding public spaces—those who, on the one hand, celebrate the potential of such spaces and those who, on the other, claim no such spaces truly exist. How can we reconcile this difference? We want to begin by suggesting that there seems to be two coherent and consistent views of public spaces.

The first mode is that we shall call the *bright* view of space. This is the view of writers like Hannah Arendt and other democratic theorists [29]. It is the view that insists that space, but especially public space, is a site and way to empower people. As such, writers of this point of view argue that these spaces provide the opportunity for people to gather together and to share their views with one another. It is based upon the notion that in ancient Greece people could assemble together and discuss their common concerns. Having engaged in lengthy and deliberate discussions they could then arrive at a common and consensual view, one that represented the results of their collaboration. The key here is one of deliberation: those who engaged in the debate and discussion may have held one view upon entering the space, like the forum, but through discussion they arrive at one that represents their common ground. Moreover, as a result of the discussion they effectively have made a public out of themselves.

We might call this the democratic view of public space and how it can be used by groups who share different perspectives in order to arrive at some kind of common ground. It is an ideal of course, but like all ideals it furnishes the elements of a vision towards which people can work and strive. Presumably by being able to engage in open and free exchange of ideas the groups of people will be able to air their differences, and thus to arrive at some kind of common solution to the issue before them—whatever the nature of that issue. But there are suppositions that must be satisfied in order to generate a fair and satisfactory consensus: (1) the public space must be open to all parties with a view on the particular issues; and (2) the public space not only must be open, but it must also be accessible to those parties. If restricted on either of these grounds the resulting decision will itself not be a truly fair and democratic one. For many people this bright view of public space is the ideal that provides a purpose to their lives and their engagement in political life.

There is a second view, however, that takes a very different perspective on the nature of public space. This is the *dark* view of such space. This view insists that the bright view is thoroughly naïve and unrealistic. It argues that public space is not a forum at all, but more like a prison. Drawing in recent times its energies from the insightful writings of Michel Foucault this perspective insists that there is no such thing as free and open public space, and therefore there is no opportunity to arrive at any kind of fair and just solution among groups of people with different points of view. Rather, public spaces today are spaces completely under the control of public (as well as private) authorities. Thus, while public parks might appear to be safe and open, they are, in fact, anything but; instead, there is always some form of surveillance at work in such spaces. Thus, no discussion, apparently open and free, is, in fact, continuously being monitored, sometimes by actual police figures who are present, sometimes by cameras that are used to identify both the talk and the participants.

In effect, then, there is no such thing as open, free, and fair discussion among people nor will there ever be. Big Brother is always watching and recording what happens. The result is that people must always and everywhere be wary of what they say and do. Like a prison there are guards and there is surveillance everywhere. Nothing, no one, goes untouched and unidentified. Among other things, as Foucault pointed out, the effect of such monitoring is that people engage in self-monitoring, always being wary and cautious about what they do and say. The possibility always exists that even in the private spaces of our lives, like our homes, we will be watched and monitored.

Now many people will argue with a good deal of evidence that, in fact, this dark view of space is, indeed, the realistic view of such space. The new world of technology possesses ways of spying on us not only in public spaces like parks, but also through various news outlets, without us even being aware of such surveillance.

Nevertheless, those who argue on behalf of the bright view of public space counter as follows. Politics in governments, like local governments, seem to offer individuals and groups the chance to express their point of view to their representatives. Moreover, those who choose not to take this opportunity can always vote for people who represent their point of view and thus are able to have their voice heard. Still, critics—often those who espouse the dark perspective— argue that institutions like government often are biased and thus there are no guarantees that voting or even the forceful expression of one's point of view will make much different to those in positions of authority. The fact that people can freely express their views in democratic societies furnishes the hope and the opportunity to register their voice, and thus have some chance of making a difference within the places where decisions are made.

When all is said and done these two perspectives offer dramatically different readings of our world today and the nature of public spaces—as well as of public authority. Moreover, no evidence it would seem exists that can fully confirm or substantiate one or the other view. In fact, they seem to generate fundamentally different sets of questions about the kind of evidence we would want to gather, and how we might gather it.

Moving past the irreconcilable views

Given these equally compelling views how might we move beyond them? In fact, how can we use them to deepen our understanding of power and space in our world today? There appear to be several directions that we can take.

Let me suggest the first of several moves. While I believe the dark view of public space is a coherent and comprehensive view, owing, in part, to a good deal of recent empirical research, I think the bright view may be too restrictive. Indeed, I think it concentrates too much on one element—that of talk and of deliberation—an element that can be traced to some of the original thinking about public spaces as democratic. If such spaces are, indeed, public they should not only be accessible to everyone, but they also ought to include the variety of activities that may take place in such sites. Such variety would include various forms like that of performance activities like dancing or singing, but also merely groups of people who are chatting with one another. In effect, as Nancy Fraser correctly suggests, such spaces can involve different collective activities of people together, therefore the constitution of different kinds of publics. This is central to the underlying element of a democratic, or free and open, space. By allowing the possibility of more activities, and thus more publics, we make the bright view a more comprehensive view but one that remains true to the notion of a democratic, and thus open, space. I believe, therefore, the bright view needs to be amended to take fuller account of the range of activities that can occur in public space.

But there is a second move that one might make. Some could argue that the bright view of public space is, in fact, only an idealized version of how such space can and should work. In contrast, the dark view represents the reality of how it works today, and how such space has become less and less open to all people. Being like a prison then such space is never truly open and people are always under surveillance. Therefore, no genuine and true deliberation can take place nor can any genuine public activities occur; people always will be wary of who is watching and recording what they do because they never believe themselves to be free. Hence, those who espouse the bright view may relish their ideals but it is truly unlikely that those ideals will ever be realized anywhere.

Frankly, this is not an intellectually satisfying answer at all. It simply claims that there are the two camps and that both camps rely on evidence and argumentation in support of their views. To any informed person this seems like an intellectual surrender and totally unsatisfactory. One might argue that given this particular move the idealistic vision of public space may always be morally correct but can, in fact, never be realized. And by the same token the same observer might argue that the dark view is the realistic one, and therefore we should dispense with the romantic and idealistic vision altogether. Realism trumps moral authority.

There is yet a third criticism that can be made of these arguments, and a third move. We have suggested that the bright view is an idealized view of democratic public space. By contrast we have also claimed that the dark view is a realistic view of the world today based upon various pieces of evidence. But perhaps the dark view is not realistic at all? Perhaps it, too, is a mere fiction, although a different kind of fiction than the bright view. Consider that over the past several decades a vast literature of dystopian novels and claims have emerged, a literature that by itself paints a very dark portrait of the world. Consider the various motion pictures that have appeared over this time, among them *The Hunger Games*. This is a stark picture of a world undergoing great change. Indeed, anyone who wishes to watch movies on American television nowadays is struck by the various dystopian images among popular movies, for example. It is not only movies, but also literature that paints such a view.

Thus, it is entirely possible that a new narrative has emerged to counter the old ones, for example, about the positive features of democratic governments. Such a fictional narrative, in fact, takes on many of the features I have used to portray the dark view of public space. Such space is like a prison—consider, for example, the movie *Blade Runner*. In the end, one really does not know whether the dark view is simply an argument based on a variety of fictional pieces of work or rather a view grounded in more substantial claims, like those of Foucault, for instance [30]. But, regardless of whether the dark view is based on fact or fiction, it is an overpowering and compelling view—and it just so happens to show up in various kinds of social science literature, certainly more often the bright view.

Thus, in the worst of all cases the two instances, the bright and the dark view of public spaces, may both be certain kinds of fictions: one a fiction to which an ideal world aspires but only approximates at best, the other a fiction that gives a view of the world of the future that is inevitably dismal, bleak, and filled with chaos of all sorts and forms.

Here then we seem to find ourselves on the horns of a dilemma. Two perfectly clear and coherent versions of the nature of public space but one we dismiss because it seems too unrealistic; and we keep the other one because the evidence—regardless, perhaps, of its factual foundations—keeps on piling up to support it. This is the kind of dilemma, I believe, that inspired Immanuel Kant to fashion arguments on behalf of moral reason, on the one hand, and scientific reason, on the other. Otherwise, the two views seem entirely incompatible, and yet what grounds could one use to keep one and dismiss the other? They may both be wrong in some factual sense, or fictions in a narrative sense. But could they both be right?

Maybe they simply describe different yet prevailing forms public space in the entire array of public spaces in a particular place?

In the end the only way to resolve the differences between the two views of public spaces and how they are used is to conduct systematic empirical research. The bright view of public spaces suggests that such spaces are used by a variety of people for a variety of purposes, and that the groups of people who use them are thereby empowered. The dark view suggests, to the contrary, that public spaces are really spaces of enclosure, that people using them are constantly under surveillance, and that therefore such spaces truly are dismal and bleak. All the things to which the bright view aspires really do not exist at all. Instead, public spaces, even spaces like airlines, are spaces where authority can be exercised and is exercised in ways that mistreat people and do not treat them with dignity. Here, I do not have the space to lay out the details of such research, but I recommend that readers consult recent writings on these matters [31–33].

References

1. **Weber M.** *The City* (translated and edited by Don Martindale and Gertrud Neuwirth). New York: The Free Press, 1958.
2. **Simmel G.** The metropolis and mental life. In: K Wolff (ed.) *The Sociology of Georg Simmel*. Glencoe, IL: The Free Press, 1950, pp. 409–426.
3. **Park R, Burgess EW.** *Introduction to the Science of Sociology.* Chicago, IL: University of Chicago Press, 1924.
4. **Park RE.** Human ecology. *American Journal of Sociology* 1936; **43**: 1–15.
5. **Burgess EW.** The growth of the city: an introduction to a research project. In: RE Park, E Burgess, RD McKenzie (eds) *The City.* Chicago, IL: University of Chicago Press, 1925, pp. 47–62.
6. **Bethke Elshtain J** (ed.) *The Jane Addams Reader.* New York: Basic Books, 2002.
7. **DuBois WEB.** *The Philadelphia Negro.*Philadelphia, PA: University of Pennsylvania Press, 1899).
8. **Wirth L.** Urbanism as a way of life. *American Journal of Sociology* 1938; **44**: 1–24.
9. **Castells M.** *The Urban Question* (translated by Alan Sheridan). Cambridge, MA: M.I.T. Press, 1972.
10. **Harvey D.** *Social Justice and the City.* Oxford: Basil Blackwell, 1973/1988.
11. **Portes A, Castells M, Benton LA** (eds). *The Informal Economy: Studies in Advanced and Less Developed Countries.* Baltimore, MD: Johns Hopkins, 1989.
12. **Logan J, Molotch H.** *Toward A Political Economy of Place.* Berkeley, CA: University of California Press, 1987.
13. **Molotch H.** The city as a growth of machine. *American Journal of Sociology* 1976; **82**: 309–332.
14. **Lees L.** A re-appraisal of gentrification: towards a geography of gentrification. *Progress in Human Geography* 2000; **24**: 389–408.

15. **Smith N.** *The New Urban Frontier: Gentrification and the Revanchist City*. London and New York: Routledge, 1996.

16. **Orum AM.** *City-Building in America*. Boulder, CO: Westview Press, 1995.

17. **Sassen S.** *The Global City: New York, London, Tokyo*, 2nd ed. Princeton, NJ: Princeton University Press, 2001.

18. **Florida R.** *The Rise of the Creative Class and How It's Transforming Work, Leisure, Community and Everyday Life*. New York: Basic Books, 2002.

19. **Zukin S.** *The Cultures of Cities*. Oxford: Blackwell, 1995.

20. **Zukin S.** *Landscapes of Power*. Berkeley, CA: University of California Press, 1991.

21. **Parnell P, Robinson J.** (Re)theorizing cities from the Global South: looking beyond neo-liberalism. *Urban Geography* 2012; **33**: 593–617.

22. **Robinson J.** Cities in a world of cities: the comparative gesture. *International Journal of Urban and Regional Research* 2011; **35**: 1–23.

23. **Goheen PG.** Public space and the geography of the modern city. *Progress in Human Geography* 1998; **22**: 479–496.

24. **Carmona M.** Re-theorizing contemporary public spaces: a new narrative and a new normative. *Journal of Urbanism* 2015; **8**: 373–405.

25. **Low S.** *On the Plaza: The Politics of Public Space and Culture*. Austin, TX: University of Texas Press, 2000.

26. **Lefebvre H.** *The Production of Space*. Oxford: Basil Blackwell, 1991.

27. **Mitchell D.** *The Right to the City: Social Justice and the Fight for Public Space*. New York: Guilford Books, 2003.

28. **Crawford M.** Contesting the public realm: struggles over public spaces in Los Angeles. *Journal of Architectural Education* 1995; **49**: 4–9.

29. **Calhoun C** (ed.). *Habermas and the Public Sphere*. Cambridge, MA: M.I.T. Press, 1992.

30. **Foucault M.** *Discipline and Punish: The Birth of the Prison*. New York: Vintage Books, 1995.

31. **Orum AM, Neal ZP** (eds) *Common Ground? Readings and Reflections on Public Space*. New York: Routledge, 2010.

32. **Orum AM.** Public man and public space in Shanghai today. *City & Community* 2009; **8**: 369–389.

33. **Orum AM, Li JC.** Life in public spaces: a theater of the streets, social exclusion, and a safe zone in Shanghai. *Perspectives on Global Development and Technology* 2017; **16**: 241–259.

Chapter 3

Urban design and mental health

Layla McCay

Introduction

There is an intriguing parallel between the components of good mental health and the components of a thriving city: a thriving city depends on the good mental health of its population. The World Health Organization defines mental health as 'a state of well-being in which every individual realizes his or her own potential, can cope with the normal stresses of life, can work productively and fruitfully, and is able to make a contribution to her or his community' [1]. In addition to referring to personal mental well-being, these components could be extracted to define a city's state of well-being: a state that is essential for achieving the 'inclusive, safe, resilient and sustainable' city to which the United Nations' (UN) Sustainable Development Goal 11 aspires.

If mental health is important for thriving cities, the current statistics ought to catch the attention of citymakers across the world, not least because so many people live in urban settings. Today, half of the world's population is in cities, and by 2050, the UN believes this proportion will rise to two-thirds of the population [2]. Of those people, most will experience some symptoms of mental health problems in the course of their lives, and one out of every four people will develop a diagnosable mental disorder. This risk increases as the population ages [3]. However, these are the general statistics that apply regardless of where a person lives. For people who live in cities, the risk of developing various mental disorders seems to be higher than those who live in the countryside. Estimates vary, but compared to rural settings, people who live in cities seem to have an almost 40% increased risk of depression, over 20% more anxiety, and double the risk of schizophrenia [4]. Research tells us that even being simply born into an urban environment increases the odds of developing schizophrenia in 28–34.3% of all cases [5]. The scale and potential impact of urban mental health problems means that city populations will experience a substantial burden of disease due to mental disorders. It also means that the remit for improving mental health can no longer be simply relegated to mental health professionals. Nor should it be.

It would be folly to simply blame the city for people's mental health problems: it is widely understood that genetic, biological, psychological, social, and environmental factors can all contribute to the development of mental disorders. And yet it is also clear that the city must be implicated in some way. The differences that have been noted in mental disorder prevalence must have an explanation. Just as the causes of mental health problems are multifactorial, so, too, are the solutions. The myriad of opportunities for urban planners and designers to improve mental health have, until recently, been a sparsely considered afterthought; the full potential of this approach to public mental health is just beginning to be understood. If good mental health is a prerequisite for a thriving city, then in this rapidly urbanizing world, good mental health must be a priority that extends far beyond the health sector. Urban planners, architects, and other citymakers have an important role to play in designing good mental health into cities. This chapter will explore several mechanisms by which the city can exert negative effects on mental health, and use these to consider potential solutions that can be implemented by urban planners and designers.

Four ways in which cities may be implicated in mental health

Good mental health is more than simply the absence of a mental disorder: it is a feeling of mental well-being and ability to conduct one's life: the ability to have strong relationships, to work or study, to enjoy leisure activities, to make decisions. This can be affected by our social circumstances and our surroundings, which are partially determined by where we live.

Life in the city, as with life anywhere, comes with factors that exert both positive and negative influences on mental health. The factors driving the city's positive impact on mental health are often among the incentives that draw an increasing number of people to make their home in the urban setting. Cities offer education and economic opportunities, and cultural enrichment; they can supply a wide variety of housing and transport options to suit different incomes and needs; they can have more diversity, more health and social services, and more support services for people with drug and alcohol addictions. Cities certainly offer a diversity of opportunities that may be less accessible in the countryside, and can contribute to good mental health.

However, there are also some specific factors that increase the prevalence of mental illness in the city. How can so-called 'citymakers' play a role in promoting and supporting people's mental health? It is illuminating to consider these factors through a lens of urban planning and design.

Vulnerability: pre-existing risk factors in the city

The determinants that make a person vulnerable to mental disorders involve complex interactions between individual predisposition, social and economic circumstances, and environmental factors. Even before considering city-specific environmental factors, the individual, social, and economic circumstances of people who live in cities can be particularly likely to elevate their pre-existing risk factors. This effect is sometimes termed 'social drift'.

Several of the reasons that draw people to live in the city are also factors that predispose them to mental health problems. Low income, poverty, unemployment, and homelessness are important risk factors for mental illness. These are also drivers for people to move to the city in pursuit of better employment, affordable housing, social support, and economic opportunities. People with a history of mental health problems, parental mental health problems, and, indeed, those with physical health problems all often gravitate towards living in the city, due partly to their need to access health and social care, which are often centred in the city. The same is true for people with harmful use of alcohol and/ or illicit drugs; in addition, they may be attracted by increased supply and demand for substances.

Being in a minority group is another important risk factor for mental health problems. The cultural diversity, education, and employment opportunities makes cities particularly attractive places for immigrants who often choose to settle in the city initially or in the longer term. Choice is, of course, not always available: many asylum seekers and refugees are temporarily or permanently settled in cities, where supportive infrastructure is often based. Exposure to violence, war, and disaster, another risk for mental disorders, is particularly likely in this population group. Finally, the trend of people from other countries gravitating to the city is also relevant because research indicates that first- and second-generation migrants seem to be at increased risk of developing schizophrenia compared with the rest of the population, although the mechanisms remain unclear [6].

Disparities and segregation in the city

People with socio-economic disadvantages encounter particularly pronounced disparities in the city. Evidence of differences between the rich and the poor are often more blatant in cities, with physical and social segregation imposed. People may live in neighbourhoods that are determined by socio-economic status, which may have higher rates of crime and violence, which reduces the protective feelings of safety and security, and the positive feelings of belonging and trusting the local community. However, the answer is not so simple as imposing mixed housing: this can play a particular role in highlighting income differences, the so-called 'poor door effect.' The exposure of poorer people to the additional opportunities enjoyed by richer people, alongside experiences of stigma and discrimination, including racism, and social exclusion, can have a negative impact on people's mental health. They may experience frustration, lower self-esteem, and feelings of hopelessness and helplessness. For young boys in particular, the response to this effect is often antisocial behaviour.

Overload

Living in the city exposes people to a mass of humanity at close quarters and can result in a level of stimuli that may feel overwhelming, with crowding, noise, smells, sights, polluted air, disarray, and the need to maintain a certain level of vigilance for personal security. These factors can combine to create a sense of overstimulation from which people may try to retreat. In the pursuit of private space and quiet, social withdrawal may occur, meaning that people might miss out on developing and maintaining social connections, leisure, exercise, and spending time in positive environments such as parks. The ecological hypothesis for schizophrenia is also relevant here. The hypothesis proposes that overt psychotic symptoms can be directly triggered by failure to cope with constant demands of the urban environment, from social demands to those of urban design. Golembiewski [7] describes this effect thus: 'An ecological maelstrom of demands constantly acts on everyone, but it is only when our natural ability to appropriately inhibit the demand/action pathway is limited that we start to suffer symptoms. This typically occurs as a failure to cope with the pressing demands of the urban environment.'

Stripping away protective factors for mental health

There is an implication that when it comes to urban life, people experience more inputs. However, cities do not only add, they also take away. A wide range of factors are protective for mental health, and the very nature of cities can often strip these away, leaving people more vulnerable to the development of mental health problems. People who live in cities can find themselves with less access to nature than those living in the countryside; similarly, they may find themselves exercising for less time in the course of their regular routine. Light, noise, crowding, and other disturbances may affect sleep. And the all-important social connection and social capital can be lost in the city. People who move to the city may leave their social networks behind and have to develop new networks, and people feeling overwhelmed in the city may form less strong social networks, reducing social capital and resilience, particularly when they are marginalized from community activities due to barriers such as lack of access or fear of neighbourhood crime. Social isolation is a particular risk factor for older adults.

Figure 3.1 conceptualizes the complexity of relationships between the commonly studied hypothetical aetiological factors for schizophrenia, and illustrates the influences that the urban environment may exert on mental health.

Targets for urban design to promote better mental health

The complexity of mental disorder aetiology tends to give urban designers implicit permission to dismiss any mental health promotion responsibilities. People come to the city with their own personal combination of genetics, past experiences, health status, social, and socio-economic status. But once they are there, in the city, urban planning and design can mitigate and modify risk factors to create a setting that exerts potential positive impact on people's mental health.

Clearly, some of the risk factors for mental illness that are prominent in city living (e.g. genetics) cannot be addressed by urban design. And yet, with creative thinking, the opportunities are wider and more diverse than they may at first appear. It may seem at first glance, for instance, that urban design cannot address someone's unemployment status (other than directly employing them in the design and building process); however, delivering an affordable, reliable, and safe public transport system may widen their opportunities and facilitate a successful search for employment in different parts of the city. One might argue that urban design cannot remove a person's previous traumatic exposure to violence during war, a risk factor for developing mental disorders. Certainly that may be true, but urban design can be applied creatively to help deliver some of the determinants of recovery: delivering settings that facilitate relaxation, and the development of social support, community trust, and a sense of security and belonging that will support and promote that person's mental health.

The Centre for Urban Design and Mental Health summarizes the four main evidence-based targets for urban design to promote good mental health. In the *Mind the GAPS* framework, GAPS refers to Green, Active, Pro-social and Safe Places. This framework, while not fully inclusive of every emerging opportunity, summarizes the primary targets. It can be applied to both individual projects and to a wider assessment of the city's basic current readiness to support good mental health through urban planning and design—and, importantly, to identify further opportunities.

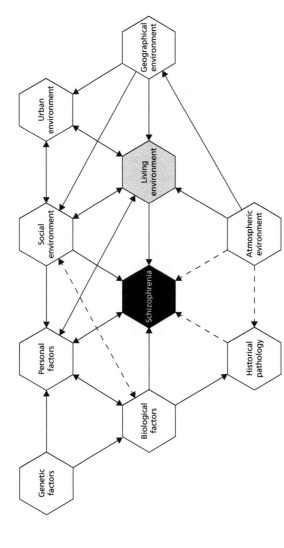

Figure 3.1 Relationships between the commonly studied hypothetical factors that contribute to the development of schizophrenia.

Green space and mental health

The vegetated land and water in the urban environment includes parks, gardens, sports facilities, woods, and anywhere in the city where plantlife is thriving. People who live in the city tend to have less regular exposure to green space; increasing access represents one of the most promising opportunities for mental health promotion through urban design.

Numerous associations have been found between green space and mental health, spanning from views of greenery from an office window to full immersion in natural settings, such as in a park or urban woods. If green space is likely protective for good mental health, restricted access to green space has been posited as a risk factor for mental health problems in the city. In the UK, communities living in greener urban areas were found to be less likely to report mental distress and more likely to report mental well-being; this effect persisted even after adjusting for individual and regional socio-economic variation [8]; when people move from a greener to less green neighbourhood, deterioration in several measures of mental health have been noted [9]. Associations have also been found between tree density and antidepressant prescriptions as a proxy measure of depression [10]. Other studies focusing on specific impacts of green space have identified likely associations with stress [11], depression, social and cognitive functioning, and mood and aggression in dementia [12].

There is a range of explanations for why designing green space into urban environments seems to have such a marked effect on people's mental health and well-being. The full impact is surely a combination of several mechanisms working together to deliver a concentrated benefit for urban mental health. Part of the explanation may be found in the theories surrounding the specific benefits of green space for mental well-being.

Considered in isolation, the experience of simply being in green space seems in itself to have positive benefits for mental well-being. Three principal theories offer different explanations for our positive mental response to green space. The biophilia theory (Edward Wilson) proposes a special relationship between humans and the natural world, such that we have a subconscious biological urge to seek contact with other species that is sated when we access green space [13]. The stress reduction theory (Roger Ulrich) has a more practical premise, proposing that green space triggers physiological and psychological stress reduction responses by providing a venue that distances us from everyday demands, alongside opportunities for aesthetic appreciation and interest [14]. Finally, the attention restoration theory (Rachel and Stephen Kaplan) proposes that urban and work environments demand that we perform tasks that require prolonged maintenance of attention; green spaces physically and psychologically distance people from that environment and counteract 'attention fatigue' by facilitating our use of attention without the need for concentration [15]. Elements of these theories may combine to help explain the positive effects of green space and mental well-being. (The other mechanisms, providing a setting for exercise and positive social interactions, will be explored in the next section.)

One of the most common questions asked by designers is whether there is a 'dose' of green space for mental health: how can they integrate green space into their designs in a way that will maximize positive impact on mental well-being? In fact, current evidence suggests that there is no one-size-fits-all re-commended approach [16]. However, some principles are emerging that may be useful. Firstly, there seems to be a 'dose'–response relationship between the amount and quality of green space exposure and its impact on mental health. Even minimal exposure to green space, such as views from an office window seems to help reduce mental fatigue, aggression, and stress. In terms of in-dividual green spaces, the greatest positive impact is most likely to be from (1) spaces that people encounter in the course of their daily routines, and (2) immersive, walkable green spaces, such as parks and wide, natural walk-ways. The greatest benefits seem to come when location-appropriate local green spaces facilitate exercise, solitude, relaxation, and natural, positive social inter-actions. In particular, green spaces can act as venues to facilitate exercise and prosocial interaction, both of which have clear and substantial positive impact on mental health [17].

However, while more research is needed, it seems that, overall, consistent 'greenness' of a place may be more important than occasional green pockets in an otherwise non-green built environment [18]. This means that one large, won-derful park has the potential to deliver mental health benefits, but achieving full benefits means a commitment to integrate greenery all over the city. For these reasons, gardens placed near offices for lunch breaks, and street greenery such as trees and flowers have the potential to play an important role in enhancing overall 'greenness' and promoting good mental health alongside larger green spaces that allow people to become more immersed in a natural setting (see Figure 3.2).

However, there is no guarantee than simply installing green space will have a positive impact on anyone's mental health. Poorly managed green spaces can become neglected, overgrown, dirty, and filled with trash, leading to people avoiding the green spaces, feeling unsafe, and developing negative feelings about their neighbourhood; certain poorly managed green spaces also risk be-coming the settings for illegal and/or threatening activities such as illicit drug use, which further increase people's anxiety and negative thinking about the space. Particular risk factors for illicit drug transactions and use are green

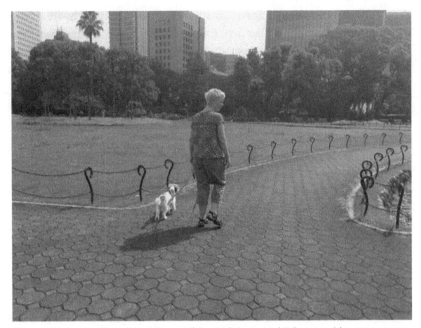

Figure 3.2 Amidst the tall buildings, Hibiya Park in central Tokyo provides easy access to green space for city dweller. Its paths are configured to provide shortcuts between stations, offices, restaurants, and other buildings, incentivizing commuters to walk through the green space as part of their daily routine.

spaces where entrances are disorganized and confused, dilapidated park furniture, and dark, shady areas with plant overgrowth and limited sightlines. Good design and provisions for good upkeep are essential to avoid these pitfalls and achieve the potential mental health benefits of green space.

Physical activity and mental health

Exercise and mental health are closely correlated. Regular exercise can substantially affect people's mood and can be as effective as antidepressant medication in treating mild-to-moderate depression [19]. Exercise is particularly effective in addressing depression that is associated with chronic physical illness, and in reducing symptoms of stress and anxiety, and symptoms associated with attention deficit disorder, dementia (mood), and schizophrenia (blunted emotions, loss of drive, and thinking difficulties). Exercise can be further helpful for improving the physical health of people who are taking certain common medications to manage mental disorders, which can have a side effect of weight gain [20].

There are almost limitless opportunities to design cities in ways that facilitate physical activity. Clearly, green space plays an important role. Well-designed and managed parks, woods, playing fields, and other 'walkable' green spaces all facilitate physical activity for those who choose to access them. However, reaping the full benefit from such facilities often requires people to set aside time and travel to a park or sports facility; urban design can intervene to develop active options that integrate exercise opportunities into people's daily routines to improve both physical and mental health.

Other than green spaces, a major opportunity for urban planners and designers is active transport. This is a broad term that for the purposes of this chapter refers to the various methods of moving around a city—with the key exception of driving a car from the start to end location. In many cities, cars have become king, and their dominance can have an important negative impact on people's mental health. This is particularly the case for those who commute: noise, crowds, unpredictable traffic, and traffic congestion can directly exert negative effects on people's mental well-being, particularly if commutes take more than 30 minutes. Direct negative effects can include an increase in frustration, anxiety, and hostility; further, a long commute has the effect of consuming time that could otherwise be spent on leisure, social activities, including time with family and friends, physical activity, and sleep [21–24].

There are also indirect effects of the dominance of car infrastructure on people's mental health. When roads and parking lots command primary use of a city's land, walkability and cycling are impeded, green space opportunities are reduced, communities are often split with physical road dividers, and noise, pollution, and physical danger are added to the urban experience.

If certain facilities, such as education, work opportunities, and social venues, are poorly connected by public transport, bike lanes, and walking routes, people without cars will experience reduced access and therefore reduced opportunities. In these various ways, non-car-users may feel like second-class citizens, and experience frustration, discrimination, and reduced confidence and potential as city users. If road infrastructure dominates, the traditional public meeting spaces and grouping of facilities in the city centre are often diminished as people drive between distant shops and facilities that are not within easy walking distance, reducing people's opportunities to socialize naturally, and to feel part of a community. Those who are unable to drive, such as older people, those with certain illnesses, including some mental illnesses, or those who cannot afford a car, become particularly disadvantaged in this case, creating a vicious cycle of vulnerability to mental illness, and reduced protective factors.

Urban design efforts should focus on reducing commute duration and stressfulness; increasing leisure, social and sleep time; increasing physical activity; and increasing connectivity and public gathering spaces. This may involve walkways and bikeways to enable safe, convenient, efficient, and cost-effective transit around the city; it may involve improving pedestrian plazas and the interestingness of main commuting streets to encourage their use; it may mean implementing bikeshare schemes or introducing more convenient routes. Each city will have different solutions that should be developed according to individual circumstances, closely involving users of the city to ensure local ownership, and to ensure that the solutions meet local needs.

Prosocial interaction and mental health

If positive, natural social interaction in the city is essential to help promote good social cohesion, belongingness, social capital, and thus better mental health, urban planning, and design can play an important role in its facilitation. Indeed, social interaction is one of the key mechanisms by which green spaces deliver their positive impact on mental health, particularly anxiety and depression. Social belongingness and social capital are important for building resilience, with strong social relationships delivering confidantes that people can turn to when they are distressed. However, moving to the city often removes people from their original social support systems, and urban design is often poorly configured to facilitate the development of new social networks, leading to isolation and loneliness, even in a crowd.

Public open spaces are the classic setting for urban design to facilitate cooperative community activities from chess tournaments to festivals [25]. Such spaces facilitate safe social gathering, natural social interactions, and even volunteering opportunities that deliver the mental health benefits of altruistic donation of time and skills. They provide settings for the neighbourhood to get together and experience feelings of community and belonging.

However, public open spaces are not the only opportunity for urban design. Other targets for prosocial design within the wider streetscape include street furniture and fittings from bus shelters to benches to planters, which encourage people to stop and chat. Streets with lively, diverse shops and cafes, as well as housing and offices, allow people to walk between their errands or other activities, are more likely to project positive perceptions of a neighbourhood and facilitate spontaneous social interactions, an effect that is lost when people have to drive alone between each stop on their errand route, or when they are compelled to walk along the unremitting, monotonous façades of giant shops or offices that take up entire city blocks and predispose people to boredom, negative ruminations, and a lack of interest in interacting with their environment.

Again, there is the risk that if these spaces are poorly managed and allowed to fall into disrepair or become the setting for illegal or intimidating activity that they will cease to be prosocial spaces. Instead, they risk exerting the converse impact on mental health, potentially increasing distress, alienation, and isolation, and even increased alcohol consumption.

Those living in neighbourhoods with dilapidated and deteriorating buildings have been found to be 150% more likely to report heavy drinking than those who live in neighbourhoods in better condition, and more likely to use illicit drugs, including drug overdose, even after individual factors have been taken into account [26, 27]. The density of locations that sell alcohol is also associated with amount of alcohol consumed, binge drinking, and alcohol-related violence [28].

Public spaces offer particular opportunities for prosocial experience in different age groups. For children, places to play, socialize, and explore are particularly important for their cognitive development and mental health. For adolescents, age-appropriate public spaces facilitate the development of social capital, social support, peer competence, and improved mood [29].

Older people who do not experience social isolation or feelings of disconnection have been found to be half as likely to experience rapid cognitive decline in a range of functional domains [30]. However, in practice this can be challenging to achieve. Older people often find that a combination of retirement and physical and mental health problems can start to narrow their geographical and social reach. This puts them at risk of social isolation and reduced quality of life. Accessible, high-quality public spaces can contribute to their independence, autonomy, self-esteem, and physical and mental well-being, providing settings for social interaction and activities of daily living.

Two factors that help prevent depression in older people are living in a home that is clean, well-decorated, and has at least two rooms [31], and having access to diverse amenities [32]. The ability to leave the house is particularly important, providing access to nature, physical activity, natural social interactions, and a sense of independence, self, and quality of life.

However, people who have dementia with disorientation and confusion are at particular risk of becoming largely restricted to their homes, contributing to their development of low mood. Owing to the risk of becoming lost or getting into unsafe situations when they go out alone, these people can find themselves rapidly losing independence, with dramatically narrowing geographical reach. Given the increasing number of people with dementia living in the city, this should be a specific priority for urban planners and designers.

There are two major opportunities in urban design to support the continuing independence and quality of life of people with dementia: facilitating social engagement and delivering simple, accessible navigation aids. In particular, key opportunities lie with design that incorporates familiarity, legibility, distinctiveness, accessibility, comfort, and safety [33], an approach currently being taken by the movement to create safe, confident navigation around 'dementia-friendly neighbourhoods'. Some examples include promoting and preserving clear environmental navigation cues (varied architecture with distinctive, recognizable features such as a church with a steeple, a grocery store with fruit in front); clear, simple navigation signs placed perpendicular to walls, and using realistic symbols; open public spaces with welcoming seats; good lighting; and avoidance of startling loud noises.

Of course, the aim of urban design should not be unremitting prosocial contact for anybody. Alongside the need for positive social interaction is the need for privacy. Furthermore, people need to feel they have the agency to control when to be social and when to have more solitary time. Architects designing mental health facilities have considered this in detail, and lessons can be extrapolated to the wider urban environment, from designing welcoming entry features like porches to encourage social interaction to the choices of taking different routes to reach a particular location and flexible ways of using spaces to provide opportunities to avoid interactions [33].

Safety in the city as a determinant of mental health

Safety is an essential part of feeling comfortable and secure in the city. And yet absolute safety risks creating an atmosphere of such sanitization and lack of choice that it loses some of the very factors that give a thriving, bustling city its personality and people their autonomy.

In particular, the risk of crime is important to address if people are to feel safe in the city. Those who have their property stolen, experience, or even witness violent crime experience poorer mental health, even a year after the incident occurs [34]. There are a vast number of ways in which urban design can help prevent crime and increase people's feelings of safety and security. The key principles are surveillance, access control, and maintenance.

As people are more likely to commit crimes when they believe themselves to be unobserved, creating the feeling that they are being watched is a powerful deterrent, and thus presents an obvious opportunity for urban design. Stationary surveillance involves simple measures such as designing windows into building walls that overlook pedestrian areas, avoiding walls that limit sightlines, and ensuring that lighting is designed to illuminate faces (but avoiding brightness that casts glare and shadows). Mobile surveillance, however, means increasing the likely witnesses in risky places, for instance improving pedestrian and cyclist infrastructure to not only reduce the risk of injury, but by encouraging more people to use a particular area, they provide natural surveillance.

Access control means ensuring clear demarcations between public and private space in a way that discourages encroachment by public space users onto private space. Examples include dissuading access by limiting the number of entry points into private spaces; using impediments like thorny plantation underneath windows; reducing public-facing access to upper levels; and using lighting and signs to clearly demarcate whether the public is welcome in a particular space.

Again, the question of maintenance arises. The very appearance of a neglected space can lead people to feel unsafe, and this can become a self-fulfilling prophecy. A dilapidated, deteriorating space implies tolerance of disorder and lack of oversight and management, and thus encourages further disorder, increasing the risk that the space will attract criminal behaviour. Good maintenance gives the message of oversight and can reduce the risk of a space becoming threatening, exclusive, or developing features that make people feel unsafe.

Promoting and supporting good mental health through the means of urban design often incorporates several of these key principles (see Figure 3.3).

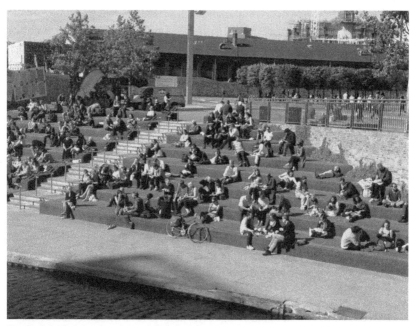

Figure 3.3 The Granary Square development in Kings Cross, London, provides opportunities for social interaction in public open spaces, integrating natural elements such as trees and water, plus accessibility for walkers, cyclists, and public transport users. It offers good sightlines and surveillance to enhance safety. It is also near a university and many offices, providing an important place for lunch and relaxation.

Conclusion

The urban environment can have a wide range of effects on people's mental health and well-being, many of which have long been understood, and some of which are just emerging. The city can create conditions for better mental health; it can also strip away protective factors and provide a setting for mental health deterioration.

Green, active, prosocial, and safe spaces contribute to people's mental health. More research will further illuminate the mechanisms by which cities can affect mental health, and opportunities to leverage cities to promote and support good mental health. However, whether the city is able to promote and support good mental health, or not, cannot be dismissed as a matter of happenstance; nor can it be dismissed as the remit of public health or mental health professionals. Just as citymakers are starting to assert their responsibility in improving physical health, so, too, must they assume their role in mental health. Opportunities abound for urban planners and designers to have impact here: they can help mitigate existing risk factors, provide settings that help build resilience, and foster protective factors for good mental health. The World Health Organization defines public health as 'the art and science of preventing disease, prolonging life and promoting health through the organized efforts of society'. Perhaps urban public mental health is a clunky term, but its meaning is precise: in an urbanizing world, it is incumbent on those involved in the design and management of cities to organize prioritization of the promotion of mental health and well-being for their citizens. This is important at the individual level; it is also essential for a thriving, resilient city.

References

1. **World Health Organization**. Mental health: a state of wellbeing. Available at: http://www.who.int/features/factfiles/mental_health/en/ (accessed 25 January 2017).

2. **UN Habitat**. World Cities Report 2016. Available at: http://wcr.unhabitat.org/ (accessed 25 January 2017).

3. **Whiteford HA, Degenhardt L, Rehm J, Baxter AJ, Ferrari AJ, Erskine HE**, et al. Global burden of disease attributable to mental and substance use disorders: findings from the Global Burden of Disease Study 2010. *The Lancet* 2013; **382**: 1575–1586.

4. **Peen J, Schoevers RA, Beekman AT, Dekker J**. The current status of urban-rural differences in psychiatric disorders. *Acta Psychiatrica Scandinavica* 2010; **121**: 84–93.

5. **Kelly BD, O'Callaghan E, Waddington JL, Feeney L, Browne S, Scully PJ**, et al. Schizophrenia and the city: a review of literature and prospective study of psychosis and urbanicity in Ireland. *Schizophrenia Research* 2010; **116**: 75–89.

6. **Cantor-Graae E, Selten JP**. Schizophrenia and migration: a meta-analysis and review. *American Journal of Psychiatry* 2005; **162**: 12–24.

7. Golembiewski J. Architecture, the urban environment and severe psychosis: aetiology. *Journal of Urban Design and Mental Health* 2017; **2**: 1.

8. White MP, Alcock I, Wheeler BW, Depledge MH. Would you be happier living in a greener urban area? A fixed-effects analysis of panel data. *Psychological Science* 2013; **24**: 920–928.

9. Alcock I, White MP, Wheeler BW, Fleming LE, Deplege MH. Longitudinal effects on mental health of moving to greener and less green urban areas. *Environmental Science & Technology* 2015; **48**: 1247–1255.

10. Taylor MS, Wheeler BW, White MP, Economou T, Osborne NJ. Research note: urban street tree density and antidepressant prescription rates—a cross-sectional study in London, UK. *Landscape and Urban Planning* 2015; **136**: 174–179.

11. Grahn P, Stigsdotter UA. Landscape planning and stress. *Urban Forestry and Urban Greening* 2003; **2**: 1–18.

12. Dannenberg AL, Jackson RJ, Frumkin H, Schieber RA, Pratt M, Kochtitzky C, et al. The impact of community design and land-use choices on public health: a scientific research agenda. *American Journal of Public Health* 2003; **93**: 1500–1508.

13. Wilson EO. *Biophilia—the Human Bond with Other Species.* Cambridge, MA: Harvard University Press, 1984.

14. Ulrich RS. Aesthetic and affective responses to natural environment. In: I Altman, J Wohlwill (eds) *Behaviour and the Natural Environment.* New York: Plenum Press, 1983, pp. 85–125.

15. Kaplan R, Kaplan S. *The Experience of Nature. A Psychological Perspective.* Cambridge: Cambridge University Press, 1983.

16. World Health Organization. *Urban Green Spaces and Health: A Review of Evidence.* Bonn: World Health Organization European Centre for Environment, 2016.

17. Sugiyama T, Leslie E, Giles-Corti B, Owen N. Associations of neighbourhood greenness with physical and mental health: do walking, social coherence and local social interaction explain the relationships? *Journal of Epidemiology and Community Health* 2008; **62**: e9.

18. Alcock I, White M, Wheeler P, Fleming LE, Depledge MH. Longitudinal effects on mental health of moving to greener and less green urban areas. *Environmental Science & Technology* 2014; **48**: 1247–1255.

19. Stathopoulou G, Powers MB, Berry AC, Smits JAJ, Otto MW. Exercise interventions for mental health: a quantitative and qualitative review. *Clinical Psychology* 2006; **13**: 179–193.

20. Morgan AJ, Parker AG, Alvarez M, Jimenez AF, Jorm AF. Exercise and mental health: an Exercise and Sports Science Australia commissioned review. *JEP Online* 2013; **16**: 64–73.

21. Fong G, Frost D, Stansfeld S. Road rage: A psychiatric phenomenon? Social *Psychiatry & Psychiatric Epidemiology* 2001; **36**: 277.

22. Sygna K, Aasvang GM, Aamodt G, Oftedal B, Krog NH. Road traffic noise, sleep and mental health. *Environmental Research* 2014; **131**: 17–24.

23. Christian TJ. Automobile commuting duration and the quantity of time spent with spouse, children, and friends. *Preventive Medicine* 2012; **55**: 215–218.

24. Hansson E, Marrisson K, Bjork J, Ostergren PO, Jakobsson K. Relationship between commuting and health outcomes in a cross-sectional population survey in southern Sweden. *BMC Public Health* 2011; **11**: 834.

25. Francis J, Wood LJ, Knuiman M, Giles-Corti B. Quality or quantity? Exploring the relationship between Public Open Space attributes and mental health in Perth, Western Australia. *Social Science & Medicine* 2012; **74**: 1570–1577.

26. Bernstein KT, Galea S, Ahern J, Tracy M, Vlahov D. The built environment and alcohol consumption in urban neighborhoods. *Drug and Alcohol Dependence* 2007; **91**: 244–252.

27. Hembree C, Galea S, Ahern J, Tracy M, Piper TM, Miller J, Tardiff KJ. The urban built environment and overdose mortality in New York City neighborhoods. *Health and Place* 2005; **11**: 147–156.

28. Pereira G, Wood L, Foster S, Haggar F. Access to alcohol outlets, alcohol consumption and mental health. *PLOS ONE* 2013; **8**: e53461.

29. Aneshensel CS, Sucoff C. The neighborhood context of adolescent mental health. *Journal of Health and Social Behavior* 1996; **37**: 293–310.

30. Mitchell L, Burton E. Neighbourhoods for life: designing dementia-friendly outdoor environments. *Quality in Ageing and Older Adults* 2006; **7**: 26–33.

31. Chan A, Malhotra C, Malhotra R, Østbye T. Living arrangements, social networks and depressive symptoms among older men and women in Singapore. *International Journal of Geriatric Psychiatry* 2011; **26**: 630–639.

32. Gillespie S, LeVasseur MT, Michael YL. Neighbourhood amenities and depressive symptoms in urban-dwelling older adults. *Journal of Urban Design and Mental Health* 2017; **2**: 4.

33. Evans GW. The built environment and mental health. *Journal of Urban Health* 2003; **80**: 4.

34. Clark C, Myron R, Stansfeld S, Candy B. A systematic review on the effect of the built and physical environment on mental health. *Journal of Public Mental Health* 2006; **6**: 14–27.

Chapter 4

Globalization and urbanization

Debby Darmansjah, Gurvinder Kalra,
and Dinesh Bhugra

Introduction

Globalization affects health directly and indirectly in a number of ways. Globalization has led to an increase in the movement of people and resources. The variations reported in rates of various psychiatric and physical illnesses are often ignored and the focus is often on similarities, thereby creating a homogeneous global culture with an emphasis on the premise of universalizing the provision of health treatment for all people in a Westernized allopathic care model, ignoring local models of care. It is important to bear this in mind because with urbanization as a direct correlate of globalization and resulting industrialization social, economic, and political transitions are taking place, which at one level are increasing economic growth and also discrepancies, but on the other changing expectations of the individual patients and their families.

There is no doubt that globalization has become an oft-used and abused term to describe a collection of processes all involving social, economic, and cultural *exchanges*. The abuse of the term is related to its negative aspects and political interpretations, leading to xenophobia and nationalism. However, the term retains a wide currency and usage that focuses on debates about economics, development, international relations, and, increasingly, health, but there remain problems in clarifying what is understood by the term itself. Definitions of globalization have often tended to emphasize the material impacts of development, and downplayed dynamic processes affecting the movement of people, goods, services, and ideas, including those ideas that pertain to health care. There is no doubt that the processes related to globalization have influenced health care, resources, policy making, and provision in global circles of influence for much of the past 30 years.

For mental health, the impact of changing economic and social relations introduces particular problems, including those of external and inter-cultural validity of diagnosis, rapidly changing circumstances within which people live,

Box 4.1 The links between various factors and mental ill health

- ◆ Social determinants.
- ◆ Urbanization overcrowding.
- ◆ Poverty.
- ◆ Unemployment.
- ◆ Mental ill health.

age, and work, and specificity—factors that influence the occurrence of mental health problems, which may at times be similar to those affecting physical illness. Even though mental health should be an integral part of health, reality is often different. Those who experience mental ill health also carry with them specific concerns and, indeed, challenges for understanding the impact of globalization on living and functioning. How globalization itself influences mental health is poorly characterized, but it can be argued that urbanization may play a mediating role in this development. Patterns of causation are necessary to understand so that appropriate interventions can be employed and policies developed (see Box 4.1).

Social determinants and urbanization

Social conditions are fundamental causes of ill health [1]. Although other forms of causation, especially in epidemiological studies, have been causal and often uni-directional, increasing emphasis is being placed on 'web of causation', which makes much more sense in our understanding of mental ill health. Marmot [2] lays out a series of ways in which social and economic environments influence health. Social stratification, along lines of ethnicity, geographical location, sexual identity, and economic and political power is presented as a dynamic process, interrelating with an individual's development. The psychosocial environment at work is considered crucial. Although evidence is strong for the social determinants of health, evaluating and intervening on such determinants (e.g. education, employment, job opportunities, living conditions, access to healthy food) there are political and economic barriers, which are often very difficult to cross. Using bereavement as an example, it is clear that depth of grief is very strongly influenced by a number of factors, including the type of loss, preparedness of the event, the meaning attached to the deceased, and the broader social, economic, and cultural expressions, as well as repercussions of the bereavement—similar arguments can be made about drastic changes to one's work, family life, food availability, sex life, and recreational pattern.

Life events, life experiences, and resilience all play a role in managing stresses and violence which is often higher in urban areas. Understanding the process of identity formation in the context of these issues is likely to be crucial. The incorporation of conceptions of selfhood and mental wellness are necessary to understand the local elaboration and occurrence of mental disorder. Increasing rates of attention deficit–hyperactivity disorder diagnosis, the construction of intermittent explosive disorder and dangerous and severe personality disorder as psychiatric problems, and the changing relevance of dependence diagnoses for understanding the global use of drugs such as alcohol and opiates, are all examples of how disease constructs are arrived at through a complicated prism of economic and socio-cultural-political concerns.

Development affects not only definitions of illness, but also of wellness; angry disagreement over the utility and ethics of various policymakers and the State in defining sickness and sick benefits allows a population to recognize what it is to be well enough to work, above and beyond what it means to be ill. There are clear and apparently increasing tensions within popular notions of illness, work capability, and well-being. Both within the workforce and outside it, there is good evidence that economic downturn in many parts of the world and austerity has negatively affected mental health. Theoretical approaches to the effect of global social and economic shifts on mental health require sensitivity to issues of definition, and how stakeholders engage with these definitions. These notions are left unexamined by World Health Organization (WHO) pronouncements on global health, such as the definition cited at the beginning of this chapter.

The question of culture-sensitive definitions not only applies to what constitutes mental health in low- and middle-income countries, but also relates to reference point categories like violence and trauma—the development and establishment of cross-cultural concepts of trauma and trauma-related mental health problems is crucial.

The number and areas of various cities in the world are growing as a result of globalization and migration of people from rural areas, this growth being largely limited to the developing countries, but also seen in the developed ones. Cities have thus been aptly described as the culmination of globalization. The level of urbanization is expected to increase worldwide. According to the 2014 *World Urbanization Prospects* by the United Nations, 54% of the world's population resides in urban areas. This has almost doubled compared to 30% in 1950, and has been predicted to increase to 66% by 2050. Africa and Asia are expected to be urbanizing faster than other continents, and are projected to become 54% and 64% urban, respectively, by 2050. Particularly, three combined countries (India, China, and Nigeria) are expected to account for 37% of the projected growth between 2014 and 2050 [3]. Cities that were once considered centres of trade, science, education, and progress have transformed into scenes of crime, traffic congestion, and pollution, and in recent times, terrorism. Owing to increasing populations and moves into cities from rural areas, cities are continuing to expand often in a very haphazard fashion, without proper planning and infrastructure in place. Even cities that had started in a planned way have often produced rather ill-organized expansion with increasing demands on basic amenities such as water supplies and sewage. One could argue that these cities are now becoming hyper-cities, with multiple centres and increased pressures on space, threatening their basic sustainability.

Changing geographies and demographics

Cities around the world are changing for a number of reasons: first and perhaps the most important is the increase in population. With over 7.5 billion people on the planet it is inevitable that people will move into cities and towns, but reasons for this movement are many and need better understanding, especially in the context of health. A move to urban areas may also create poverty and other issues for people who are left behind in rural areas and may contribute to poverty if there is not adequate submission of finances from those who are urban migrants. Rural economies may be affected and thus influence this migration into cities.

Urbanization has been defined as 'the process by which towns and cities are formed and become larger as more and more people begin living and working in central area' [4]. It can also refer to 'the change in size, density and heterogeneity of cities' [5]. A large number of people migrating from rural to these urban setups may bring with them poverty, hoping to turn it into riches as cities are seen as potential sources for financial rewards. As accommodation may be too expensive, migrants from rural areas will stay initially (and this may well become permanent) in poor-quality shared settlements with resulting overcrowding and limited amenities. There may be a large social divide as the original population moves on to better houses in suburban parts of the city and migrants settle in inner-city areas, which are run down with dilapidated buildings. Thus, parts of the city are populated by the rich, whereas the others are inhabited by the poor, creating a clear social and a structural divide. Furthermore, as noted in the previous section, a rapid, uncontrolled, and unplanned growth of these shanties and ghettos leads to the formation of 'mini-villages within cities'. There are several examples of such growth—*Favellas*, as seen in Brazil, and *Dharavi* in Mumbai, Asia's biggest slum area. The population residing in such urban 'villages' are prone to physical and psychiatric disorders directly or indirectly due to hazardous environmental conditions that give rise to different patterns of morbidity and mortality, marginalizing them in terms of health [6].

There are a number of hazards that these populations face, including unhygienic and over-crowded living conditions, poor sanitation with lack of waste and sewage disposal, inadequate water supplies, pollution, drug use, limited job opportunities, exposure to occupational hazards, and accidents [7]. All these factors contribute to a general degradation of the environment and a decline in the quality of life in the urban populace. These factors also affect people across all ages, including the old and the young alike, who may have to continue working in order to earn a decent livelihood. It may lead to increased morbidity in this already vulnerable population. For instance, a cross-sectional study in India found that the incidence of falls in the elderly is three times higher in urban areas than rural [8]. It has been argued that the number of street children in urban areas has risen manifold, especially in developing countries, with the additional impact of issues such as child labour and malnutrition, among others [9].

The urban population mix of rich and the poor can thus be viewed as a double burden of health problems, with the rich suffering from the more chronic diseases, accidents, and lifestyle diseases, and the poor suffering from infectious diseases, for example [10, 11]. It has been shown that longevity within the same city varies dramatically [12]. Diabetes is one of the few chronic diseases that is being fueled by rapid urbanization, and the increasingly sedentary lifestyles associated with it [13]. Other risk factors for non-communicable diseases such as obesity and hypertension predominate in an urbanized population. A study in sub-Saharan Africa found a higher prevalence of diabetes and hypertension in urban men and women [14]. Residing in an urban area was also associated with higher odds of a body mass index (BMI) > 25 [14, 15].

Urbanicity refers to 'the impact of living in urban areas at a given time' [5]. Allender et al. [16] developed an 'urbanicity' scale and found a clear relationship between urbanicity and common modifiable risk factors for chronic disease in Sri Lankan adults. It was shown that urban-dwelling women were almost three times as likely to have an increased BMI and more than twice as likely to have diabetes mellitus than rural dwellers. In addition, migration has a significant influence on an individual having high blood pressure. Research among Asian immigrants in Canada has highlighted the relationship between duration of residence and prevalence of hypertension after adjusting for all other variables such as age and BMI. In this particular population, the prevalence of hypertension increases with the longer duration of residence [17].

The detrimental physical implications of urbanization on an individual or population that have been described may also coexist with impaired mental health. A Danish study implied a dose–response relationship between degree of urbanization at birth and the incidence of psychiatric disorders in general, as listed in the *10th Revision of the International Classification of Diseases* (ICD-10) [18]. This is consistent with the findings from a meta-analysis of urban–rural prevalence of psychiatric disorders in developed countries [19]. In a Chinese population moving from rural to urban regions, prevalent depressive symptoms and insomnia have particularly been noted. This could be reflected in the string of suicide and suicidal attempts by several young 'rural–urban workers' at a low-paying factory in southern China [20]. More recently, lack of access to 'green space' has been investigated in terms of its relation to mental health. A twin study concluded that greater access to 'green space' is associated with less depression [21].

As well as communication difficulties and culture shock, it is not unexpected to infer that migrants may be at a higher risk of developing mental health problems. A significant proportion of Burmese people that have migrated to Australia reported symptoms of anxiety, depression, and somatization, which have been correlated with post-migration living difficulties [22]. Similarly, schizophrenia was noted to be of a higher relative risk in Danish immigrants than in non-immigrants [23]. In another Danish study, Pedersen and Mortensen [24] found that the risk for schizophrenia was more than twofold for individuals who had spent their first 15 years in a major city versus those who had grown up in rural areas.

Learnings

As alluded to previously, one of the negative outcomes of urbanization is a surge in homelessness. According to the 2011 Australian Census, approximately 44,000 young people are homeless and a quarter of this population includes those in the 12–24 year old group [25]. More particularly, it has been demonstrated that homeless young people who identify as a sexual minority (i.e. as lesbian, gay, bisexual, or transgender) report higher levels of depressive symptoms, somatic complaints, delinquency, and aggression [26]. According to Rice et al. [27], a significant protective factor for depression in these young people is contacting their friends through social networking. The importance of fostering these relationships may be highlighted in community-based programmes and agencies serving homeless young people.

A pivotal learning point can also be adopted from the WHO's Healthy Cities Project, which first started in 1985. On its first review of progress from 1987 to

1990, it has grown to include 30 projects in European cities and has also sparked interest in developing countries. It puts health on a pedestal during the process of urban planning and policy making. The ultimate aim is to maximize the physical, mental, social, and environmental well-being of people who live and work in cities. Simply put, it believes that the improvement of environments and expansion of its resources will lead to people living healthier lives. Some examples of the initiatives include the implementation of healthier food project and nutrition contest for schools and kindergartens in Munich, regular testing of bathing water to monitor pollution in Stockholm, and strong publicizing to raise awareness about the project around European cities [28].

Throughout the decades, this project has grown and continues to be evaluated. More recently, an evaluation of Phase V of the WHO Health Cities Network was summarized in 2014. This was a review of progress from 2009 to 2013, which involved 99 cities in the WHO European National Healthy Cities Network. A 'health impact assessment' has been applied in certain European cities prior to starting projects, programmes, or policies. Additionally, case studies have demonstrated that citizen participation in programme planning leads to more targeted interventions, and hence enhance overall service satisfaction. Although theoretical and methodological plans have been carefully laid out to promote healthy cities, one of the main challenges is to get approval and support from local governments [29].

As a result, many non-governmental organizations have started working in various countries to ensure equitable healthcare services to all with increased community participation. There are many examples of good practice, for example SCARF, which stands for Schizophrenia Research Foundation. It is a non-governmental, non-profit organization in Chennai that aims to 'implement structured psychosocial rehabilitation services to individuals with mental health problems'. SCARF prescribes minimum standards of care for individuals with schizophrenia focusing not only on continuity of care across different interventions, including psychosocial and pharmacological, but also across different age groups [30]. A part of their services includes a monthly caregiver psychoeducation programme that serves a very important purpose. SCARF is also affiliated with the WHO for their contribution in mental health research and training within a multidisciplinary team. 'Harmony Place', a non-governmental, community-based multicultural organization in Australia provides culturally sensitive mental health services to people from diverse cultural and language backgrounds. By employing professional staff members who are bilingual or migrants and/or have also experienced mental health issues, they are also able to offer peer support services, as well as professional counselling and other group activities [31]. It has been shown that the involvement of peer support workers in mental health services helps in reducing admission rates and in promoting 'hope and belief in the possibility of recovery' [32].

Conclusion

Under the impact of urbanization, rapidly growing cities, rather than becoming symbols of power and growth, have become symbols of poverty, socio-ecological deterioration, congestion, and a lack of basic health care for a number of reasons. While the rapid urbanization can not necessarily be stopped, whether there is any mileage in slowing it down so that adequate preparations can be made to improve physical and mental health needs to be discussed as a matter of urgency. It is critical to address issues of inequalities in health care distribution in urban areas that is happening as a result of the sheer speed of this process, overpopulation, and overcrowding; Active cooperation between policymakers, healthcare providers, community groups, and neighbourhood associations is required in helping to create more healthier and liveable cities. Being able to negotiate newer resources for health promotion by building up stronger alliances for public health is the need of the hour.

References

1. **Link BG, Phelan JC.** McKeown and the idea that social conditions are fundamental causes of disease. *American Journal of Public Health* 2002; **92**: 730–732.
2. **Marmot M.** *The Health Gap: The Challenge of an Unequal World.* London: Bloomsbury, 2016.
3. **United Nations.** *World Urbanization Prospects: The 2014 Revision.* New York: United Nations, 2014.
4. **Merriam-Webster.** Urbanization. 2017 Available at: https://www.merriam-webster.com/dictionary/urbanization (accessed 5 November 2018).
5. **Vlahov D, Galea S.** Urbanization, urbanicity, and health. *Journal of Urban Health* 2002; **79**: 51–59.
6. **Harpham T, Stephens C.** Urbanization and health in developing countries. *World Health Statistics Quarterly* 1991; **44**: 62–69.
7. **Satterthwaite D.** The impact on health urban environments. Environment and Urbanization 1993; **5**: 87–111.
8. **Thakur N, Banerjee A, Nikumb VB.** Health problems among the elderly: a cross sectional study. *Annals of Medical and Health Science Research* 2013; **3**: 19–25.
9. **Woan J, Lin J, Auerswald C.** The health status of street children and youth in low-and middle-income countries: a systematic review of the literature. *Journal of Adolescence Health* 2013; **53**: 314–321.
10. **Crompton DW Savioli L.** Intestinal parasitic infections and *urbanization. Bulletin* of the World Health Organization 1993; **71**: 1.
11. **Stephens C.** Healthy cities or unhealthy islands? The health and social implications of urban inequality. *Environment and Urbanization* 1996; **8**: 9–30.

12. **Marmot MG.** Geography of blood pressure and hypertension. *British Medical Bulletin* 1984; **40**: 380–386.

13. **Hu FB.** Globalization of diabetes. *Diabetes Care* 2011; **34**: 1249–1257.

14. **Sobngwi E, Mbanya JC, Unwin NC, Porcher R, Kengne AP, Fezeu L,** et al. Exposure over the life course to an urban environment and its relation with obesity, diabetes, and hypertension in rural and urban Cameroon. *International Journal of Epidemiology* 2004; **33**: 769–776.

15. **Oyebode O, Pape UJ, Laverty AA, Lee JT, Bhan N, Millett C.** Rural, urban and migrant differences in non-communicable disease risk-factors in middle income countries: a cross-sectional study of WHO-SAGE data. *PLOS ONE* 2015; **10**: e0122747.

16. **Allender S, Wickramasinghe K, Goldacre M, Matthews D, Katulanda P.** Quantifying urbanization as a risk factor for noncommunicable disease. *Journal of Urban Health* 2011; **88**: 906.

17. **Kaplan MS, Chang C, Newsom JT, McFarland BH.** Acculturation status and hypertension among Asian immigrants in Canada. *Journal of Epidemiology and Community Health* 2002; **56**: 455–456.

18. **Vassos E, Agerbo E, Mors O, Pedersen CB.** Urban–rural differences in incidence rates of psychiatric disorders in Denmark. *British Journal of Psychiatry* 2016; **208**: 435–440.

19. **Peen J, Schoevers RA, Beekman AT, Dekker J.** The current status of urban-rural differences in psychiatric disorders. *Acta Psychiatrica Scandinavica* 2010; **121**: 84–93.

20. **Mou J, Griffiths SM, Fong H, Dawes MG.** Health of China's rural–urban migrants and their families: a review of literature from 2000 to 2012. *British Medical Bulletin* 2013; **106**: 19–43.

21. **Cohen-Cline H, Turkheimer E, Duncan GE.** Access to green space, physical activity and mental health: a twin study. *Journal of Epidemiology and Community Health* 2015; **69**: 523–529.

22. **Schweitzer RD, Brough M, Vromans L, Asic-Kobe M.** Mental health of newly arrived Burmese refugees in Australia: contributions of pre-migration and post-migration experience. *Australia and New Zealand Journal of Psychiatry* 2011; **45**: 299–307.

23. **Sørensen HJ, Nielsen PR, Pedersen CB, Benros ME, Nordentoft M, Mortensen PB.** Population impact of familial and environmental risk factors for schizophrenia: a nationwide study. *Schizophrenia Research* 2014; **153**:214–219.

24. **Pedersen CB, Mortensen PB.** Evidence of a dose-response relationship between urbanicity during upbringing and schizophrenia risk. *Archives of General Psychiatry* 2001; **58**: 1039–1046.

25. **Australian Bureau of Statistics.** Census of population and housing: estimating homelessness, 2011. Available at: http://www.abs.gov.au/AUSSTATS/abs@.nsf/DetailsPage/2049.02011?OpenDocument (accessed 5 November 2018).

26. **Cochran BN, Stewart AJ, Ginzler JA, Cauce AM.** Challenges faced by homeless sexual minorities: comparison of gay, lesbian, bisexual, and transgender homeless adolescents with their heterosexual counterparts. *American Journal of Public Health* 2002; **92**: 773–777.

27. **Rice E, Kurzban S, Ray D.** Homeless but connected: the role of heterogeneous social network ties and social networking technology in the mental health outcomes of street-living adolescents. *Community Mental Health Journal* 2012; **48**: 692–698.

28. **World Health Organization (WHO).** *Healthy Cities Project: A Project Becomes a Movement, Review of Progress 1987 to 1990.* Milan: WHO Regional Office for Europe, 1997.

29. **World Health Organization (WHO)**. Healthy Cities: Promoting Health and Equity—Evidence for Local Policy and Practice, Summary Evaluation of Phase V of the WHO European Healthy Cities Network. Copenhagen: WHO Regional Office for Europe, 2014.

30. **Bhugra D.** Mental health for nations. *International Review of Psychiatry* 2016; **28**: 342–374.

31. **Harmony Place**. Multicultural youth peer mentoring program. Available at: http://www.harmonyplace.org.au (accessed 12 August 2017).

32. **Repper J, Carter T.** A review of the literature on peer support in mental health services. JMH. 2011;**20**(4):392–411.

Chapter 5

Internal migration and internal boundaries

Antonio Ventriglio and Dinesh Bhugra

Introduction

Migration occurs across nations, as well as within a nation, for example from rural to urban centres, as well as from urban to rural areas, although the latter seems to be rarer. International migration is often attributed to political and economic reasons, from escaping poverty to escaping persecution against religious, political beliefs, and sexual orientation. Both internal and external migration are associated with globalization and its consequences, especially rapid industrialization and urbanization. Migration is not a recent phenomenon, but the speed with which it occurs and our awareness of it became more pronounced in the twentieth century. The movement of people from rural areas to urban areas has occurred since the Industrial Revolution in Western Europe in late eighteenth and early nineteenth centuries. The scale and the speed of urbanization, especially in low- and middle-income countries has been truly amazing, which has meant that there are significant challenges for not only the provision of public infrastructure, but also affordable and safe housing and affordable health care. While many urban dwellers benefit from the opportunities that city life provides, large numbers of people often live in desperation and deprivation. The large socio-economic inequality within cities can be attributed to the heterogeneous nature of urban living and employment, which, in an interconnected world, are also affected by global inequalities. One's place of residence within a city also determines one's health and well-being. In Chapter 6, Peter Schofield discusses specific issues related to refugees and asylum seekers, so our focus in this chapter will be on migrants who migrate for educational or economic reasons.

People move across geographical areas, cultures, societies, nations, and cities for all types of reasons. Migration has been defined as a process of social change where an individual, either alone or with others, leaves one geographical area for another for a number of reasons [1]. Migration can be in either direction, but in this chapter we will focus on moving from rural to urban areas. Migration can be defined according to purpose of migration, perceived duration of migration, and time to prepare will affect post-migration adjustment. Therefore, the actual response to the process of migration will depend upon a number of factors, such as the age at which migrant moves, their gender, whether they move alone or in a group, their educational and socio-economic status, distances travelled, and social support available. Different cultural groups may respond to the actual act of migration in different ways [2]. The three angles of the triangle of globalization are (1) interconnectedness of people, (2) raw materials and (3) products; these processes have led to major movements across the globe. The International Organization for Migration (IOM) [3] has estimated that there are 1 billion migrants in the world at the present time. It is inevitable that the impact of movement of materials and products will affect the mental state of people—those who are migrating, those they leave behind, and those who are struggling to move. Each of these groups will have a number of stressors, which can contribute to developing mental illness and thus need to be identified.

When people move across national borders they face a number of challenges. However, migration into cities also brings with it a series of stressors at both individual and familial levels. There will be social, political, and cultural changes that are likely to influence economic expectations and aspirations not only of the individual migrant, but also of those who have been left behind. The aspiration and achievement on the part of the individual and those who have been left behind will play a role in helping the self-esteem of the individual. If these expectations are not met, then it is quite likely that any discrepancy between aspiration and achievement will affect their mental health and also that of family members left behind. An associated complication is that this disparity may add to alienation and a sense of disaffection, leading to stress.

Among social determinants, unemployment, poverty, overcrowding, and lack of education at a personal level and urbanicity at a familial or social level mediate and affect rates of mental disorders. Even within the same broader cultures, cultures are dynamic and these alter over the years in response to many factors such as economic pressures, rapid urbanization with varying quality of housing, unaffordable overcrowded living, and direct or indirect exposures to other cultures through the media—written and visual—through the Internet, television, newspapers, magazines, social media, and journals. Political aspects of globalization need to be borne in mind, too. The exposure of the individual to other cultures directly or indirectly will influence individuals, their kinships, and support systems. Another possible impact of exposure to other cultures will affect language, dress codes, and dietary habits, but, in the long run, attitudes and behaviours.

Reasons for migration

The reasons leading to internal migration are most likely to be economic, although in a small number it may be educational. Reasons for migration into urban areas may be affected by political persecution. Intra-national migration is likely to be attractive to people who wish to seek employment, which may or may not be supported by housing.

Migration as a process can be broadly divided into three stages, even when it is an internal (within the country) process. These three stages are (1) pre-migration, (2) migration, and (3) post-migration. It must be emphasized that these are not discrete stages and can often run into one another. The pre-migration stage involves preparations and identifying resources needed for movement and survival, modes of travel needed, and contacts in the new place. In case of forced migration due to natural or man-made disasters, this preparation stage may be shortened and inadequate preparations can contribute to development of psychological problems, such as adjustment disorders.

For intra-national migration the phase of physical migration may be short. The post-migration stage may commence with arrival into the city without knowing anyone, or knowing a few people, and each such experience may well contribute to a degree of isolation or alienation. Social support and financial stability will also affect the experience of settling down. The post-migration phase is a long one and it may take years for the individual to settle down and adjust.

We know that life events (especially negative ones) can lead to depression. Migration itself is a significant life event and may be negative and may be accompanied by other events, thereby producing a cumulative effect. The aspiration–achievement gap has recently been identified as a possible contributor to mental health problems. However, potential stress related to the expectation of the family and the kinship of the individual will also play a role, although this has not been studied as extensively.

It must be recognized that even if the migration is in the same country, the broad culture of the country is unlikely to be entirely homogenous and micro-cultures may well exist, which will be affected by the micro-identities of the individuals, therefore ensuring that adjustment to new settings can be complex. The individual characteristics of the migrant will also play a role.

Acculturation

In many countries, especially in low- and middle-income countries or those with cultures-in-transition, migrants into urban areas may need to adjust and learn the characteristics of the urban culture and reduce the dissonance between their own and the new cultures (assimilation). This is a complex process of re-defining one's own identity with retaining, as well as giving up, some characteristics of the culture of one's origin. Thus, there may occur cultural contraction (giving up some of one's cultural characteristics) and cultural expansion (taking on other culture's values and characteristics). Some migrants may find it difficult to adjust and may end up distancing themselves (separation) from one or both the cultures, thereby further alienating themselves, whereas some may be able to maintain their own cultural identities at the same time as becoming part of the new urban culture (biculturalism). Acculturative stress can lead to decompensation and produce psychopathology in vulnerable individuals. Cultural identities can be misunderstood on both sides, from the migrant's side and from that of the larger urban populace.

Cultural identity

Cultural identity helps define a person's uniqueness and is a composite of gender, ethnicity, race, religion, occupation, and so on. It distinguishes a person from others by their attitudes, world view, social behaviour, clothes, food, lifestyle, religious beliefs, and so on. Each of these characteristics can lead to what has been described as micro-identities [4]. Attempts at preservation of personal and cultural identity, especially in the face of an unwelcoming environment may cause considerable conflict. Institutional discrimination (real and perceived) based on one's racial and cultural identities can affect social standing contributing to stigma, which will, in turn, influence help-seeking for mental ill health. Holding traditional values in a more modern society may contribute to alienation and conflict, especially if the younger members of the same family hold less traditional values, leading to an element of culture conflict.

Prevalence of mental disorders

Studies over the past century have repeatedly identified migration as an important factor in the development of mental disorders in migrant communities (see Chapters 10 and 11) and we do not aim to expand on these findings. Discrimination, social disadvantage, underachievement, and ethnic density all have been linked to this.

The data from urban areas have their own problems in that often cities are not defined in a uniform way, creating problems in the comparability of the city-related data. Although recognized for decades, a significant improvement in data collection has not yet been seen [5].

Addressing health issues in the context of migration to cities is paramount, as migration and mobility are determinants of the health of migrants, as well as of the health of non-migrants both at places of origin and destination [6]. In addition to natural population growth, urbanization is driven mainly by rural–urban migration and migration between cities. Urban migrants form a hugely diverse group that comprises internal migrants originating from rural areas in search of better employment and education opportunities in cities, cross-border migrants, internally displaced persons, and urban refugees, as well as victims of trafficking and forced labour. Half of the world's refugees now live in cities [7]. Certain migration paths are more likely to affect physical and psychological vulnerabilities and add to the stress experienced by the migrants, as is the case for minors who travel unaccompanied [8]; refugees and internally displaced people [9] escaping from wars, conflicts, natural disasters and famine, forced migrants [10]; and those who end up in exploitative situations [11] or in detention [12]. Migration to urban areas can be for all these reasons and the pathways may well differ creating different levels and types of stress.

Rapid and unplanned urban growth threatens sustainable development when the necessary infrastructure is not developed or when policies are not implemented to ensure that the benefits of city life are equitably shared [13]. Urban poverty is increasing, although in many countries millions of people have come out of poverty[14] for a number of reasons, which further adds to the likelihood of mental illness. There is considerable evidence suggesting that income inequalities are affecting rates of poverty in urban areas with people living in favelas, and in slums and informal settlements with inadequate infrastructure. Their numbers are increasing and are currently estimated at some 863 million; this means that every third urban dweller lives in a slum. These rapid urbanization processes pose severe challenges, in particular for public health authorities. UN-Habitat [15,16] has identified a 'triple threat' that consists of infectious diseases that thrive in poor and overcrowded urban environments; non-communicable diseases, which are exacerbated by unhealthy lifestyles that are available in urban areas and are taken up in the course of settling in cities; and injuries and violence that stem from dangerous road traffic and unsafe working and living conditions. When discussing non-communicable or even communicable disease often the mental ill health aspects get ignored. Death as a result of violence or road traffic accidents will influence the mental health of the survivors and the family, but these are also often ignored.

Greater globalization leading to increased movement of people within a country has highlighted the need for more epidemiological studies in this area. And some data are beginning to emerge from China, although the findings are not entirely clear.

It is inevitable that the reasons for migration and preparation will act as potential stressors or support. It is highly likely that those who have migrated for educational or economic advancement may well be better motivated and pre-pared to adjust, whereas those who have been pushed out for political or dis-criminatory reasons may find themselves further alienated and find it difficult to adjust.

In addition to the migration itself and its nature, it is also important that per-sonality systems, ideologies, commitments, aspirations, and role performance are taken into account because these may add to the stress [17].

Furnham and Bochner [18] have described eight theoretical constructs that must be taken into account while trying to understand the impact of migration. These include loss, fatalism (embedded in a sense of control), and expectations of and from the new society, negative life events, and social support, along with loss of or clash of values and skills deficit. The migrant may have lost specific objects and relationships, as well as cultural values. Unresolved grief and mourning may produce depression in vulnerable in-dividuals. Grief under the circumstances may be extreme, exaggerated, or internalized. This has been attributed to cultural bereavement as discussed later in this chapter.

Vulnerable groups, such as women, LGBTQ+ (lesbian, gay, bisexual, trans-gender, and queer/questioning), children, or the elderly, may face additional stresses. They may feel isolated in the new culture, especially if the patriarchal values in the family are strong and keep these groups from mixing with others. Another complicating factor for women is gender-role expectations, which may put them under a tremendous amount of strain. Chandra [19] points out that the feminization of migration work force is increasing with globalization and work opportunities, and that women face a differential impact on their mental health as a result of migration. However, within-country migration may have very different patterns and needs. The gender role and expectations, along with demarcation of such a role, produce health risks. Poor economic security, isola-tion, and lack of language skills may lead to women becoming more vulnerable to social stresses. Gender and gender-role expectations may have an additional impact on children and adolescents, as well as on child bearing. Female ado-lescents may feel pressure to conform from their family and from the larger society, thereby producing additional stress. Female migrants may get stuck in low-status, low-paid jobs in spite of their skills, and family pressures may con-tribute to vulnerability to depression.

Social and economic factors are likely to play a significant role in the gen-esis of depression among migrants to urban areas. There may be specific social factors that influence the individual's functioning soon after arrival, but other factors may emerge after moving into the city.

Housing

Poor housing in inner city areas and overcrowding with material poverty may cause individuals to develop psychiatric disorders. Uncertainty of tenancy and the inability to purchase or rent suitable properties will place an additional burden on individuals, contributing to a discrepancy between aspiration and achievement.

Employment

Migrants even from within the same country often end up in unpopular, difficult-to-fill jobs in unpopular settings and may have low-status, poorly paid jobs in spite of their superior educational attainments and skills. This discrepancy may further add to feelings of underachievement, thereby affecting their self-esteem (see Chapter 23).

Other factors, especially perceived or real discrimination against new arrivals in urban areas, may contribute to the genesis of depression by generating feelings of persecution, producing a real or perceived lack of opportunity, and, once again, discrepancy between aspiration and achievement.

The concept of culture conflict relates to a degree of conflict between the two members of the same culture, often across generations. It is possible that even within the same broader culture exposure to factors such as social media, which is more likely in urban areas, some aspects of an individual's cultural identity may become more rigid in the context of the migration experiences; those who are born and brought up in the urban areas may hold less traditional values and such tension may lead to further altercations, leading to culture conflict.

Culture conflict is an affective and cognitive dissonance as a consequence of attempts to assimilate values of the new culture, and reflects dilemmas experienced by the individual in trying to integrate two cultures that may hold extreme and differing views on a specific issue [20]. Such conflicts will lead to emotional and psychological distress in both parties and may go on to produce a sense of isolation, alienation, and a sense of abandonment, producing depression.

Culture shock was used as a term to explain the shock experienced by some migrants after their move to new cultural settings [21]. Bock [22] uses the term culture shock to describe an emotional reaction related to a lack of familiarity, which produces a stress reaction. It may have both negative and positive aspects to it. Resulting anxiety and feelings of helplessness and impotence may confirm feelings that the new culture is not only remarkably different, but also unwelcoming and alien. This alienation may produce further anxiety. Culture shock does dissipate with time, but high levels of culture shock are associated with high levels of dysphoria, which may be seen as a variant of depression. Availability of social support is thus critical in managing culture shock. Females tended to experience higher levels of culture shock, which may be related to gender and gender roles, both of which are social constructs and thus liable to be affected by social and cultural factors. Culture shock may be seen as a short-lived experience, but this may not always be the case as it may linger and contribute to non-acceptance and delayed acculturation.

Cultural bereavement as a concept was described as a response to a series of losses experienced by the migrant individual as a result of migration. Even when they are moving within the country, from rural to urban areas, they will be leaving networks and relationships behind and perhaps some of their cultural values too. Working with refugees, Eisenbruch [23, 24] described cultural bereavement as occurring as a result of the loss of social structures, cultural values, and (cultural) identity, and highlighted by an almost unnatural attachment to the past. This may also be considered as idealization of the past and seeing the culture left behind as perfect and both ideal and idealized. Particularly after disaster, individuals may experience survivor guilt. Western constructs of bereavement may have only a limited value in explaining expressions of grief and its management in other cultures [25]. The migrant may not only experience physical losses, but also losses related to skills, social status, and so on, which may produce a delayed reaction [26].

Challenges and the way forward

As internal migration patterns are often not noted, it is difficult to know the exact numbers of internal migrants, although the estimates are said to be around 740 million globally [27]. These numbers include seasonal migrants, students, and many others [28]. Urbanization is constantly rising and will be a global challenge in the coming years [29]. In 2015, 27.8 million individuals were internally displaced [30]. These numbers parallel the populations of New York City, London, Paris, and Cairo combined. Of those, 8.6 million were fleeing conflict and violence in 28 countries and these numbers are likely rising on a daily basis. Another 19.2 million were displaced as a result of natural disasters in 113 countries, in the same year [30]. It is not surprising that low- and middle-income countries end up bearing the brunt of migration, but for many reasons the focus of discussion in media and political circles are high-income countries. The most affected country was Yemen, where 2.2 million individuals—8% of the population—had to flee their homes [30]. As in previous years, the South East Asia and the Pacific regions faced the largest internal displacement associated with natural disasters. Low- and middle-income countries were most affected across the world as a whole [31]. In South/Latin America there are said to be nearly 26 million migrants moving from one poor country to another.

Particularly vulnerable migration pathways, both in terms of internal and international migration, are related to sex trafficking of children and women. In many settings children are sent with traffickers who may pose as travel agents. Unaccompanied or separated minors are at particular risk. A victim of trafficking is an individual—who has been convinced to migrate either internally or externally with false information; or kidnapped, through the use of force or threat, or the abuse of their vulnerability for the purpose of being exploited sexually—in domestic servitude or as part of a workforce in different industries. It has been argued that in many settings people have been trafficked for purposes of organ harvesting [32]. A rough estimate reports that around 700,000 people are trafficked every year [33], but, unsurprisingly, these data are not entirely reliable. Also, it is possible that only a small proportion of victims of trafficking are identified or seek help. Their position and vulnerability makes it extremely difficult for them to be open about their experiences. For example, only 7000 trafficked individuals in 115 countries were assisted by the IOM [34]. Unaccompanied minors are recognized as children who have been separated from either parent or other adults who carry responsibility for their care due to natural or manmade disasters or other reasons and are not being taken care of by an adult who would be responsible to do so by law or custom [35]. 'Separated children' are identified as those children who have been separated from both parents, or from their previous legal or customary primary caregiver, but not necessarily from other relatives. These may therefore include children accompanied by other adult family members [35]. Again, the numbers of such children may well vary. For example, in 2014 alone, more than 23,000 asylum applicants in the European Union were registered as unaccompanied and separated children [36]. However, with internal migration from rural to urban areas it is much more difficult to ascertain the exact figures. Mass communication and social media can further contribute to social inequalities and contribute to a sense of isolation and alienation [37].

There is no doubt that migratory experiences combined with an exposure to physical, sexual, and political violence, along with dangers related to the likelihood of exploitation as a result of internal or external migration, are likely to contribute to the possibility of developing mental illness. Vulnerability factors also apply to non-migrants, but this group may have better resilience and social capital and social support.

It can be argued that good mental health is a basic human right, whether living in rural areas or urban areas. It is therefore important that the general focus on high rates of mental illness of certain groups of migrants should move away towards understanding resilience and strengths rather than weaknesses.

Box 5.1 Assessing the mental health needs of migrants to urban areas

1. Different explanatory models between clinicians and patients
2. Unwillingness to seek help due to potential costs
3. Unwillingness to disclose symptoms
4. Variations in clinical symptoms related to social factors
5. Language and cultural barriers
6. Use of metaphors
7. Inefficient explanation of symptoms
8. Clinician's knowledge of cultural differences
9. Patient's presentation itself and their understanding of distress

Thus, human rights and social and health justice for mental health may have a better outcome. Even when the legal right to remain is granted, problems of outreach, information, language, cultural relevance, stigma, and education remain [38], especially for those who are moving across nations, but may not necessarily apply to those moving from rural to urban areas.

Even within the same country, actual physical act of migration can be stressful. In urban areas after internal migration most mental disorders in migrants are correlated with social problems and social discrimination. Furthermore, their educational, social care, and health care needs, along with the supportive role of religion, can require a carefully balanced approach.

There is no doubt that migration is a regular feature of today's citizenship around the globe and is not likely to diminish as urbanization progresses at a fast pace. Migrants even within the same country tend to have problems in accessing existing services for a number of reasons, including a lack of information and understanding of mental distress, using different idioms of distress, and stigma. Box 5.1 illustrates how to assess the mental health needs of migrants to urban areas.

It is important to ascertain the discrepancy between achievement and aspiration after migration. A number of domains can be explored. This part of the assessment may be seen as less threatening and more facilitatory, and people may find it easier to answer these questions. Some of the questions are illustrated in Box 5.2.

It is important to recognize that not all migrants will have the same reasons for migrating to urban areas or have similar experiences in migration or settling

---

Box 5.2 Assessing achievement and aspiration in various domains, e.g. education, social status, financial status, and social standing

What was your status (on a scale of 1–10)?
Where are you at present (on a scale of 0–10)?
What level did you think you would achieve (on a scale of 0–10)?
Have you achieved this? Yes/No
If not, how far would you want to go?
Do you feel let down? Yes/No
If yes, how? Explain.
Do you feel content with this level? Yes/No
If yes, how?
If no, what is missing?

---

down. Clinicians need to be aware that the migrants will carry certain expectations and aspirations, which may not be met, and individuals may feel let down or develop low self-esteem. However, a move to the city may help them blossom without restrictions on their activities. However, migrants may successfully cross geographical boundaries but may not have the ability, capability, or possibility of crossing internal borders. The clinician in first contact and assessment must make the migrant feel welcomed and valued, and understand their experiences.

Conclusions

With globalization leading to rapid industrialization and consequent urbanization, increasing numbers of people are moving from rural to urban areas. Although the majority are likely to be young, children and the elderly may well have to migrate largely as secondary migrants. Acculturation even within the same country means that people may well have to change language, behaviours, and so on, in order to be part of the larger culture. This adjustment may also involve changing patterns of thinking, clothing, and dietary habits. Assimilation is influenced by a number of factors and clinicians must explore these in their interactions. It is important that assumptions are not made that because it has been an internal migration there are no stressors. Pressures related to overcrowding, poverty, unemployment, and poor social support may all play a role in contributing to the genesis of mental illness. Resilience and individual strength must be nourished properly in order to help the individual settle down well and flourish. Additional facilities such as the option of meeting others, spaces that are non-threatening and green, and possible opportunities for physical activity, including exercise, can help develop resilience and enable reduction in rates of mental illness.

References

1. **Bhugra D.** Migration, distress and cultural identity. *British Medical Bulletin* 2004; **69**: 129–141.

2. **Sashidharan S.** Afro-Caribbeans and schizophrenia. *International Review of Pyschiatry* 1993; **5**: 129–144.

3. **International Organization for Migration (IOM).** *Global Migration Trends 2015 Factsheet.* Geneva: IOM, 2016

4. **Wachter M, Vaentriglio A, Bhugra D.** Micro-identities, adjustment and stigma. *International Journal of Social Psychiatry* 2015; **61**: 436–437

5. **Schultz C.** *Migration, Health and Cities. Migration, health and urbanization: interrelated challenges.* International Organization for Migration (IOM) background paper 2014.

6. **Mosca D, Rijks B, Schultz C.** Health in the post-2015 development agenda: the importance of migrants' health for sustainable and equitable development. In: F Laczko, LJ Lönnback (eds) *Migration and the United Nations Post-2015 Development Agenda.* Geneva: IOM.

7. **UNHCR.** UNHCR viewpoint: 'refugee' or 'migrant' – which is right? Available at: http://www.unhcr.org/55df0e556.html (accessed 31 July 2016).

8. **Jensen TK, Skårdalsmo EMB, Fjermestad KW.** Development of mental health problems—a follow-up study of unaccompanied refugee minors. *Child and Adolescent Psychiatry and Mental Health* 2014; **8**: 29.

9. **Salah TT, Abdelrahman A, Lien L, Eide AH, Martinez P, Hauff E.** The mental health of internally displaced persons: an epidemiological study of adults in two settlements in central Sudan. *International Journal of Social Psychiatry* 2013; **59**:782–788.

10. **Siriwardhana C, Stewart R.** Forced migration and mental health: prolonged internal displacement, return migration and resilience. *International Health* 2013; **5**: 19–23.

11. **Zimmerman C, Hossain M, Yun K, Roche B, Morison L, Watts C.** Stolen Smiles: A Summary Report on the Physical and Psychological Health Consequences of Women and Adolescents Trafficked in Europe. London: The London School of Hygiene and Tropical Medicine, 2016.

12. **Robjant, K., Hassan, R., Katona C.** Mental health implications of detaining asylum seekers: systematic review. *The British Journal of Psychiatry* 2009; **194**: 306–312.

13. **UNDESA.** *International Migration Report 2015: Highlights (ST/ESA/SER.A/375).* New York: UN, 2016.

14. **Baker JL.** Impacts of financial,food and fuel crises on the urban poor. Directions in Urban Development. Urban Development Unit Report, World Bank. Available at: www.openknowledge.worldbank.org (accessed 12 November 2018).

15. **UN-Habitat.** *Prosperity of Cities: State of the World's Cities.* Nairobi: UN-Habitat, 2013.

16. **UN Habitat**. *Urban Development: Emerging Future. World Cities Report*. Nairobi: UN Habitata, 2016.

17. **Shaw RP**. *Migration Theory and Fact: A Review and Bibliography of Current Literature*. Philadelphia, PA: RSSI, 1975.

18. **Furnham A** and **Bochner S**. *Culture Shock*. London: Routledge, 1986.

19. **Chandra P**. Mental health issues related to migration in women. In D Bhugra, S Gupta (eds) *Migration and Mental Health*. Cambridge: Cambridge University Press, 2011, pp. 209–219.

20 **Inman A, Ladany N, Constantine MG, Morano CK**. Development and preliminary validation of the cultural values conflict scale for South Asian women. *Journal of Counseling Psychology* 2001; **48**: 17–27.

21 **Oberg K**. Culture shock, adjustment to new culture environments. *Practical Anthropology* 1960; **7**: 177–182.

22 **Bock P** (ed.) *Culture Shock*. New York: Knopf, 1971.

23. **Eisenbruch M**. The cultural bereavement interview: a new clinical research approach for refugees. *Psychiatric Clinics of North America* 1990; **13**: 715–735.

24. **Eisenbruch M**. From post-traumatic stress disorder to cultural bereavement: diagnosis of Southeast Asian refugees. *Social Science & Medicine* 1991; **33**: 673–680.

25. **Bhugra D, Becker M**. Migration, cultural bereavement and cultural identity. *World Psychiatry* 2005; **4**: 18–24.

26. **Wojcik W, Bhugra D**. Loss and cultural bereavement. In D Bhugra, T Craig, K Bhui (eds) *Mental Health of Refugees and Asylum Seekers*. Oxford: Oxford University Press, 2010, pp. 211–223.

27. **UNDP**. Human development report. Available at: http://hdr.undp.org/en/content/human-development-report-2009 (accessed 24 July 2016).

28 **ILO**. *International Labour Migration*. A Rights-based Approach. Geneva: ILO, 2010.

29. **ILO**. Unemployment threatens world cities; jobs are needed to check growth in urban poverty. Available at: http://www.ilo.org/global/about-the-ilo/newsroom/news/WCMS_008055/lang--en/index.htm (accessed 24 July 2016).

30. **International Detention Coalition (IDC)**. What is immigration detention? Available at: http://idcoalition.org/aboutus/what-is-detention (accessed 20 July 2016).

31. **Bilak A, Cardona-Fox G, Ginnetti J, Rushing EJ, Scherer I, Swain M**, et al. Global Report on Internal Displacement. Geneva: IDMC.

32. **OHCHR**. **Migration and Human Rights**. *Improving Human Rights-based Governance of International Migration*. New York: UN.

33 **IOM**. Counter trafficking. Available at: https://www.iom.int/infographics/iom-2015-counter-trafficking-statistics (accessed 31 July 2016).

34 **IOM**. Migration key terms. Available at: https://www.iom.int/key-migration-terms (accessed 5 April 2016).

35 **IOM**. International migration law information note. The protection of unaccompanied migrant children. Available At: https://unofficeny.iom.int/sites/default/files/InfoNote-Unaccompanied-Migrant-Children-Jan2011.pdf (accessed 31 July 2016).

36 OECD. International migration outlook 2015. Available at: https://www.oecd-ilibrary.org/social-issues-migration-health/international-migration-outlook-2015/summary/english_767accc1-en (accessed 6 November 2018).

37. **Calhoun C, Rojek C, Turner BS.** *The SAGE Handbook of Sociology.* London: Sage Publications.

38. **Mosca D, Rijks B, Schultz C.** A role for health in the global migration and development debate? Looking ahead at the UN High-Level Dialogue on Migration and Development (HLD) and other forums. *Migration Policy Practice* 2013; 3: 19–24.

Chapter 6

Why urban environments matter for refugee mental health

Peter Schofield

Introduction

A defining feature of most urban environments is that they are receptive to migrants of one kind or another. With cities now inextricably linked across vast global networks the refugee experience, at least in the global north, is largely an urban experience [1]. In this chapter, I outline why the kind of urban environment where refugees eventually find themselves can play an important role in their subsequent mental health. This is a pressing concern as we are in the midst of a global refugee crisis, with the numbers displaced as a result of conflict or persecution increasing at an unprecedented rate [2]. Across much of Europe, government agencies are now tasked with accommodating those fleeing conflict and persecution, typically adopting dispersal policies aimed at avoiding their accumulation in particular urban areas and ostensibly 'spreading the burden' across municipalities [3]. The potential consequences of these policies are one of the themes I address. There is often little we can do about circumstances in those countries from which refugees are fleeing that might impact on their mental health. However, as I show, the neighbourhood environment into which they are received is one relevant, and potentially modifiable, risk factor over which we have some influence.

Refugee mental health

So, firstly, what do we know about the mental health of refugees? Often, studies have shown refugees to be more resilient to mental health problems than might be expected given their exposure to severe trauma [4]. However, research has consistently demonstrated an overall increase in their rate of mental disorders compared to not only the general population, but also other migrants. Refugee status has long been associated with an increased risk of depression and anxiety disorders [5, 6], with one review estimating around 9% (99% confidence interval (CI) 8–10%) of refugees suffering from post-traumatic stress disorder [7]. More recently, studies have also highlighted an increased risk of psychotic illness, such as schizophrenia and bipolar disorder [8–10]. One Swedish population cohort study found the rate of psychotic disorders among refugees was nearly three times that of the Swedish born population (adjusted hazard ratio (aHR) 2.9, 95% CI 2.3–3.6) and this was also greater than that of other migrants (aHR1.7, 95% CI 1.3–2.1) [8].

Given the traumatic circumstances from which they are fleeing it may, perhaps, not be surprising that refugees are more likely to suffer mental health problems. However, while explanations for these increased rates have in the past largely focused on trauma pre-migration, it is increasingly argued that post-migration risk factors play an important, if not equal, role [11–13]. For example, one wide-ranging review found a range of post-migration factors made a difference to refugee mental health equal to or greater than the experience of war and exposure to violence. This conclusion was arrived at after comparing studies of refugees with those of similar non-refugee migrant groups who had also been exposed to war and violence [11]. The authors of this review cite restricted economic opportunities and living in institutional accommodation as major post-migration risk factors. They conclude that mental ill health is not an inevitable consequence of trauma pre-migration, but instead reflects contextual factors in the host country that are, importantly, amenable to intervention.

However, studies of refugee populations are often very limited in what they can tell us about the impact of these post-migration risk factors. Whereas for migrant groups, in general, there is now a wealth of research evidence about relevant mental health risk factors, for refugees this is a mostly under-developed field. This is, in part, because refugees are a largely hidden population, absent from health records and other administrative data that is usually made available for research [14]. Whereas ethnic group or country of origin is now routinely coded in health records in the UK and in many other European countries, it is unusual for refugee status to be recorded, both because this is administratively burdensome and because these are often highly sensitive data. Also, where large-scale surveys have been attempted they have been prone to a very high rate of attrition. For example, the UK Survey of New Refugees, to date the most comprehensive attempt to survey refugees in the UK, began with 5678 refugees at the first wave, whereas only 867 (15%) remained at the fourth wave [15].

What we can learn from the migrant experience

While research on post-migration factors for refugees is limited there is much we can learn from what is already known about the experience of migrants in general that can point to relevant contextual factors that are likely to be relevant to the mental health of refugees. Migrants have long figured disproportionally among those diagnosed with severe mental illness, since it was first shown in the 1930s that Scandinavian immigrants to the US were more likely to be diagnosed with schizophrenia [16, 17]. The original explanation was that that this was due to selective migration; that is, those with a predisposition to psychosis were more likely to migrate, although this has been subsequently discounted in the light of evidence from large-scale cohort studies [18, 19]. International comparison studies have also failed to show any corresponding increased incidence in the country of origin, therefore ruling out genetic explanations [20, 21]. More recently, reviews have highlighted how the elevated risk persists from the first to the second generation, which suggests that explanations are likely to be found in the post-migration context [17, 22]. There is now increasing evidence that the neighbourhood environment itself can play an important role in the mental health of migrant and minority ethnic groups. For example, an ethnic density effect has been consistently shown where psychosis incidence is reduced for members of minority ethnic groups living in areas where their ethnic group is well represented [23–26]. While this effect is clearest for psychotic disorders, such as schizophrenia, a similar effect has also been demonstrated for other, more common mental disorders [27–29]. Although the underlying mechanism behind the ethnic density effect is still unclear, it is thought likely that those living in high co-ethnic density neighbourhoods benefit from improved social support and access to social capital in a way that is protective against mental illness [24, 28]. There is also evidence that these factors, in turn, can act as a buffer against discrimination which might otherwise be a significant risk factor [30].

Neighbourhood ethnic density and refugee dispersal

This is likely to be particularly relevant to refugees, who are often allocated housing in widely dispersed locations far from neighbourhoods where migrants from their country of origin have previously settled [3, 31, 32]. International comparison studies have demonstrated how this can lead to a reduction in social capital and social networks and a corresponding weakening of refugees' own cultural identity [33, 34]. Dispersal is also a problem because dispersal areas typically lack a history of migration and therefore do not have relevant services available to cater for refugees [35]. Furthermore, it is now recognized that hostility to immigration is more likely in areas with little experience of diverse ethnic groups [36]. It has also been shown that accommodating refugees in low co-ethnic density neighbourhoods can have the effect of severely reducing opportunities for employment [37, 38]. This has been demonstrated in a series of Danish studies that take advantage of the way that refugees are, in effect, randomly assigned to different types of neighbourhood, thus creating a natural experiment. The study authors argue that the lower employment rates in low ethnic density neighbourhoods is a consequence of restricted access to social networks that would otherwise be relied on for employment opportunities. Paradoxically, the resulting lack of economic activity serves to hinder integration into the host society, one of the primary aims of the Danish dispersal policy. In this way, they argue, living in an 'ethnic enclave' can ultimately lead to better integration into the wider community [39]. While the overall mental health consequences of this are still unclear, the authors of a recent large-scale cohort study of refugee psychosis in Sweden cite neighbourhood ethnic density as one, possibly key, explanatory factor for their increased psychosis risk [13]. However, to date, only one study has explicitly examined the effect of neighbourhood ethnic density on the mental health of refugees. This large [2, 28] survey of South East Asian refugees in California found that areas of greater ethnic density served as a buffer against demoralization for some of the refugee groups they looked at [40]. Interestingly, one group, refugees from Cambodia, showed the opposite effect: living in an ethnically dense area served to reinforce feelings of demoralization.

There is, however, a paucity of research looking at the mental health consequences of dispersal policies in Europe. What we do know, from recent studies, is that one of the more obvious consequences of 'no choice' dispersal has been a steady stream of onward migration to other urban areas with established ethnic minority communities [3, 33, 34, 41]. One example is Denmark, where the adverse effects of a rigorously applied dispersal policy have been well documented [33, 42]. As a result, large numbers of Somali refugees have left Danish cities to move to urban areas in the UK, claiming they feel more at home, despite moving to relatively deprived neighbourhoods with often poorer-quality housing [3]. A similar process has also been clearly observed in the Netherlands, where Somali refugees who were originally dispersed and isolated also moved to areas in the UK with large Somali communities [34]. However, that is not to say that the UK itself is immune to this phenomenon, with onward migration also well-documented in the UK [33]. While we know that onward migration is common, little is known of the mental health consequences for those who remain behind and there remains a large gap in the research evidence on the mental health impact of refugee dispersal.

Other neighbourhood factors

Other neighbourhood factors are also important. Migrants, in general, and refugees, in particular, are mostly concentrated in deprived urban areas that have long been associated with increased rates of mental disorder, even when individual socio-economic circumstances are taken into account [43–45]. Urban environments themselves are also associated with a greater risk of psychosis, with increasing levels of urbanicity related to increased incidence in a dose–response fashion [46]. Furthermore, refugees are often settled in urban neighbourhoods typified by low levels of social cohesion, comprising transient and often fragmented populations with little sense of involvement in the local community. Studies have found a high correlation between low levels of neighbourhood social cohesion and rates of psychosis independent of area deprivation and urbanicity [47–49].

Neighbourhood and refugee mental health studies

While these neighbourhood studies are relevant it is still unclear exactly how these risk factors might apply to refugees. There are, however, a few refugee studies that look directly at the mental health impact of neighbourhood factors. Warfa et al. [50] set out to address the lack of research evidence for the role of the post-migration environment using a cross-national comparison design. They compared a similar population of refugees from Somalia in two contrasting areas, London and Minneapolis, with the same data collection methods in both sites, combining in-depth qualitative data from focus groups with larger-scale surveys. They found that access to labour markets was a key contextual factor, contributing to an increased risk of mental disorders, including major depression.

Research on the mental health of migrant groups has benefited from studies using large cohort designs. However, this is relatively rare in research looking specifically at refugees. One exception is a large cohort study conducted in Ontario, Canada that looked at both refugees and first-generation migrants [9]. This followed a retrospective design using health records over a 10-year period covering just over 95,000 refugees. The results showed a higher rate of psychosis among refugees and the study authors point to the protective effect of neighbourhood income levels as one relevant contributory factor. Unfortunately, much of the report conflates refugees and other migrants when presenting the study results.

Another large-scale refugee study in the USA used a survey approach to examine mental health outcomes, covering a nationally representative sample of 656 Latino and Asian refugees [51]. This found that experience of pre-resettlement trauma failed to make a statistically significant difference to post-migration mental health outcomes. However, having a good perception of the neighbourhood environment, based on items covering levels of social cohesion and physical safety, was strongly associated with positive self-rated mental health. The authors conclude that the resettlement environment can play a central role in the mental health of refugee populations.

Neighbourhood environment and residential instability

As well as the type of neighbourhood environment, residential instability itself can also be an important risk factor. A UK study investigated the accommodation histories of a large (n = 142) group of Somali refugees in London over a 5-year period using in-depth and semi-structured interviews [52]. Once again, the authors failed to find a relation between past experiences of traumatic events and current psychiatric disorders. However, they did show that number of moves post-migration was a risk factor with this depending on whether moves were by choice and also the existence of a strong friendship network whether moves were by choice and also existence of a strong friendship network. They conclude that choosing to move to areas where there is better social support is associated with better mental health outcomes for refugees.

Future research priorities

What we currently know about the mental health impact of the neighbourhood environment from studies of refugee populations is therefore relatively limited. However, what we know from the wider migrant mental health literature, and neighbourhood studies in general, suggests that these factors are likely to play an important role in the mental health of refugees. Further research is now needed to better determine the extent to which these factors are relevant and how they might affect different groups in different contexts. Ideally, studies would look at both a broad population level while also examining specific groups in a local context using more in-depth qualitative approaches. For example, the kind of population register data available for research in Scandinavian countries could be used to assess the impact of dispersal policies on subsequent mental health outcomes for refugees. As we have seen, one by-product of a rigorously applied dispersal policy is that neighbourhood can, under certain conditions, be considered randomly allocated. This has already been successfully utilized in quasi-experimental study designs in refugee research and this approach could equally well be used in a mental health context [37, 38]. Where relevant administrative data are lacking, for example in the UK, survey approaches could be adopted. Future surveys should incorporate information about the neighbourhood in which refugees are living at a detailed area level, including area deprivation indices and census ethnicity profiles. At a micro-level, further qualitative research could address the specific priorities of different refugee groups in different local contexts to gain a deeper understanding of contextual factors perceived to be important and the mechanisms through which these impact on mental health.

Conclusions

The refugee experience is one of involuntary displacement and as a result the urban spaces in which refugees eventually find themselves are typically not of their choosing and may contribute to poor mental health. What we understand of migrants, in general, is that the post-migration context is central to explanations for increased rates of mental disorder. Some neighbourhood-level factors, such as ethnic density, may be particularly salient for refugees, subject to 'no-choice' dispersal policies and therefore potentially isolated and vulnerable to mental ill health. To conclude, we have a responsibility to ensure that the urban environments in which refugees live allow them to thrive and not be detrimental to their mental health and future research is therefore needed to better inform these decisions.

References

1. **Darling J.** Forced migration and the city: irregularity, informality, and the politics of presence. *Progress in Human Geography* 2016; **41**: 178–198.
2. **UN Refugee Agency (UNHCR).** Forced Displacement in 2015. Available at: http://www. unhcr.org/uk/statistics/unhcrstats/576408cd7/unhcr-global-trends-2015.html (accessed 12 November 2018).
3. **Wren K.** Refugee dispersal in Denmark: from macro- to micro-scale analysis. *International Journal of Population Geography* 2003; **9**: 57–75.
4. **Simich L, Andermann L** (eds). *Refuge and Resilience: Promoting Resilience and Mental Health Among Resettled Refugees and Forced Migrants.* Cham: Springer Nature, 2014.
5. **Bogic M, Njoku A, Priebe S.** Long-term mental health of war-refugees: a systematic literature review. *BMC Int Health Hum Rights* 2015; **15**: 29.
6. **Lindert J, Ehrenstein OS von, Priebe S, Mielck A, Brähler E.** Depression and anxiety in labor migrants and refugees—a systematic review and meta-analysis. *Social Science & Medicine* 2009; **69**: 246–257.
7. **Fazel M, Wheeler J, Danesh J.** Prevalence of serious mental disorder in 7000 refugees resettled in western countries: a systematic review. *The Lancet* 2005; **365**: 1309–1314.
8. **Hollander A-C, Dal H, Lewis G, Magnusson C, Kirkbride JB, Dalman C.** Refugee migration and risk of schizophrenia and other non-affective psychoses: cohort study of 1.3 million people in Sweden. *BMJ* 2016; **352**: i1030.

9. Anderson KK, Cheng J, Susser E, McKenzie KJ, Kurdyak P. Incidence of psychotic disorders among first-generation immigrants and refugees in Ontario. *Canadian Medical Association Journal* 2015; **187**: E279–E286.

10. Parrett NS, Mason OJ. Refugees and psychosis: a review of the literature. *Psychosis* 2010; **2**: 111–121.

11. Porter M, Haslam N. Predisplacement and postdisplacement factors associated with mental health of refugees and internally displaced persons: a meta-analysis. *JAMA* 2005; **294**: 602–612.

12. Anderson KK, Flora N, Archie S, Morgan C, McKenzie K. A meta-analysis of ethnic differences in pathways to care at the first episode of psychosis. *Acta Psychiatrica Scandinavica* 2014; **130**: 257–268.

13. Norredam M, Garcia-Lopez A, Keiding N, Krasnik A. Risk of mental disorders in refugees and native Danes: a register-based retrospective cohort study. *Social Psychiatry and Psychiatric Epidemiology* 2009; **44**: 1023–1029.

14. Enticott JC, Shawyer F, Vasi S, Buck K, Cheng I-H, Russell G, et al. A systematic review of studies with a representative sample of refugees and asylum seekers living in the community for participation in mental health research. *BMC Medical Research Methodology* 2017; **17**: 37.

15. Cebulla A, Daniel M, Zurawan A. Spotlight on refugee integration: findings from the Survey of New Refugees in the United Kingdom. Available at: https://assets.publishing. service.gov.uk/government/uploads/system/uploads/attachment_data/file/116062/ horr37-report.pdf (accessed 12 November 2018).

16. Ødegård Ø. *Emigration and Insanity: A Study of Mental Disease Among the Norwegian Born Population of Minnesota*. Copenhagen: Levin & Munksgaard.

17. Cantor-Graae E, Selten JP. Schizophrenia and migration: a meta-analysis and review. *American Journal of Psychiatry* 2005; **162**: 12–24.

18. van der Ven E, Dalman C, Wicks S, Allebeck P, Magnusson C, van Os J, et al. Testing Ødegaard's selective migration hypothesis: a longitudinal cohort study of risk factors for non-affective psychotic disorders among prospective emigrants. *Psychological Medicine* 2015; **45**: 727–734.

19. Pedersen CB, Mortensen PB, Cantor-Graae E. Do risk factors for schizophrenia predispose to emigration? *Schizophrenia Research* 2011; **127**: 229–234.

20. Jablensky A, Sartorius N, Ernberg G, Anker M, Korten A, Cooper JE, et al. Schizophrenia: manifestations, incidence and course in different cultures. A World Health Organization ten-country study. *Psychological Medicine Monograph Supplement* 1992; **20**: 1–97.

21. Bhugra D, Hilwig M, Hossein B, Marceau H, Neehall J, Leff J, et al. First-contact incidence rates of schizophrenia in Trinidad and one-year follow-up. *British Journal of Psychiatry* 1996; **169**: 587–592.

22. Bourque F, van der Ven E, Malla A. A meta-analysis of the risk for psychotic disorders among first- and second-generation immigrants. *Psychological Medicine* 2010; **41**: 897–910.

23. Boydell J, van Os J, McKenzie K, Allardyce J, Goel R, McCreadie RG, et al. Incidence of schizophrenia in ethnic minorities in London: ecological study into interactions with environment. BMJ 2001; **323**: 1336–1338.

24. **Kirkbride JB, Morgan C, Fearon P, Dazzan P, Murray R, Jones PB.** Neighbourhood-level effects on psychoses: re-examining the role of context. Psychological Medicine 2007; **37**: 12.

25. **Veling W, Susser E, van Os J, Mackenbach JP, Selten J-P, Hoek HW.** Ethnic density of neighborhoods and incidence of psychotic disorders among immigrants. *American Journal of Psychiatry* 2008; **165**: 66–73.

26. **Schofield P, Thygesen M, Das-Munshi J, Becares L, Cantor-Graae E, Pedersen C,** et al. Ethnic density, urbanicity and psychosis risk for migrant groups—a population cohort study. *Schizophrenia Research* 2017; **190**: 82–87.

27. **Das-Munshi J, Becares L, Dewey ME, Stansfeld SA, Prince MJ.** Understanding the effect of ethnic density on mental health: multi-level investigation of survey data from England. *BMJ* 2010; **341**: c5367–c5367.

28. **Shaw RJ, Atkin K, Bécares L, Albor C, Stafford M, Kiernan KE,** et al. Impact of ethnic density on adult mental disorders: narrative review. *British Journal of Psychiatry* 2012; **201**: 11–19.

29. **Schofield P, Das-Munshi J, Mathur R, Congdon P, Hull S.** Does depression diagnosis and antidepressant prescribing vary by location? Analysis of ethnic density associations using a large primary-care dataset. *Psychological Medicine* 2016; **46**: 1–9.

30. **Becares L, Das-Munshi J.** Ethnic density, health care seeking behaviour and expected discrimination from health services among ethnic minority people in England. *Health Place* 2013; **22**: 48–55.

31. **Stewart ES.** UK dispersal policy and onward migration: mapping the current state of knowledge. *Journal of Refugee Studies* 2012; **25**: 25–49.

32. **McColl H, McKenzie K, Bhui K.** Mental healthcare of asylum-seekers and refugees. Advances in Psychiatric Treatment 2008; **14**: 452–459.

33. **Valentine G, Sporton D, Nielsen KB.** Identities and belonging: a study of Somali refugee and asylum seekers living in the UK and Denmark. *Environment and Planning D: Society and Space* 2009; **27**: 234–250.

34. **van Liempt I.** From Dutch dispersal to ethnic enclaves in the UK: the relationship between segregation and integration examined through the eyes of *Somalis Urban Studies* 2011; **48**: 3385–3398.

35. **Boswell C.** Burden-sharing in the European Union: lessons from the German and UK experience. *Journal of Refugee Studies* 2003; **16**: 316–335.

36. **Kaufmann E, Harris G.** *Changing Places: Mapping the White British Response to Ethnic Change.* London: Demos.

37. **Damm AP.** Neighborhood quality and labor market outcomes: evidence from quasi-random neighborhood assignment of immigrants. *Journal of Urban Economics* 2014; **79**: 139–166.

38. **Damm AP, Rosholm M.** Employment effects of spatial dispersal of refugees. *Review of Economics of the Household* 2009; **8**: 105–146.

39. **Damm AP.** Ethnic enclaves and immigrant labor market outcomes: quasi-experimental evidence. *Journal of Labor Economics* 2009; **27**: 281–314.

40. **Ying Y, Akutsu PD.** Psychological adjustment of Southeast Asian refugees: the contribution of sense of coherence. *Journal of Community Psychology* 1997; **25**: 125–139.

41. **Hammar T.** The 'Sweden-wide strategy' of refugee dispersal. In: Black R, Robinson V (eds) *Geography and Refugees: Patterns and Processes of Change*. London: Belhaven Press, 1993, pp. 104–117.

42. **Larsen BR.** Becoming part of welfare scandinavia: Integration through the spatial dispersal of newly arrived refugees in Denmark. *Journal of Ethnic Migration Studies* 2011; **37**: 333–350.

43. **Kirkbride JB, Jones PB, Ullrich S, Coid JW.** Social deprivation, inequality, and the neighborhood-level incidence of psychotic syndromes in East london. *Schizophrenia Bulletin* 2014; **40**: 169–180.

44. **Werner S, Malaspina D, Rabinowitz J.** Socioeconomic status at birth is associated with risk of schizophrenia: population-based multilevel study. *Schizophrenia Bulletin* 2007; **33**: 1373–1378.

45. **Harrison GL, Gunnell D, Glazebrook C, Page K, Kwiecinski R.** Association between schizophrenia and social inequality at birth: case-control study. *British Journal of Psychiatry* 2001; **179**: 346–350.

46. **Pedersen CB.** Evidence of a dose-response relationship between urbanicity during upbringing and schizophrenia risk. *Archives of General Psychiatry* 2001; **58**: 1039–1046.

47. **Allardyce J, Gilmour H, Atkinson J, Rapson T, Bishop J, McCreadie RG.** Social fragmentation, deprivation and urbanicity: relation to first-admission rates for psychoses. *British Journal of Psychiatry* 2005; **187**: 401–406.

48. **Newbury J, Arseneault L, Caspi A, Moffitt TE, Odgers CL, Fisher HL.** Why are children in urban neighborhoods at increased risk for psychotic symptoms? Findings from a UK longitudinal cohort study. *Schizophrenia Bulletin* 2016; **42**: 1372–1383.

49. **Kirkbride JB, Fearon P, Morgan C, Dazzan P, Morgan K, Murray RM,** et al. Neighbourhood variation in the incidence of psychotic disorders in Southeast London. *Social Psychiatry and Psychiatric Epidemiology* 2007; **42**: 438–445.

50. **Warfa N, Curtis S, Watters C, Carswell K, Ingleby D, Bhui K.** Migration experiences, employment status and psychological distress among Somali immigrants: a mixed-method international study. *BMC Public Health* 2012; **12**: 749.

51. **Kim I.** Beyond trauma: post-resettlement factors and mental health outcomes among Latino and Asian refugees in the United States. *Journal of Immigrant and Minority Health* 2016; **18**: 740–748.

52. **Bhui K, Mohamud S, Warfa N, Curtis S, Stansfeld S, Craig T.** Forced residential mobility and social support: Impacts on psychiatric disorders among Somali migrants. *BMC International Health and Human Rights* 2012; **12**: 4.

Chapter 7

Urbanization and mental health

Mauro G. Carta and Dinesh Bhugra

Introduction

The growth of the urban population worldwide is one of the current critical issues for public health and global mental health [1]. The trend of urbanization is well recognized in that in 1950 only 30% of the world population lived in urban areas, but in 2014 it had increased to 54% and is further estimated to rise to 66% of the world's population living in cities by 2050 [2]. It is inevitable that this shift will influence not only the longevity of the population, but also affect social determinants of mental health as older people may be left behind while younger generations move into cities [2].

Urban living means that populations are exposed to several factors that may play a role in the modification of the profile of mental health risks. These can be summarized into macro-social; relational/support; macro-environment; and evolutive/(eu)genetic. It must be emphasized that these factors are strongly interlinked and although considered separately their effects are cumulative.

In this chapter we present a synthesis of some of the research findings related to urbanization and increased psychopathological risks.

Community surveys

Several studies over the past few decades have looked at relationships between urban living and mental health of these community surveys give a clearer picture into prevalence of psychiatric disorders and into association of higher rates with living in cities.

A meta-analysis of urban–rural residence and prevalence on overall psychiatric disorders, focusing specifically on mood, anxiety, and substance use disorders, using data from 20 population survey studies published between 1985 and 2010 [3], reported a significant association with urban living for all psychiatric disorders, and for mood disorders and anxiety disorders. However, this contrary to expectations report showed no association with substance use disorders.

Later studies from some Latin American countries such as Cuba, Dominican Republic, Venezuela, Mexico, and Peru [4] showed a similar association with anxiety disorders. In the megacity of São Paulo, Brazil, in comparison with the other Latin American sites of the Mental Health Survey consortium [5], India and China [4], Timor Lest [6], and Iran [7], as well in later studies in the UK [8], similar observations have emerged.

However, data on mood and depressive disorders are controversial, as are the findings on substance abuse/dependence disorders.

Mood disorders were found more frequently among urban German residents (13.9% vs 7.8% in rural areas) [9], and depressive disorders more frequently in São Paulo, Brazil [5] and in elderly urban people from Sardinia, Italy [10]. However, several studiesfrom China [11–13] and Vietnam [14] seem to indicate a different trend, with a higher prevalence of depression in rural areas, particularly in the elderly. These may reflect changes in cultures, as they are in transition from traditional to different values.

Interestingly a survey in Italy aimed at studying the perception of quality of life, a factor strictly associated with the risk of depressive disorders, showed that men are more sensitive to urban/rural residence than women. Young men live better in cities and elderly men better in rural areas [15]. This may indicate aspirations, as well as social networks of support, which may well vary across generations.

Higher rates of addiction, especially related to online gambling, have been observed in young university graduates living alone in French cities [16]. Higher rates of substance use disorders were found in São Paulo, Brazil, than in other Latin American sites of the Mental Health Survey consortium [5]. In contrast, in a study from China, rural residents were found to have higher alcohol dependence than urban residents [11]. In a study aimed at exploring rural/urban, sex, and racial differences in substance use in college students in USA, the authors reported that rural students were less likely to use alcohol and marijuana than their urban counterparts at the start of their studies, but their use increased within a few years to meet the rates of urban students [17]; however, this observation, which concerns a specific range of young people with a high level of education and coming from high-income families, contrasts with other findings. In a study of a large sample of young people from the USA, in the National Survey on Drug Use and Health (2008–14), the authors reported a narrower association of addiction disorders with rural residence and, not surprisingly, higher levels of unmeet needs for treatment in young people living in rural areas [18].

The association between those living in cities and the risk of schizophrenia is now a well-established finding. A meta-analysis of Vassos et al. [19] reported that the risk for developing schizophrenia in the urban environment was 2.37 times that of the rural population. Similar measures of risk were seen in non-affective psychosis. The association between schizophrenia and urban living increases proportionally with rising levels of urbanity, determined in terms of population size and density [19]. The risk seems proportional to the years of childhood and early adolescence spent in the city, with a dose–response relationship: the more years spent in cities in the early years, the higher the risk of schizophrenia [20–22].

Social determinants in cities

The association between macro social factors and mental health in cities has been studied by consistent lines of research from the milestone study of Faris and Dunham from Chicago in 1939 [23]. However, it must be considered that association is not causation. These authors reported that selective migration may lead to social drift to deprived areas, even if, in the last 80 years, some cohort and case–control studies have helped, in part, to better understand the interaction between social drift and (socio) environmental risks.

Living in deprived areas of the city was found to be associated with mental illness. This association was the result of a concentration of people with low socio-economic status in such areas [24]. The poverty in a neighbourhood, as reflected by the proportion of residents in a local neighbourhood living on social security or public welfare, explained significantly more variance in mental health among migrants and those with minority background (in respect of people without this condition), beyond individual effects of age and income [25]. An interaction between family vulnerability to mental illness and living in deprived urban areas has also been reported [26], suggesting some kind of interaction between the two. However, people who have a low health status and then go on to experience stressful life events, such as poverty, low income, or unemployment, may well move from lower to even more deprived areas [27].

A recent study in Sweden suggested that living in deprived neighbourhoods was substantially heritable and that the association between schizophrenia and neighbourhood deprivation may be entirely explained by genetic influences [28]. However, these findings are not totally confirmed, as in the Danish cohort study the association between time spent in childhood living in cities and schizophrenia seems to be independent to some well-known genetic factors linked to the risk of schizophrenia [29]. However, a recent study reported significant interactions between childhood changes of residence towards urbanization in the first 10 years of life and the level of IQ with regard to risk for the development of schizophrenia in adulthood, and it is postulated that there is a risk of developing schizophrenia within the critical time window of childhood sensitivity, when response to urbanization happens, and may also be linked to IQ level [30]. Thus, environmental and genetic factors (not only related to the risk of schizophrenia, but also with IQ as the protective factor) seems to interplay in really complex and still unclarified models.

In a study of healthy participants, Haddad et al. [31] found a strong inverse correlation between living in cities in early life and grey matter volume in the right dorsolateral prefrontal cortex in Brodmann area 9, and also a negative correlation with grey matter volumes in the perigenual anterior cingulate cortex (but, intriguingly, this was only seen in men). They go on to suggest that a mechanism influenced by stimuli due to early-life urbanity could affect brain architecture, which may be linked to the increased of risk of schizophrenia.

The interaction between social drift and environmental disorders is well recognized in the increased risk for schizophrenia in people who have lived in cities 5 years after disease onset [20]. This seems to underline an environment risk factor, but this effect in itself is not sufficient to explain the excess. Thus, environmental factors may appear to be synergic to the impact of urbanization in early life, as noted earlier in this section [32]. However, further research is required to understand the interaction between social and biological factors.

There is no doubt that social support, whether it is at the personal level or at the community level, can play a significant role in the genesis or prevention of mental illness of certain types. In urban areas people may have difficulties in building and maintaining effective social relationships. Some people move to urban areas seeking anonymity. A recent comment underlined the persistent relevance of the research borne by the milestone study of Berkman and Syme [33], which, firstly, 'demonstrated that social networks were related to the risk of early mortality' [34]. It is worth noting that the importance of physical social networks may well give in to more social media-based interactions [34]. It is intuitive that the city favours and facilitates the use of the Internet due to the ease and extent of online access and availability of free WiFi spaces, but cities do not favour the use of direct interaction in people with severe mental disorders. In fact, rural living is associated with greater frequency of social contact in patients with schizophrenia versus patients with schizophrenia living in cities [35]. However, the role of the city in the use of online social networks and their impact on an individual's mental health is poorly studied, as are generational and age differences. Therefore, the city is a key element that should be studied to understand and explore the importance of both online and offline networks for population health today.

A key point that concerns social direct interaction in cities is the perception of security and violence. A study from the European Schizophrenia

Cohort Study found that urban living is associated with subjective perception of insecurity in people with schizophrenia contributing to increased stress and anxiety [36]. This effect may be further amplified in socially disorganized neighbourhoods; therefore, the risk for mental health problems may be influenced by insecurity and potential exposure to violence and trauma. In fact, studies show a higher presence of stressors in neighbourhoods with a higher likelihood of mental disorders [37]. Neighbourhood economic conditions may also affect well-being and thus can be a source of stress, with a high frequency of violence and criminality and availability of alcohol and drugs, which may mediate the effect of neighbourhood economic contexts. However, neighbourhood stress-buffering mechanisms (e.g. average household occupancy and churches per capita) seem to be associated with a lower likelihood of disorders [37].

Studies on migration and mental health, especially schizophrenia and mood disorders, are numerous (see also Chapter 6). Hospital admission rates for schizophrenia in the UK are highest for people with a Caribbean, Irish, Indian, Pakistan, or Polish background [38–40], with a particularly high incidence in 16–29-year-olds from the Caribbean. In England, African-Caribbeans were also shown to be at increased risk for mania [41]. The impact of migration may determine high levels of stress, but the risk of schizophrenia is even higher in the second generation, suggesting that other social factors and genetic vulnerability may interact, also bearing in mind that only sub-groups of migrants show higher rates of psychosis [39].

Studies carried out in the Netherlands have confirmed UK evidence that the incidence [42] and prevalence [43] of schizophrenia were shown to be increased in some groups of migrants (from Morocco, Suriname, and The Netherlands Antilles), but other immigrants groups seem not to show that association (people from Turkey and people from Western countries). The relative risk of schizophrenia in Suriname-born immigrants was higher than Suriname resident-born population [42].

The interaction of the genetic hypothesis (selective migration according to Ødegaard's definition) [44] and stress of migration is, however, really complex. Both Sardinian migrants in Buenos Aires and Sardinian residents (especially in rural areas) seem to be affected in terms of depressive risk, in response to two waves of crisis in Argentina in 2001 and in Italy in 2015 [45]. However, Sardinians resident in Buenos Aires showed higher levels of lifetime manic episodes [46]. In Sardinian migrants (in Paris) and Greek Cypriots in London, migration was shown to be associated with a higher risk of both anxiety (as people living in Sardinia or Greece) and depressive disorders (as Parisians and Londoners) [47, 48].

In new countries with a focus on migration to the cities by migrants in addition to urban factors, these migrants also face difficulties regarding adaptation, cultural barriers, communication difficulties, resulting isolation, economic disadvantage, and high levels of violence [1]. In contrast, a stimulating environment could offer many opportunities to change the lives of people who have previously lived in deprivation or war. It should not be forgotten that asylum seekers who flee the theatres of violence are not truly isolated in the current world, and constitute a large mass of people moving to cities of high-income countries, as well as those of low-and-middle-income countries. In many parts of the world, such as Asia and Latin America (but also, in part, in Western cities), exodus to the city often occurs from areas strongly deprived of economic opportunities. In this case, according to the theory of goal-striving stress [49], the city, although frequently seen as a deprivation or unfavourable condition for those who have lived there for generations, could offer riches and opportunities for newcomers.

Studies replicated over time in mining villages with strong outbound emigration, as a consequence of mine closures, reflect that in many settings people will migrate to cities, and those who are poor, deprived, and have mental illness may remain in these villages, raising various psychopathological issues [50]. Thus, differences in access to social, family, and human resources make it possible to survive in villages, but not necessarily in cities, even with a minimal economic level and psychosocial disability. A further factor that may well play a role is the individual temperament, which in some cases will affect functioning, especially among migrants [46].

In this framework of great complexity, to affirm that emigration and the impact of the city may expose those at risk is too reductive [51]. Various aspects of migrant health may illuminate risk and protective factors, which may be at stake in relation to each specific situation [52, 53]. For example, living in predominantly ethnic neighbourhoods can cause segregation and the risk of depression and anxiety in some conditions compared with living in less segregated neighbuorhoods [54]. However, in some other settings, ethnic density (defined as the proportion of people of the same ethnic group) may play a protective role with regard to risk of mental illness owing to protective cultural-borne networks [55].

Determinants and urban physical environment

Some determinants of the physical environment itself may play a role in increasing the risk for mental illness in cities. These include high levels of pollution (soil, air, water), noise and light pollution, traffic, and urban architecture.

Urban outdoor pollution deserves special attention for the impact it can have on the structures of the brain, as also mentioned in the previous section [56]. In fact, fine and ultrafine particulate matter are capable of reaching the brain, leading to neuroinflammation and oxidative brain stress. Thus, a case can be made that epidemiological, cognitive, behavioural, and mechanistic studies need to be integrated into exploring an association between exposure to air pollution and the development of central nervous system damage. These factors are a pressing and major concern for public health, to address measures to prevent or reduce further exposure [56].

An epidemiological study reported an association between short-term exposure to nitrogen dioxide and sulphur dioxide and suicide in Salt Lake County [57]. Madrigano et al. [58] found an association between DNA methylation, a potential pathway linking air pollution and psychological functioning, with ambient particulate matter less than 2.5 μm in diameter (PM 2.5). Methylation in a large sample of elderly residents was shown to have declined after acute exposure to both black carbon and PM 2.5. Participants with low optimism and high anxiety had exposure to PM 2.5 that was 3–4 times larger than those with high optimism or low anxiety. These results have not been confirmed in other studies, such as that of Wang et al. [59], from Boston, who studied a sample of elderly individuals [59]. These authors found no evidence of association between depressive symptoms and long-term exposure to traffic pollution, concluding that there is no evidence that air pollution is associated with depressive symptoms in older adults living in a metropolitan area in the USA [59].

A study of 6630 older people (aged > 60 years) from the database of the China Health and Retirement Longitudinal Survey, after controlling for social demographic variables, reported an association between air pollution (sulphur dioxide emission), and, consequently, rural–urban residence, and depressive symptoms (as measured by the Center for Epidemiologic Studies Depression Scale (CES-D) score) [60]. A review by Tzivian et al. [61]. summarized the evidence of air pollution on mental health in adults from 15 studies and showed that the long-term effects of air pollution are associated with several measures of cognitive functioning and memory, and depressive and anxiety symptoms. They concluded that there was clear existing evidence that supported the association of environmental factors with mental health.

Consistent research evidence collected in the past few years has indicated an association between perinatal exposures to ambient air pollution (hazardous air toxics, ozone, particulate, and traffic-related pollution) with an increased risk of autism spectrum disorder (ASD) [62]. An association between urban residential proximity to industrial facilities emitting air pollutants (arsenic, lead, or mercury) and a higher prevalence of ASD has been noted [63]. A recent study suggests that green spaces, specifically tree cover in areas with a high road density, may also affect rates of autism in elementary school children and may, indeed, be beneficial [64]. It has been argued that socio-economic status and place of residence may play a role in affecting the rates and observations of these studies [65]. These authors concluded that there is a specific association with perinatal air pollution exposure during the third, but not the first, trimester of pregnancy. Given the consistency of findings across studies and the exposure-window-specific associations, evidence for a causal association between air pollution and ASD is increasingly compelling.

A review of the literature found a detrimental effect of noise on mental health in a consistent manner [66], including traffic noise pollution [67] and living in areas close to airports [68]. Noise seems to impair cognitive functioning and mental health (especially mood and anxiety disorders), but results from epidemiological surveys need to be strengthened with evidence of dose and times of exposure that can produce damage [66]. Road traffic noise seems to be associated with poorer mental health, specifically in those who experience poor sleep. Thus, individuals with poor sleep quality seem to be more vulnerable to the effects of road traffic noise on mental health [69]. It is difficult to know whether their poor sleep is the result of the noise or they were previously poor sleepers for other reasons. The impact of pollution on sleep is not only related to noise, but also to artificial light, which may disrupt the circadian rhythm and influence the normal patterns of sleep, and be a risk factor for breast cancer [70], but has not been studied for potential increases in vulnerability to mood disorders, especially bipolar disorders.

The impact of noise and light pollution is further complicated by inappropriate and inadequate architecture and design of cities. It has been argued that natural features and architectural design, irrespective of the humans living in urban areas, can help to improve well-being and reduce stress associated with urban life [71]. These authors go on to propose that public health could benefit from street trees, green roofs, community gardens, parks and open spaces, and extensive connective pathways for walking and biking. Access to daily exercise in relaxing and aesthetically pleasing surroundings may further benefit the physical and mental heath of people. In fact, urban design and structure is integral to the mental health of citizens [72, 73].

Conclusions

A considerable amount of research has focused on the risk conditions associated with city living. Given the hectic, haphazard, and rapid processes of global urbanization, robust research mixing qualitative and quantitative data and prospective approaches are needed to explore and clarify the causal links of the associations so far highlighted and the interactions between environmental and genetic factors. Studies on positive adaptation factors to the city are not yet sufficient. Urban rehabilitation interventions need to be studied over time in the wake of the welfare of populations. These approaches should take a multidisciplinary collaborative approach involving skills and knowledge, ranging from architecture to urban planning to anthropology and to human wellness and mental health.

References

1. **Srivastava K.** Urbanization and mental health. *Indian Journal of Psychiatry* 2009; **18**: 75–76.
2. **United Nations.** World Urbanization Prospects. The 2014 Revision. Available at: https://esa.un.org/unpd/wup/Publications/Files/WUP2014-Highlights.pdf (accessed 12 November 2018).
3. **Peen J, Schoevers RA, Beekman AT, Dekker J.** The current status of urban-rural differences in psychiatric disorders. *Acta Psychiatrica Scandinavica* 2010; **121**: 84–93.
4. **Prina AM, Ferri CP, Guerra M, Brayne C, Prince M.** Prevalence of anxiety and its correlates among older adults in Latin America, India and China: cross-cultural study. *British Journal of Psychiatry* 2011; **199**: 485–491.
5. **Andrade LU, Wang YP, Andreoni S, Silveira CM, Alexandrino-Silva C, Siu ER,** et al. Mental disorders in Megacities: findings from the São Paulo megacity mental health survey, Brazil. *PLoS One* 2012; **7**: e31879.
6. **Silove D, Ivancic L, Rees S, Bateman-Steel C, Steel Z.** Clustering of symptoms of mental disorder in the medium-term following conflict: an epidemiological study in Timor-Leste. *Psychiatry Research* 2014; **219**: 341–346.
7. **Sharifi V, Amin-Esmaeili M, Hajebi A, Motevalian A, Radgoodarzi R, Hefazi M, Rahimi-Movaghar A.** Twelve-month prevalence and correlates of psychiatric disorders in Iran: the Iranian Mental Health Survey 2011. *Archives of Iranian Medicine* 2015; **18**: 76–84.
8. **Jenkins R, Lewis G, Bebbington P, Brugha T, Farrell M, Gill B, Meltzer H.** The National Psychiatric Morbidity Surveys of Great Britain—initial findings from the household survey. *International Review of Psychiatry* 2003; **15**: 29–42.
9. **Jacobi F, Höfler M, Siegert J, Mack S, Gerschler A, Scholl L,** et al. Twelve-month prevalence, comorbidity and correlates of mental disorders in Germany: the Mental Health Module of the German Health Interview and Examination Survey for Adults (DEGS1-MH). *International Journal of Methods in Psychiatric Research* 2014; **23**: 304–319.
10. **Carpiniello B, Carta MG, Rudas N.** Depression among elderly people. A psychosocial study of urban and rural populations. *Acta Psychiatrica Scandinavica* 1989; **80**: 445–450.
11. **Phillips MR, Zhang J, Shi Q, Song Z, Ding Z, Pang S,** et al. Prevalence, treatment, and associated disability of mental disorders in four provinces in China during 2001-05: an epidemiological survey. *The Lancet* 2009; **373**: 2041–2053.

12. Li N, Pang L, Chen G, Song X, Zhang J, Zheng X. Risk factors for depression in older adults in Beijing. *Canadian Journal of Psychiatry* 2011; **56**: 466–473.

13. He G, Xie JF, Zhou JD, et al. Depression in left-behind elderly in rural China: prevalence and associated factors. *Geriatrics and Gerontology International* 2016; **16**: 638–643.

14. Fisher J, Tran T, La BT, Kriitmaa K, Rosenthal D, Tran T. Common perinatal mental disorders in northern Viet Nam: community prevalence and health care use. *Bulletin of the World Health Organization* 2010; **88**: 737–745.

15. Carta MG, Aguglia E, Caraci F, Dell'Osso L, Di Sciascio G, Drago F, et al. Quality of life and urban/rural living: preliminary results of a community survey in Italy. *Clinical Practice and Epidemiology in Mental Health* 2012; **8**: 169–174.

16. Achab S, Nicolier M, Mauny F, Monnin J, Trojak B, Vandel P, et al. Massively multiplayer online role-playing games: comparing characteristics of addict vs non-addict online recruited gamers in a French adult population. *BMC Psychiatry* 2011; **11**: 144.

17. Derefinko KJ, Bursac Z, Mejia MG, Milich R, Lynam DR. Rural and urban substance use differences: effects of the transition to college. *American Journal of Drug and Alcohol Abuse* 2018; **44**: 224–234.

18. Chavez LJ, Kelleher KJ, Matson SC, Wickizer TM, Chisolm DJ. Mental health and substance use care among young adults before and after Affordable Care Act (ACA) implementation: a rural and urban comparison. *Journal of Rural Health* 2018; **34**: 42–47.

19. Vassos E, Pedersen CB, Murray RM, Collier DA, Lewis CM. Meta-analysis of the association of urbanicity with schizophrenia. *Schizophrenia Bulletin* 2012; **38**: 1118–1123.

20. Pedersen CB, Mortensen PB. Evidence of a dose-response relationship between urbanicity during upbringing and schizophrenia risk. *Archives of General Psychiatry* 2001; **58**: 1039–1046.

21. Heinz A, Deserno L, Reininghaus U. Urbanicity, social adversity and psychosis. *World Psychiatry* 2013; **12**: 187–197.

22. Gruebner O, Dr. Rapp MA, Adli M, Kluge U, Galea S, Heinz A. Cities and mental health. *Deutsch Ärzteblatt International* 2017; **114**: 121–127.

23. Faris REL, Dunham HW. *Mental Disorders in Urban Areas: An Ecological Study of Schizophrenia and Other Psychoses.* Chicago, IL: University of Chicago Press. 1939.

24. Reijneveld SA, Schene AH. Higher prevalence of mental disorders in socioeconomically deprived urban areasin The Netherlands: community or personal disadvantage? *Journal of Epidemiology and Community Health* 1998; **52**: 2–7.

25. Rapp MA, Kluge U, Penka S, Vardar A, Aichberger MC, Mundt AP, Schouler-Ocak M, et al. When local poverty is more important than your income: Mental health in minorities in inner cities. *World Psychiatry* 2015; **14**: 249–250.

26. Binbay T, Drukker M, Alptekin K, Elbi H, Aksu Tanik F, Özkinay F, et al. Evidence that the wider social environment moderates the association between familial liability and psychosis spectrum outcome. *Psychological Medicine* 2012; **42**: 2499–2510.

27. Tunstall H, Shortt NK, Pearce JR, Mitchell RJ. Difficult life events, selective migration and spatial inequalities in mental health in the UK. *PLoS ONE* 2015; **10**: e0126567.

28. Sariaslan A, Fazel S, D'Onofrio BM, Längström N, Larsson H, Bergen SE, et al. Schizophrenia and subsequent neighborhood deprivation: revisiting the social drift

hypothesis using population, twin and molecular genetic data. *Translational Psychiatry* 2016; **6**: e796.

29. Paksarian D, Trabjerg BB, Merikangas KR, Mors O, Børglum AD, Hougaard DM, et al. The role of genetic liability in the association of urbanicity at birth and during upbringing with schizophrenia in Denmark. *Psychological Medicine* 2018; **48**: 305–314.

30. Toulopoulou T, Picchioni M, Mortensen PB, Petersen L. IQ, the urban environment, and their impact on future schizophrenia risk in men. *Schizophrenia Bulletin* 2017; **43**: 1056–1063.

31. Haddad L, Schäfer A, Streit F, Lederbogen F, Grimm O, Wüst S, Deuschle M, et al. Brain structure correlates of urban upbringing, an environmental risk factor for schizophrenia. *Schizophrenia Bulletin* 2015; **41**: 115–122.

32. March D, Hatch SL, Morgan C, Kirkbride JB, Bresnahan M, Fearon P, Susser E. Psychosis and place. *Epidemiology Reviews* 2008; **30**: 84–100.

33. Berkman LF, Syme SL. Social networks, host resistance, and mortality: a nine-year follow-up study of Alameda County residents. *American Journal of Epidemiology* 1979; **109**: 186–204.

34. Aiello AE. Invited commentary: evolution of social networks, health, and the role of epidemiology. *American Journal of Epidemiology* 2017; **185**: 1089–1092.

35. Schomerus G, Heider D, Angermeyer MC, Bebbington PE, Azorin JM, Brugha T, Toumi M; European Schizophrenia Cohort. Residential area and social contacts in schizophrenia. Results from the European Schizophrenia Cohort (EuroSC). *Social Psychiatry and Psychiatric Epidemiology* 2007; **42**: 617–622.

36. Schomerus G, Heider D, Angermeyer MC, Bebbington PE, Azorin JM, Brugha T, Toumi M. Urban residence, victimhood and the appraisal of personal safety in people with schizophrenia: results from the European Schizophrenia Cohort (EuroSC). *Psychological Medicine* 2008; **38**: 591–597.

37. Stockdale SE, Wells KB, Tang L, Belin TR, Zhang L, Sherbourne CD. The importance of social context: neighborhood stressors, stress-buffering mechanisms, and alcohol, drug, and mental health disorders. *Social Science & Medicine* 2007; **65**: 1867–1881.

38. Littlewood R, Lipsedge M. Psychiatric illness among British Afro-Caribbeans. *BMJ* 1988; **296**: 950–951.

39. Bhugra D. Migration and schizophrenia. *Acta Psychiatrica Scandinavica* 2000; **407**: 68–73.

40. Carta MG, Bernal M, Hardoy MC, Haro-Abad JM; Report on the Mental Health in Europe Working Group. Migration and mental health in Europe (the state of the mental health in Europe working group: appendix 1). *Clinical Practice and Epidemiology in Mental Health* 2005; **1**: 13.

41. Sharpley M, Hutchinson G, McKenzie K, Murray RM. Understanding the excess of psychosis among the African-Caribbean population in England. Review of current hypotheses. *British Journal of Psychiatry* 2001; **40**: 60–68.

42. Selten JP, Cantor-Graee E, Slaets J, Kahn RS. Odegaard's selection hypothesis revisited: schizophrenia in Surinamese immigrants to the Netherlands. *American Journal of Psychiatry* 2002; **159**: 669–671.

43. Schrier AC, van de Weterin BJ, Mulder PJ, Selten GP. Point prevalence of schizophrenia in immigrants groups in Rotterdam: data from outpatients facilities. *European Psychiatry* 2001; **16**: 162–166.

44. **Ødegaard Ø**. Emigration and Insanity. A study of mental disease among the Norwegian born population of Minnesota. *Acta Psychiatrica Neurologica Scandinavica* 1932; (Suppl 4): 1–206.

45. **Carta MG, Perra A, Atzeni M, D'Oca S, Moro MF, Kurotschka PK**, et al. An evolutionary approach to mania studying Sardinian immigrants to Argentina. *Revista Brasileira de Psiquiatria* 2017; **39**: 147–153.

46. **Carta MG, Atzeni M, D'Oca S, Perra A, D'Aloja E, Brasesco MV**, et al. Depression in Sardinian immigrants in Argentina and residents in Sardinia at the time of the Argentinian default (2001) and the Great Recession in Italy (2015). *BMC Psychiatry* 2017; **17**: 59.

47. **Mavreas V, Bebbington P.** Acculturation and psychiatric disorder: a study of Greek Cypriot immigrants. *Psychological Medicine* 1990; **20**: 941–951.

48. **Carta MG, Kovess V, Hardoy MC, Morosini PL, Murgia S, Carpiniello B.** Psychiatric disorders in sardinian immigrants in Paris: a comparison with parisians and sardinians resident in Sardinia. *Social Psychiatry and Psychiatric Epidemiology* 2002; **37**: 112–117.

49. **Parker S, Kleiner RJ, Needelman B.** Migration and mental illness. Some reconsiderations and suggestions for further analysis. *Social Science & Medicine* 1969; **3**: 1–9.

50. **Carta MG, Carpiniello B, Kovess V, Porcedda R, Zedda A, Rudas N.** Lifetime prevalence of major depression and dysthymia: results of a community survey in Sardinia. *European Neuropsychopharmacology* 1995; **5**(Suppl.): 103–107.

51. **Bhugra D.** Migration and mental health. *Acta Psychiatrica Scandinavica* 2004; **109**: 243–258.

52. **Bhugra D.** Cultural identities and cultural congruency: a new model for evaluating mental distress in immigrants. *Acta Psychiatrica Scandinavica* 2005; **111**: 84–93.

53. **Bhugra D, Gupta S, Schouler-Ocak M, Graeff-Calliess I, Deakin NA, Qureshi A**, et al. EPA Guidance mental health care of migrants. *European Psychiatry* 2014; **29**: 107–115.

54. **Meyer OL, Castro-Schilo L, Aguilar-Gaxiola S.** Determinants of mental health and self-rated health: a model of socioeconomic status, neighborhood safety, and physical activity. *American Journal of Public Health* 2014; **104**: 1734–1741.

55. **Schrier AC, Peen J, de Wit MA, van Ameijden EJ, Erdem O, Verhoeff AP**, et al. Ethnic density is not associated with psychological distress in Turkish-Dutch, Moroccan-Dutch and Surinamese-Dutch ethnic minorities in the Netherlands. *Social Psychiatry and Psychiatric Epidemiology* 2014; **49**: 1557–1567.

56. **Calderón-Garcidueñas L, Calderón-Garcidueñas A, Torres-Jardón R, Avila-Ramírez J, Kulesza RJ, Angiulli AD.** Air pollution and your brain: what do you need to know right now. Prim Health Care Res Dev. 2015; **16**: 329–345.

57. **Bakian AV, Huber RS, Coon H, Gray D, Wilson P, McMahon WM**, Renshaw PF. Acute air pollution exposure and risk of suicide completion. *American Journal of Epidemiology* 2015; **181**: 295–303.

58. **Madrigano J, Baccarelli A, Mittleman MA, Sparrow D, Spiro A 3rd, Vokonas PS**, et al. Air pollution and DNA methylation: interaction by psychological factors in the VA Normative Aging Study. *American Journal of Epidemiology* 2012; **176**: 224–232.

59. **Wang Y, Eliot MN, Koutrakis P, Gryparis A, Schwartz JD, Coull BA**, et al. Ambient air pollution and depressive symptoms in older adults: results from the MOBILIZE Boston study. *Environmental Health Perspectives* 2014; **122**: 553–558.

60. Tian T, Chen Y, Zhu J, Liu P. Effect of air pollution and rural-urban difference on mental health of the elderly in China. *Iranian Journal of Public Health* 2015; **44**:1084–1094.

61. Tzivian L, Winkler A, Dlugaj M, Schikowski T, Vossoughi M, Fuks K, et al. Effect of long-term outdoor air pollution and noise on cognitive and psychological functions in adults. *International Journal of Hygiene and Environmental Health* 2015; **218**: 1–11. 3.

62. Kalkbrenner AE, Schmidt RJ, Penlesky AC Environmental chemical exposures and autism spectrum disorders: a review of the epidemiological evidence. *Current Problems in Pediatric and Adolescent Health Care* 2014; **44**: 277–318.

63. Dickerson AS, Rahbar MH, Han I, et al. Autism spectrum disorder prevalence and proximity to industrial facilities releasing arsenic, lead or mercury. *Science of the Total Environment* 2015; **536**: 245–251.

64. Wu J, Jackson L. Inverse relationship between urban green space and childhood autism in California elementary school districts. *Environment International* 2017; **107**: 140–146.

65. Weisskopf MG, Kioumourtzoglou MA, Roberts AL. Air pollution and autism spectrum disorders: causal or confounded? *Current Environmental Health Reports* 2015; **2**: 430–439.

66. Makopa Kenda I, Agoub M, Ahami AO. Noise effects on mental health: a review of literature. *Santé Mentale au Québec* 2014; **39**: 169–181.

67. Dreger S, Meyer N, Fromme H, Bolte G; Study Group of the GME cohort. Environmental noise and incident mental health problems: A prospective cohort study among school children in Germany. *Environmental Research* 2015; **143**: 49–54.

68. Hardoy MC, Carta MG, Marci AR, Carbone F, Cadeddu M, Kovess V, et al. Exposure to aircraft noise and risk of psychiatric disorders: the Elmas survey—aircraft noise and psychiatric disorders. *Social Psychiatry and Psychiatric Epidemiology* 2005; **40**: 24–26.

69. Sygna K, Aasvang GM, Aamodt G, Oftedal B, Krog NH. Road traffic noise, sleep and mental health. *Environmental Research* 2014; **131**: 17–24.

70. Cho Y, Ryu SH, Lee BR, Kim KH, Lee E, Choi J. Effects of artificial light at night on human health: a literature review of observational and experimental studies applied to exposure assessment. *Chronobiology International* 2015; **32**: 1294–1310.

71. Hartig T, Kahn PH Jr. Living in cities, naturally. *Science* 2016; **352**: 938–940.

72. Galea S, Freudenberg N, Vlahov D. Cities and population health. *Social Science & Medicine* 2005; **60**: 1017–1033.

73. Asgarzadeh M, Koga T, Yoshizawa N, Munakata J, Hirate K. Investigating green urbanism. *Building Oppressiveness* 2010; **9**: 555–562.

Chapter 8

Urbanization and marginalization

Michael Krausz, Verena Strehlau,
Fiona Choi, and Kerry L. Jang

Marginalization and urbanization

The global trend of urbanization often means that economically disadvantaged individuals living in rural areas are migrating into large metropolitan areas in search of a better life. Rapid rural-to-urban migration adds to existing poverty and marginalization in every metropolitan region in different ways. Vulnerable neighbourhoods, townships, or favelas are growing and increasingly become a challenge for communities with poor social infrastructure and insufficient housing. This represents not only a minor shift, but also a major trend in global societies, especially for the healthcare system. It also documents the impact of social determinants of health on a much larger scale of societal structure. Individuals with mental health challenges and fewer resources may end up in an environment with little or no support, with an increased likelihood of experiencing adversities such as substance use and limited opportunities.

The consequences of urbanization for the most vulnerable are multiple. They are most likely losers of a more intense competition on scarce resources and the target of violence. They have little access to public health care. The ability of communities to respond to a changing situation and growing cities is critical to addressing these problems. Are cities prepared to adapt infrastructure and wholly integrate new citizens or not?

Consequences of urbanization for the most vulnerable

Urbanization is changing circumstances of daily living and functioning of society far more than most people are aware. As an overview, the following are common difficulties of urbanization related to groups of marginalized individuals.

More vulnerable neighbourhoods

Vulnerable urbans are not equally distributed across cities. The majority of them live in special 'vulnerable' neighbourhoods, which often exist as a containment of poverty and expression of marginalization. Some came to existence spontaneously as a consequence of urbanization and the big influx of new citizens, like the favelas in Brazil. Others have long-term historical roots and evolved as a place for poor and mobile populations, often with frequent drug use, such as the downtown eastside in Vancouver.

More high-need individuals in metropolitan areas

These migrants often move because their health care and social needs are high and not met in their places of origin. They either do not have a choice to leave, for example in African conflict zones, or they move in hope for a better future, work, support, and so on.

More competition for fewer resources in health care

The existing infrastructure in these neighbourhoods is not prepared to meet the needs of the population already living there in the first place. The increase of migrants creates more competition for fewer resources. This discrepancy is a defining condition for these parts of big metropolitan areas. Without external support and a paradigm shift in healthcare delivery any improvement will be impossible.

Trauma, mental illness, and substance use among the homeless

Adverse childhood experience, childhood trauma, and childhood abuse has received increased attention in recent years, and are reported to contribute to becoming homeless [1]. These adverse childhood experiences can function as catalysts leading to increased vulnerability to substance use and mental health disorders. There is also an increased risk among those who experienced childhood abuse for adult psychological re-traumatization. All forms of traumatization can contribute to emotional distress and to difficulties in help-seeking and coming to trust authorities including healthcare providers [2].

Mental health disorders, specifically substance use disorders, are common in homeless populations. In a representative sample of 500 homeless individuals in Canada, high rates of mental health and substance use disorders were reported. Of the 500 participants, 78% suffered from at least one substance use disorder and 68% suffered from at least one mental disorder (e.g. depression, post-traumatic stress disorder, schizophrenia, bipolar disorder). A total of 55% suffered from concurrent mental disorders [3]. These prevalence rates for substance use disorders and for the concurrent diagnosis of mental and substance use disorder seemed to be higher than in most previous studies. While the ranges reported in previous studies are quite large, a recent meta-analysis found that the mental disorders with the highest prevalence in this population are alcohol and drug dependence, with random effects pooled prevalence estimates of 37.9% (95% confidence interval [CI] 27.8–48.0%) and 24.4% (95% CI 13.2–35.6%), respectively [4].

Substance use substantially contributes to morbidity and mortality in vulnerably housed individuals. A recent review indicated that of 1302 deaths among a homeless cohort in Boston, USA, 236 were tobacco-attributable, 215 were alcohol-attributable, and 286 were drug-attributable. Thus, 52% of deaths were attributable to any of these substances, with alcohol, tobacco, and illicit drugs contributing almost equally. In comparison to the general population in these regions, tobacco-attributable mortality rates were 3–5 times higher, alcohol-attributable mortality rates were 6–10 times higher, and drug-attributable mortality rates were 8–17 times higher. Disparities in substance-attributable deaths accounted for 57% of the all-cause mortality gap between the homeless population and the general population [5]. This information alone indicates the priority of substance use disorder among health concerns in this specific population (see Figure 8.1).

Substance use disorder as a risk factor for homelessness

A recent meta-analysis of American veterans reviewed risk factors for becoming homeless. The strongest and most consistent risk factors were the presence of substance use disorders and concurrent mental disorders, followed by poverty and other income-related factors. There was some evidence that social isolation, adverse childhood experiences, and past incarceration can also be considered as important risk factors [6]. Veterans are at greater risk for homelessness than non-service adults. This study supports recent smaller and methodologically weaker studies, which indicated that mental disorders are strong risk factors for homelessness and that substance use disorders top the list of mental disorders leading to homelessness.

One factor often neglected until recently and also not addressed in the aforementioned reports is the aspect of poor cognition. A review found the pooled estimate for the frequency of cognitive impairment to be 25% of the homeless, and the mean full-scale IQ score was 85, one standard deviation below

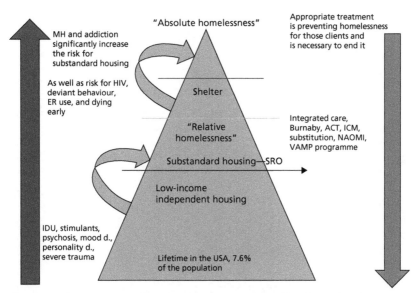

Figure 8.1 The iceberg paradigm for homelessness, mental health, and addiction. MH, mental health; ER, emergency room; IDU, injection drug use; Mood D., mood disorder; Personality D., personality disorder; SRO, single-room occupancy; ACT, assertive community treatment; ICM, intensive case management; NAOMI, North American Opiate Medication Initiative; VAMP, Vancouver Addictions Matrix Program.

the mean of the normal population [7]. The authors of the review concluded that cognitive impairment was common among homeless adults and may be a trans-diagnostic problem that potentially impedes rehabilitative efforts in this population. Homeless living conditions, prolonged substance use, and a high incidence of head trauma may contribute to these cognitive problems [8], but poor cognition is also likely to contribute to the risk of becoming homeless. Psychosocial interventions and psychotherapeutic treatments are often established in universities and in populations with average or above-average cognitive abilities. This makes it important to test the efficacy of these interventions in clinically targeted populations. Clinical practice often leads to a need to adapt manuals and treatments substantially to the needs of the specific population.

Homelessness is, in most cases, temporary, and individuals often transition and cycle through the different stages of marginalization and precarious housing. The risk factors are diverse, but mental illness most likely contributes to social destabilization to such an extreme extent. It is highly likely that mental illness and homelessness have a bidirectional relationship (Figure 8.2). To transition out of homelessness, one may need effective mental health treatment and by the same token, recovery from trauma often requires housing 'first'. To leave

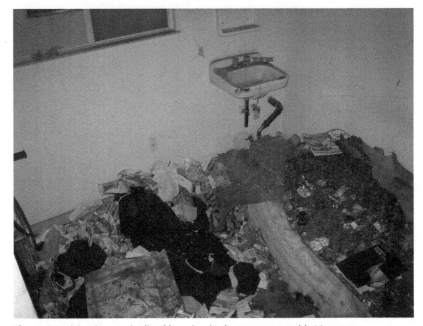

Figure 8.2 Living in marginalized housing in downtown eastside Vancouver.

a situation of being homeless, you may need treatment to recover, for example from trauma, or you need housing, 'first'.

The challenge for the system of care

Vulnerable individuals living in urban centres have, on average, higher health needs overall and more limited access to care. The combination of structural deficits, limited capacity, and individual barriers or challenges, such as a lack of health insurance or lower literacy. Being traumatized, being a severe substance user, having physical illnesses like hepatitis C, and having a mental illness also make it more complicated to find and access appropriate care regardless of where one lives across the globe.

Treatment and access to care

Access to care is a major issue and, frequently, individuals who are waiting for more specific treatment approaches or for treatment of more complex conditions are required to have some form of stable housing in order to be referred, treated, and followed by a respective service [9]. This presents as a serious barrier to receiving necessary care. In a recent qualitative European study [10], four components of good practice for treating homeless and other marginalized populations were identified: (1) establishing outreach programmes to identify and engage with individuals with mental disorders and addiction; (2) facilitating access to services that provide different, transdisciplinary components of health care, and thus reducing the need for further referrals; (3) strengthening the collaboration and coordination between different services; and (4) disseminating information on services both to marginalized groups and to practitioners in the area.

The specific psychosocial approaches effective for homeless individuals are not dissimilar to approaches for people living in housing. Aside from contingency management, which seems to be beneficial in the treatment of most substance use disorders, cognitive behavioural interventions and motivational interviewing are evidence-based treatments proven to be effective in this population [11].

These specific psychosocial interventions are generally applied within the context of community service concepts. More intensive community service concepts such as assertive community treatment (ACT) teams have proven to be effective [12]. ACT teams provide a wide variety of services, including case management, mental health services, crisis intervention, treatment, education, housing, and employment support. ACT services are available around the clock to respond to a client's immediate needs. They have shown that they can increase treatment adherence, reduce length of hospitalization, and increase housing access and stability. The original ACT treatment teams did not focus sufficiently on addiction treatment, as they were originally developed for community treatment of severe mental disorders. Still, effective addiction treatment is a major concern for ACT teams given the high incidence of comorbidity in most clients they serve.

A number of more short-term outreach concepts have been developed, such as critical time intervention or the assertive outreach team. These multidisciplinary teams focus on a time-limited adaptation of intensive case management to bring problem-solving resources, community advocacy, and motivational enhancement to clients who are homeless, specifically, during times of transition, such as those entering homeless shelters from prison, recovering from emergency treatment, and transferring to community housing resources [13].

A less resource-intensive approach is the intensive case management (ICM) approach. In a recent study, a number of substantive improvements in the quality of care and health outcomes were found by applying an ICM approach to homeless individuals in five Canadian cities; ICM had a very limited impact on substance use [14]. It seems that longer interventions and more focused approaches on substance use disorder are needed to serve this highly marginalized and highly complex client population.

Supported housing and supported employment

Supportive housing has been demonstrated to improve abstinence, stabilize living arrangements, and secure employment over time [15]. Although housing in itself is important, more often than not housing alone is insufficient to address the many facets of substance use disorder and concurrent mental health disorder.

Supportive employment assists clients in accessing, obtaining, and maintaining employment as a primary method to prevent or end homelessness. Recognizing work as a priority, Shaheen and Rio [16] note that early treatment and rehabilitation efforts often emphasize housing and supportive services, while the value of assisting clients in obtaining employment and/or education early in rehabilitation should be highlighted. They suggest that employment helps clients who are experiencing homelessness develop trust, motivation, and hope over time. Supportive employment not only aids individuals in finding job opportunities, but it also helps them achieve continued employment by teaching them skills such as problem solving, managing interpersonal conflicts, developing appropriate work-related behaviours, and managing money wisely.

Gender-specific services

Women-specific services often have the mandate to operate under a trauma-informed care approach to cater to women who often have life-long experiences of adversities, such as childhood maltreatment, household disruption in childhood, foster care, sex-work, violence, homelessness, and substance use.

Women-specific services need to account for the high complexity of their clients and also often need to consider offering services that not only focus on women themselves, but also on the women's dependents, children, or other family members. There is a substantial number of marginalized women who have children that often are not living with them but in foster care or in other settings. Nevertheless, women often wish to be involved in the lives of their children—regardless of whether they live with them or not at that given time. Women-specific services should be prepared to aid women in navigating these situations, which may mean providing legal help or access to assistance with child and family ministries.

There are both empirical evidence and anecdotal reports that homelessness and social marginalization are different for women than for men. Women have higher rates of involvement in sex work and therefore may trade sex work for a place to sleep, which may make them less visible as homeless. In some cases, involvement in sex work may mean that women are working in the sex trade during evening hours and may be sleeping during daytime hours. This could interfere with their access to health and social services and therefore specific situations like this (which is only described here as an example) need to be considered when planning a service.

Services also need to account for the fact that many marginalized women are of child-bearing age and may become pregnant during their time in contact with services. Women-specific services should have information available and staff employed that are able to educate all women accessing a service providing information on safe-sex practices, risks, testing, and treatment options for sexually transmitted infections such as hepatitis and HIV/AIDS. Further, in addition to providing information, safe-sex items, such as condoms, should be freely available to all women and men. Testing and treatment for sexually transmitted infections can either be provided as part of a service (if the mandate is medically related), or information needs to be given on where women can access these services without facing disrespect or stigma.

If a woman becomes pregnant during their time interacting with a service, every service should have basic information about healthy pregnancy behaviours, including how to stay healthy during pregnancy with a substance use disorder. Depending again on the mandate of the service, women need to have either direct or referred access to non-judgemental peri-/postnatal services, no matter if they have a concurrent substance use disorder at the time of pregnancy.

In any case, it is of highest importance—before implementing new services or restructuring existing services—to consult with the existing service providers in any given area. Despite the fact that service provides are sometimes operating under a very individual mandate/philosophy, they usually carry a wealth of knowledge with a level of detail that needs to be heard and incorporated into any new and future service planning.

Harm reduction in mental health

With limited resources and growing needs it is crucial to reconsider priorities in health care. This includes treatment paradigms and mental healthcare standards.

It is important to provide low-barrier access, especially for the most vulnerable and mentally ill. Resource allocation and structures should be supported that allow more patients to be treated and that provide access to those with the highest level of needs. Unfortunately, this is lacking, even in developed countries. Marginalized individuals have an extremely difficult time accessing appropriate care, which leads to increased morbidity and mortality.

It is also critically important to change attitudes toward the mentally ill in society and health care, and to see stigma as a serious, disabling, and dangerous attitude that places the health of thousands at risk. The approach to the HIV/ AIDS epidemic proved how important anti-stigma work was in opening doors in all directions and making a major shift possible.

Last, but not least, it is critical to prioritize treatment goals that support better functioning in daily living and foster a decent quality of life, rather than focusing simply on the elimination of symptoms.

Access to care

Many countries have legislated equal access to care as a civil right (e.g. Canada Health Act (Canada), Grundgesetz (Germany)) as a first step. Yet, there is no society in which every person has the same access. We believe it is critical for as many individuals with mental health challenges as possible to be supported. These individuals need access to care beyond what is available in emergency settings. Access may improve as e-health solutions begin to allow users direct and easy access, even if they live abroad, are in transition, or located in remote areas with no local services. In the future we will see online therapy and other solutions, improving support even to countries with low functioning healthcare systems. Important thresholds to access support are barriers of social exclusion. Individuals living on the street, in poverty, or extreme situations of social marginalization receive little attention and have a hard time accessing health care, housing, or social support. For these people, secure housing and basic social assistance within the context of a welcoming community need to be the critical components of recovery.

Taking stigma seriously

Stigma is more than just an attitude. It comes from a lack of knowledge and from inappropriate beliefs about mental illness and addiction. Stigma fosters an atmosphere of discrimination and exclusion. Acknowledging the importance of stigma and discrimination is an important first step. A systematic approach to improve mental health literacy could help to convince the public and healthcare professionals that social exclusion and stigmatization are not congruent with the rules of a democratic society and violate basic human rights for people living with disabilities, mental illness, and addiction. Anti-stigma needs to be part of professional education and training. Compassion is a critical component of high-quality health care. To work effectively with mentally ill patients, professionals need to relate to their clients in a manner that is free of stigma. Decriminalization could help to integrate people with mental illness and associated challenges such as substance use into society. Deviant behaviour should be addressed but understood as often being symptomatic or as part of the mental illness and put in this context when addressing it. Good health care and adequate social support is one of the best preventative measures against violence and crime.

Functioning and surviving

Unfortunately, resources are scarce and many health conditions currently have no cure. Much of medicine is about management of symptoms, gradual recovery, and reduction of risks and harm. Therefore, an important tool is empowerment through capacity building: supporting people with mental illness and giving them the tools to deal appropriately with their challenges will help achieve a more effective system that treats patients in a consistent and ethical manner. To this end, peers, families, and professionals must be trained to provide this empowering environment and to create a supportive atmosphere for recovery.

Experiences in addiction medicine are showing that the harm-reduction approach improves quality of care, links more clients to the system, and increases individual engagement. By addressing overdose-related deaths and serious infections it has contributed to a significant decrease in mortality rates.

Conclusions

Growing cities with growing inequalities constitute a new healthcare environment between growing demands and limited resources. This needs to lead to fundamental changes in social infrastructure and especially the way mental health care is delivered.

Harm reduction in mental health speaks to the overall need for a paradigm shift in the field of psychiatry adapting to a changing environment in societies. With standard current approaches and often ineffective structures, we are currently not providing adequate care for the most vulnerable members of society. The more we are able to prevent harm, the earlier we are able to intervene and, consequently, the higher the likelihood of recovery and reintegration into society. Patient-centred care is about addressing the needs of mentally challenged individuals in the community, in their families, and in social networks.

Addiction care has demonstrated that a harm-reduction approach is effective in preventing severe physical harm and in reducing overdose mortality. That could be a blueprint for other areas in health care too.

References

1. **Torchalla I, Strehlau V, Li K, Schütz C, Krausz M.** The association between childhood maltreatment subtypes and current suicide risk among homeless men and women. *Child Maltreatment* 2012; **17**: 132–143.

2. **Ibabe I, Stein JA, Nyamathi A, Bentler PM.** Predictors of substance abuse treatment participation among homeless adults. *Journal of Substance Abuse Treatment* 2014; **46**: 374–381.

3. **Krausz RM, Clarkson AF, Strehlau V, Torchalla I, Li K, Schütz CG.** Mental disorder, service use, and barriers to care among 500 homeless people in 3 different urban settings. *Social Psychiatry and Psychiatric Epidemiology* 2013; **48**: 1235–1243.

4. **Fazel S, Khosla V, Doll H, Geddes J.** The prevalence of mental disorders among the homeless in western countries: systematic review and meta-regression analysis. *PLoS Medicine* 2008; **5**: e225.

5. **Baggett TP, Chang Y, Singer DE, Porneala BC, Gaeta JM, O'Connell JJ, et al.** tobacco-, alcohol-, and drug-attributable deaths and their contribution to mortality disparities in a cohort of homeless adults in Boston. *American Journal of Public Health* 2015; **105**: 1189–1197.

6. **Tsai J, Rosenheck RA.** Risk factors for homelessness among US veterans. *Epidemiologic Reviews* 2015; **37**: 177–195.

7. **Depp CA, Vella L, Orff HJ, Twamley EW.** A quantitative review of cognitive functioning in homeless adults. *The Journal of Nervous and Mental Disease* 2015; **203**: 126–131.

8. **Hwang SW, Colantonio A, Chiu S, Tolomiczenko G, Kiss A, Cowan L, et al.** The effect of traumatic brain injury on the health of homeless people. *Canadian Medical Association Journal* 2008; **179**: 779–784.

9. **Palepu A, Gadermann A, Hubley AM, Farrell S, Gogosis E, Aubry T, Hwang SW.** Substance use and access to health care and addiction treatment among homeless and vulnerably housed persons in three Canadian cities. *PLoS One* 2013; **8**: e75133.

10. **Priebe S, Matanov A, Schor R, Straßmayr C, Barros H, Barry MM, et al.** Good practice in mental health care for socially marginalised groups in Europe: a qualitative study of expert views in 14 countries. *BMC Public Health* 2012; **12**: 248.

11. **Hwang SW, Burns T.** Health interventions for people who are homeless. *The Lancet* 2014; **384**: 1541–1547.

12. **Nelson G, Aubry T, Lafrance A.** A review of the literature on the effectiveness of housing and support, assertive community treatment, and intensive case management interventions for persons with mental illness who have been homeless. *American Journal of Orthopsychiatry* 2007; **77**: 350–361.

13. **Herman D, Conover S, Felix A, Nakagawa A, Mills D.** Critical Time Intervention: an empirically supported model for preventing homelessness in high risk groups. *The Journal of Primary Prevention* 2007; **28**: 295–312.

14. **Stergiopoulos V, Hwang SW, Gozdzik A, Nisenbaum R, Latimer E, Rabouin D, et al.** Effect of scattered-site housing using rent supplements and intensive case management on housing stability among homeless adults with mental illness: a randomized trial. *JAMA* 2015; **313**: 905–915.

15. **Milby JB, Schumacher JE, Wallace D, Freedman MJ, Vuchinich RE.** To house or not to house: the effects of providing housing to homeless substance abusers in treatment. *American Journal of Public Health* 2005; **95**: 1259.

16. **Shaheen G, Rio J.** Recognizing work as a priority in preventing or ending homelessness. *The Journal of Primary Prevention* 2007; **28**: 341–358.

Chapter 9

Neuroscience of mental illness in the city

Jan Golembiewski

Introduction

The way the brain processes perceptions of the physical environment is of interest in the epidemiology of mental and behavioural health because of recent discoveries that have found that the city—the locus of human endeavours—is one of the most predictable factors of the development of schizophrenia and other psychotic and mood disorders [1, 2]. The ecological model of perception is an excellent model for understanding the relationship between the mental health and the physical environment, because it asserts that perception does not commence a cognitive process, but is part of the way the brain reacts to the demands for action that are intrinsic to objects and forms within the environment.

Many studies show that the urban environment adversely affects mental health, with significant increases of incidence of severe anxiety, mood (depression and bipolar disorders), and the psychotic spectrum of disorders (paranoia through to schizophrenia), while other mental illnesses such as addictions do not appear to change significantly [3]. The negative influence of city life has been previously subdivided into 'direct' effects, such as light, ambient temperature, nature, and exposure to pollutants or parasites; and 'indirect' effects, such as how the built environment moderates the psycho-social environment by forcing people together, isolating them, and by limiting their access to amenities or exposing them to illicit drugs, and so on [4, 5]. But the distinction between direct and indirect factors appears spurious in the light of the problem, which is how the material world can so influence the mind that the brain is often permanently damaged, with no apparent causal pathways to factors such as air or noise pollution or ambient temperature. In fact, on close analysis, it is the so-called 'indirect' factors that appear to have the strongest impact, and perhaps none so strong as the urban environment itself, which in the case of schizophrenia accounts for about 30% of incidence, assuming it is a causal factor [2]. This is greater than any single genetic factor, but may be confounded

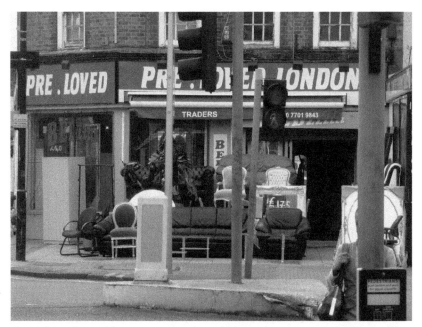

Figure 9.1 Urban environments are replete with negative messages of all kinds. This image (typical of the route of the Camberwell study of Ellet et al. [43]) offers places to sit that are simultaneously denied (the shop does not want passers by using their chairs and sofas). There are messages to walk and stop walking (walk signals); a traffic island that does not offer safety (it has been hit by vehicles); windows allow you to look in, but have mesh, suggesting a fear of thieves; a savage monster appears to hide behind a post, and even the shop name, 'Pre-loved London' has negative connotations, reminding us that love is a thing of the past.

by other suspects, such as the developmental vitamin D deficiency hypothesis [6], which may in itself be a biomarker for the urban environment, because too little vitamin D usually means too little sunlight, and for most people that means too much time indoors [7, 8].[1]

One of the current hypotheses for the deleterious effect of city life is the Ecological Hypothesis for Schizophrenia, which details a vicious circle around an inability to cope in the face of the demands that the designed environment places of a person's neural attentional system (see Figure 9.1) [9]. While this is far from obvious to designers who know little about the brain, it may in fact

---

[1] Note that studies on vitamin D-deficient rats demonstrate peculiar developmental retardation that may be analogous to schizophrenia, if such an analogy can be meaningfully made [8].

be far more direct than the so-called 'direct effects' mentioned earlier that designers do feel are controllable [10]. Indeed, this hypothesis is based on a theory called 'direct perception', a key concept of both the Ecological Theory of Perception [11] and Mirror Neuron Theory [12]. The strength of this hypothesis is that it links the external world to known neural mechanisms in the brain that are implicated in psychotic mental illness.

Extended brain theory and psychotic symptomatology

People tend to think of the brain as a knowledge-driven, probabilistic cognitive engine—as a mechanism to turn perceptual inputs (colours, sensations, sounds, etc.) into information by predicting and recognizing them as meaningful objects [13]. A hypothetical secondary process generates choice: objects are ordered and acted upon according to needs and preferences. This model of the hermetic, rational, cognitive brain was convenient for the development of functional anatomy for medicine (understanding the effects of stroke, lesions, etc.), but it fails to explain the profound impact of the environment on neural development or why people react so differently to concrete and real jungles; in short, knowledge-driven models of the brain have been very useful but fail to explain how the urban environment may be causal for psychotic mental illness.

Over the years, challenges to the traditional brain model have led to ideas about a kind of *extended mind*. In 1979 James J. Gibson published a well-reasoned body of evidence called the Ecological Theory of Perception, which finds how animal behaviour is an automatic and direct reaction to 'affordances', which are the opportunities for action that are structured into the environment, like shelters, pathways, and seats. Affordances are perceived directly (in other words, the actions that objects enable) and affordances are what stimulate behaviour, not the recognition of the object itself [11]. As Gibson put it, 'ask not what's inside your head, but what head's inside of!' [14]. Remarkably, this affordance/behaviour pathway precedes the consideration of raw sense data (qualia), such as colours, shapes, and so on [10], and furthermore, it is estimated that more than 95% of adult actions and thoughts are not the end result of deliberate cognition and planning, but are precognitive, automatic responses [15].

The actions that are triggered (or are not, if sufficient inhibition occurs) are exactly what the object or setting suggests—a chair says 'sit', a path tells us to walk, and so on, but, more alarmingly, a knife instructs us to stab and cut, a cliff says 'leap', and a gun says 'shoot' [16]. The fact that this action precedes recognition of basic sense information suggests that the impulse to action is possibly even how we actually recognize objects and our own actions. It makes sense: greater awareness and understanding occurs only with greater inhibition [10]. Totally uninhibited actions go unregistered as amnesiac events, and may be identified as symptomatic—perhaps as 'grossly disorganised behaviours'. If patients report an awareness of these very real 'commands' to act ('the cliff told me to leap'), this may well be considered hallucinatory, especially if the command is misattributed ('the TV told me to leap off the cliff'), and any post-hoc justification for these bizarre, uninhibited behaviours could very well read as delusions (I tried to leap off the cliff because it was Lover's Leap, and I'm a lover …), so it is a cogent hypothesis that the environment itself is an integral part of the psychotic symptomatology [17].

The initial research about direct perception looked at primal behaviours and animal-like instincts, but, in the human world, the ecological dynamic is more complex: we react not only to opportunities for action, but to learned actions and even beyond these. We live in a world replete with *meanings*, which in themselves solicit or inhibit reactions, depending on the nature of meaning and the context. For humans, a symbolic reading of circumstances is every bit as potent in how a basic affordance mediates behaviour. Symbolic meanings are not only in communication between people, they are embedded into the fabric of the built environment as 'behaviour settings': these are environments that either inhibit or suggest affordance-stimulated behaviours—in the way a temple or church suggests quiet contemplation and inhibits the vulgar language that can be heard in places like a sports field [18]. (Note to President Trump: in contrast, people barely speak in a locker room, and thus 'locker-room talk' is highly inhibited.)

The extended mind concept has hitherto been understood in neuroscience through the perceptual apparatus [19] and mirror neuron theory—a concept very similar to the Ecological Theory of Perception, except limited to social interactions. Like Mirror Neuron Theory, the Ecological Theory of Perception must take a step beyond the neurology of the perceptual apparatus (visual cortices, etc). Mirror Neuron Theory has identified harmonic neural networks that are stimulated in response to the actions of others, such as the premotor cortex and perigenual anterior caudal cortex (pACC) [20]. The critical neural structures that are involved in ecological perception have not been so clearly identified but must be similarly prefrontal. We know that the management of real, three-dimensional representations in real time (what is called working memory) is handled by the right dorsolateral prefrontal cortex (rDLPFC) [21], although other structures may also be involved. The rDLPFC would not be needed for well-known (learned of instinctive) representations (which will be managed subcortically—see later in this chapter), but is likely to be essential for all new or obscured ones, because prefrontal involvement is thought to be essential for all new (non-Hebbian) learning [22].

In the extended brain models, cognitive processes are not isolated, internal, and established by wilful desires alone, rather they are mediated by the phenomenal context, often in advance of associated cognitive processes. In extended brain models, the brain does not cognise and act on choice, but it reads the contextual environment, and chooses only whether or not to inhibit (and thereby refuse) an experience or opportunity. And even this ability to choose is not always there. In fact, simple life forms have no choices at all, rather the inverse: simple animals like barnacles act on an affordance without any act of choice or cognition, much less the inhibition associated with frontal lobe function that humans have [10]. Even humans with frontal lobe damage show the bizarre symptoms of utilization behaviour [23], and in more extreme cases, environmental dependency syndrome, conditions where patients lose personal autonomy and act only in ways that are prescribed by the environment [16]. In short, the more complex and functional brains are, the *less* dependence there is on the physical and chemical world for behavioural cues and the more perception and cognition takes place. The extended brain models of perception are still neural, but acknowledge that the phenomenal world triggers event potentials in the brain, and therefore that there is an intrinsic relationship between the perceptual world and the function of the brain. Just as a foundation is to hold up a building, it cannot do so without the ground.

The city's influence on the brain

This article is not a complete study of the regions involved in perception nor is it a detailed account of the entire extended brain concept. It is an introduction to the parts of the brain we currently recognize as implicated in the epidemiology of mental illness in the city. This means the neurotransmitter that is most implicated in psychosis (dopamine) and the neural anatomy that is statistically found to develop differently over a sample from an urban[2] context compared with a rural and small-town milieus. It's important to note that these data are correlational and statistical, which means they are not uniform, but bear out over an average, meaning these differences are not universal in all urban populations; however, they are likely to be more pronounced in some subgroups.

So far, the regions that have been identified have all shown significant grey-matter deficits. These are the pACC and the connective tissue of the pACC in males; and the rDLPFC. In contrast, the amygdalae are prone to significantly

---

[2] Based on studies taken from Manheim, a medium-sized German city, and the surrounding countryside.

increased activation in the same circumstances [24, 25]. Physically larger amygdalae have only been reported among bigger or more complex social groupings, which do not necessarily correlate with urban lifestyles [26].

The exploration of the functional roles of these organs goes back about 130 years to the birth of functional neuroscience, and yet findings remain inconclusive because they mostly rely on lesion studies, followed by observations of behavioural change and functional absences [27]. Most studies are of animals (usually caged laboratory rats and rhesus monkeys, but animals do not have the same cognitive functions, nor do they behave similarly to humans, especially in urban vs rural milieus). Lesion studies on humans rely on specific accidental or natural organic insults to the brains of otherwise healthy human subjects and these are rarely studied [27]. Other methodologies are easier, but weaker: currently most 'in vivo' studies rely on relevant photos being shown to participants while they pass through massive, scary, and loud magnetic resonance imaging scanners. This process provides images of 'slices' of the brain, which are analysed to identify statistically significant patterns. It is not a perfect science, because all brains are unique at the outset. The result is that we still have to speculate about what various brain regions do, albeit with reasonable information to support our postulations.

One of the areas potentially affected by city life is the pACC. This is a medial gyrus of the anterior caudal cortex (ACC), adjacent to the corpus callosum; a mass of white matter (connective tissue) that carries signals between the two hemispheres of the brain [28]. Like other brain regions, the role of the pACC is not entirely certain, but we know that it is strongly associated with declarative awareness and creativity—it is the oldest part of the frontal lobe (in terms of evolution)—and that the pACC is highly connected to the limbic 'emotional' centre of the brain [29–31]. We also know that it appears to mediate an anxiety response in regard to social standing [32]. And, importantly for our purposes, we know that it and the tissue that connects it has a tendency to atrophy with urban life and also with poor self-image, especially in males [25, 32].

The pACC is thought to be a key organ in empathetic processes, possibly to bring (or generate) awareness to feelings of love and social connectedness, notwithstanding that these emotions are generated and observed by distributed and complex processes that are also endocrinal [30, 33]. This hypothesis is supported by the finding that pACC volumes are relatively diminished in severe psychotic illnesses, which are also associated with damaged social networks and poor emotional expression [34]. When deficient, the pACC fails to bring awareness to positive emotions as it should, possibly because of a dopaminergic process described elsewhere [35]. What this urban deficiency means is that people (especially males) who live in the city are likely to be less aware of a sense of love and connectedness than those in the country.

Another area that is frequently found to be relatively small as a result of urban life is the rDLPFC. As mentioned earlier, an area that is thought to hold and manipulate spatial representations (drawn from both current circumstances and from recall) in the 'working memory'. This is where information is considered, verified, and organized before it's consciously acted upon [21]. That this area is frequently deficient in urban life is curious, because superficially it appears that city areas have much greater visual complexity than rural areas, and therefore the rDLPFC should be subject to greater growth. But this assumption may be incorrect: three-dimensional representations of space may, in fact, be far more important in rural areas where people often have to tell one tree from another as they change seasonally, or negotiate slopes and tangled organic paths just to find their way around, whereas many cities (including Mannheim, where these data were gathered) are organized along a grid and are well sign-posted. And while negotiating traffic may well be one of those skills that will improve in the city, this skill will theoretically only really improve rDLPFC mass among chronic jaywalkers! But if the rDLPFC is the organ that processes new affordances, then this atrophy might speak of a failure to recognize new affordances in the ecological context—in other words, it suggests that there is a standardization of responses to a standard set of ecological cues, as people get stuck in unchanging routines. In addition, the deficiency may speak of more time spent indoors in the city, perhaps in front of the TV, where the spatial information is that is provided is not complex, and affords the viewer no opportunities to act at all.

And although we cannot make strong assertions about why the rDLPFC atrophies with city life, the ability to maintain and assess spatial information is undeniably critical to normal activities of daily living. The atrophy may mean people find it hard to cope with the 'real world', and the increased responsibility that comes with adulthood once people step outside the spaces they know well.

Bucking the trend of decreased activation and volumetric shrinkage, the amygdalae of city folk are subject to significantly increased activation [24]. There are two amygdalae: one in either hemisphere of the brain, where they are nestled within the hippocampi (again, there are two). A significant function of the hippocampi is to recognize emergent stories that are being presented by the environment, to identify both positive and negative scenarios before they even occur. The evolutionary advantage of this process compensates for the slowness of the frontal cortex, making sure a person is able to make the most of emergent circumstances or to pre-empt disaster and organize escape [36]. One of the speculative purposes of the amygdalae within these couplings are to identify an event's relative importance to 'me' [37].[3] When an event directly concerns 'me', one of the amygdalae will signal this to draw attention to the salient event, but if the event is of no concern, the amygdalae will not signal. Thus, rats with bilateral amygdala damage show no fear of cats [38], and humans fail to care about aversive imagery [39]. There are two hippocampi/amygdala couplings because where the left brain tends to be used for immediate concerns, the right is used for broader narratives [40]. This separation allows awareness that things which appear to be good may in fact be bad—like bait in a trap, for instance [36].

Excessive amygdala activity may then mean inappropriate or excessive attribution of self-involvement within a given context. And if there is no particular social context, this over-identification may be a symptom only too common in psychotic and anxiety illness spectrums: therapists know only too well the self-centred demands of patients. Even patients who have a severely reduced sense of self often identify relevance for themselves in stimuli that could not possibly concern them—such as the conversations of strangers or TV broadcasts [41]. This kind of inappropriate identification is a feature of paranoia [42].

For most people, the increased paranoia and excessive identification that we find in an urban context is unsurprising despite a paucity of knowledge about this connection. But what people do find surprising is just how significant this impact is, especially when the urban context is particularly loaded with the subtle negative messages that we read into the hustlers, traffic dangers, obnoxious people, fumes, and demands for payment that converge in the city. What is remarkable is that statistically high significance is noted on a battery of measures for anxiety, paranoia, and other psychiatric symptoms after very small doses (10 minutes) of urban exposure [43].

The Ecological Hypothesis for Schizophrenia (which relies on Extended Brain Theory) provides a compelling reason for these findings: all messages—whether symbolic, explicit (perhaps written), or ecological (such as traffic)—are triggers for affordance-stimulated behaviours, and in urban environments, these messages are ubiquitous, meaning that people effectively go about much of their business on autopilot. What is worse is they are often negative—and need constant inhibiting: demands to spend money they do not have, or leap in front of subway trains [9].

The influence of affect—that is the positive or negative feelings about circumstances (be they architectural or social)—cannot be underplayed in this dynamic because feelings change the nature of reactions in a way that really

---

[3] The amygdalae are not single entities but are a collection of several nuclei, all of which have different functions [37]; however, most studies on the brain do not provide detail on this scale and do not differentiate which nuclei are responsible for which tasks.

separate those with mental disorders and those who do not. Reactions can be extreme at one end of the psychotic spectrum and of no consequence at the 'healthy' end, depending on the emotional quality of perceived circumstances and how much these impulses are inhibited. Whereas healthy controls are nonplussed by negative imagery (if it poses no real threat), matched cohorts of people with schizophrenia or bipolar disorder are extremely reactive—and the excessive neural excitation expresses as a range of psychiatric symptoms, including thought insertion and disorganized thought and behaviour. The inverse is less extreme, but still highly significant; whereas a group with psychiatric diagnoses will overinhibit their reactions to positive imagery, the healthy controls will not, instead allowing a laugh or smile [44]. The amygdala/hippocampus couplings are pivotal to this process, because perspectives on what's is 'good' or 'bad' depend entirely on the narrative context and the perspective of the protagonist.

Beyond this 'switching effect', the amygdala/hippocampus couplings mediate the type of attention that is given to reactive actions by stimulating one of two dopamine pathways; the anterior pathway, which is rich with D1 dopamine receptors, is thought to draw declarative (highly aware) attention to deeply considered tasks (the attention used to 'figure things out'). However, the D2 receptors that are more common in the striatum appear to trigger only latent awareness of a kind that is used for either instinctive tasks (like jumping out of the way of a car) or well-learned tasks (like driving a car) [35, 45].

In the ecological hypothesis for schizophrenia, excitation that is not inhibited turns to action, with the connections to the motor cortex, premotor cortex, and other regions determining the kind of action that eventually takes place.

Affect also determines the quality of attention that is given to these circumstances: if the stimulus is generally positive, actions will be guided, in part, by the latent awareness of the D2 receptors in the striatum and, in part, by the declaratively aware prefrontal areas of the brain, meaning that (in balance) some low level of declarative awareness is maintained. But if the stimulus is wholly negative, actions will be mostly striatal and therefore amnesiac [17, 44]. This is important because it explains why the psychiatric symptoms that are associated with unwanted actions are effectively treated by blocking the striatal D2 dopamine receptors—the central action of most effective antipsychotic medications [46].

Psychotic illness and city life

Recent findings that the urban environment correlates with an increased incidence of psychosis is echoed by further findings that the urban environment causes dose-dependent deficits in several neural regions, all of which are implicated in psychotic illness: the pACC, which is used to understand social interactions in a positive way; the amygdalae, which modulate the sense of our own involvement in circumstance; and in the organs we use to process complex spatial information and possibly even how we behave in relation to the affordances that the ecological environment offers us (rDLPFC). Taken together, these studies suggest the urban environment is causal for psychotic illness.

The correlation between psychotic illness and city life has been noted since the 1930s [5], but whereas it is usually thought that the city is a crucible for causal factors like social stress, poverty, and access to drugs, it seems the city (as a whole) has a more compelling relationship with psychosis than any of these individual factors when taken separately.

All objects that have human purpose stimulate human action, but nowhere are these objects more ubiquitous than in cities. Whereas in rural areas these demands are possibly more varied and complex, in the city they may become more routine. This shift appears to be borne out in the neuroscience of the city—with the atrophy of the rDLPFC. In classical theory, the striatum is where learned routines and instincts are managed, while the prefrontal areas, including the rDLPFC, are used for processing novelty, and conscious consideration and meaning. Therefore, this atrophy may trace a difference in the quality of awareness of those in rural areas versus—city dwellers from a generalized alertness to the kind of dim awareness.

The hypothetical actions of the deficient neural areas appear to correlate well with the very symptoms of psychosis and mood disorders, with the absences of the rDLPFC function easily explaining hallucinatory, delusional, and disorganized symptoms; the deficiencies of the pACC correlating well to diminished social networks, poor communication (disorganized speech), and low self-esteem; and the overactive amygdalae almost certainly relating to paranoid association and the distinctive ego-centric appearance of mania and some other presentations of depression.

Designing cities—and getting them right

That designers are generally unaware of the effects that their inventions have on the brain, and therefore take no responsibility of this role is deeply worrying. The world of design is like a highway, where each and every driver is asleep at the wheel [1].

Cities are designed by people for people. Every affordance is intended to trigger responses, and not always desirable ones—affordances that dangle, like bait, with expensive bills attached, affordances that come with barbs, caveats, and compromises. Designers should be very careful about how these action-triggers affect mental health. In contrast, most urban environments have a paucity of positive, delightful affordances—ones with no strings attached, which are just there to improve the environment and encourage a love of life. Designers also should attempt to create new languages for urban design, just for variation, to keep the humdrum away. These urban affordances should carefully consider interpersonal relationships—perhaps putting strangers side by side for joyful experiences. And the city should genuinely be about each and every individual; in the spirit of human-centred design, to associate those amygdaloid signals with joy, positivity, and companionship.

References

1. **Golembiewski J.** The designed environment and how it affects brain morphology and mental health. *HERD* 2016; **9**: 161–171.

2. **Krabbendam L, van Os J.** Schizophrenia and urbanicity: a major environmental influence—conditional on genetic risk. *Schizophrenia Bulletin* 2005; **31**: 795.

3. **Peen J, Schoevers RA, Beekman AT, Dekker J.** The current status of urban-rural differences in psychiatric disorders. *Acta Psychiatrica Scandinavica* 2010; **121**: 84–93.

4. **Evans GW.** The built environment and mental health. *Journal of Urban Health* 2003; **80**: 536–555.

5. **Faris REL, Dunham HW.** *Mental Disorders in Urban Areas: An Ecological Study of Schizophrenia and Other Psychoses.* Oxford: University of Chicago Press, 1939.

6. **McGrath JJ, Eyles DW, Pedersen CB, Anderson C, Ko P, Burne TH,** et al. Neonatal vitamin D status and risk of schizophrenia: a population based case-control study. *Archives of General Psychiatry* 2010; **67**: 889–894.

7. **Golembiewski J.** Are diverse factors proxies for architectural influences? A case for architecture in the aetiology of schizophrenia. *Curēus* 2013; **5**: e106.

8. **Eyles DW, Feron F, Cui X, Kesby JP, Harms LH, Ko P,** et al. Developmental vitamin D deficiency causes abnormal brain development. *Psychoneuroendocrinology* 2009; **34**: S247–S257.

9. **Golembiewski J.** Architecture, the urban environment and severe psychosis. Part I: aetiology. *Journal of Urban Design and Mental Health* 2017; **2**: 1.

10. **Bargh JA, Dijksterhuis A.** The perception-behavior expressway: automatic effects of social perception on social behavior. *Advances in Experimental Social Psychology* 2001; **33**: 1–40.

11. **Gibson JJ.** *The Ecological Approach to Visual Perception.* Boston, MA: Houghton Mifflin Company, 1979.

12. **Rizzolatti G, Fabbri-Destro M, Cattaneo L.** Mirror neurons and their clinical relevance. *Nature Clinical Practice Neurology* 2009; **5**: 24–34.

13. **Clark A.** Whatever next? Predictive brains, situated agents, and the future of cognitive science. *The Behavioral and Brain Sciences* 2013; **36**: 181–204.

14. **Mace W. James J.** Gibson's strategy for perceiving: ask not what's inside your head, but what your head's inside of. In: **RE Shaw, J Bransford** (eds) Perceiving, Acting, and Knowing. Mahwah, NJ: Earlbaum, 1977, pp. 43–66.

15. **Baumeister RF, Sommer KL.** *Consciousness, Free Choice, and Automaticity.* Mahwah, NJ: Lawrence Erlbaum Associates Publishers, 1997.

16. **Lhermitte F.** Human autonomy and the frontal lobes. Part II: patient behavior in complex and social situations: The 'environmental dependency syndrome'. *Annals of Neurology* 1986; **19**: 335–343.

17. **Golembiewski J.** Introducing the concept of reflexive and automatic violence: a function of aberrant perceptual inhibition. *Archives of Psychiatry and Psychotherapy* 2014; **16**: 5–13.

18. **Barker RG, Wright HF.** *The Midwest and its Children; The Psychological Ecology of an American Town.* Evanston, IL: Row, Peterson & Company, 1954.

19. **Phillips WA, Clark A, Silverstein SM.** On the functions, mechanisms, and malfunctions of intracortical contextual modulation. *Neuroscience and Biobehavioral Reviews* 2015; **52**: 1–20.

20. **Rizzolatti G, Craighero L.** The mirror neuron system. *Annual Review of Neuroscience* 2004; **27**: 169–192.

21. **Ramnani N, Owen AM.** Anterior prefrontal cortex: insights into function from anatomy and neuroimaging. *Nature Reviews Neuroscience* 2004; **5**: 184–194.

22. **Fletcher PC, Frith CD.** Perceiving is believing: a Bayesian approach to explaining the positive symptoms of schizophrenia. *Nature Reviews Neuroscience* 2009; **10**: 48–58.

23. **Lhermitte F.** 'Utilization Behavior' and its relation to leisons of the frontal lobes. *Brain* 1983; **106**: 237–255.

24. **Lederbogen F, Kirsch P, Haddad L, Streit F, Tost H, Schuch P,** et al. City living and urban upbringing affect neural social stress processing in humans. *Nature* 2011; **474**: 498–501.

25. **Haddad L, Schafer A, Streit F, Lederbogen F, Grimm O, Wust S,** et al. Brain structure correlates of urban upbringing, an environmental risk factor for schizophrenia. *Schizophrenia Bulletin* 2015; **41**: 115–122.

26. **Bickart KC, Wright CI, Dautoff RJ, Dickerson BC, Barrett LF.** Amygdala volume and social network size in humans. *Nature Neuroscience* 2011; **14**: 163–164.

27. **Damasio AR.** Descartes' Error: Emotion, Reason, and the Human Brain. New York: G.P. Putnam, 1994.

28. **Cheetham A, Allen NB, Whittle S, Simmons J, Yucel M, Lubman DI.** Orbitofrontal cortex volume and effortful control as prospective risk factors for substance use disorder in adolescence. *European Addiction Research* 2016; **23**: 37–44.

29. **Dietrich A, Kanso R.** A review of EEG, ERP, and neuroimaging studies of creativity and insight. *Psychology Bulletin* 2010; **136**: 822–848.

30. **Frith CD, Frith U.** Interacting minds—a biological basis. *Science* 1999; **286**: 1692–1695.

31. **Devinsky O, Morrell M, Brent A.** Contributions of the anterior cingulate cortex to behaviour. *Brain* 1995; **118**: 279–306.

32. **Gianaros PJ, Horenstein JA, Cohen S, Matthews KA, Brown SM, Flory JD,** et al. Perigenual anterior cingulate morphology covaries with perceived social standing. *Social Cognitive and Affective Neuroscience* 2007; **2**: 161–173.

33. **Bartels A, Zeki S.** The neural basis of romantic love. *Neuroreport* 2000; **11**: 3829–3834.

34. **American Psychiatric Association (APA).** *Diagnostic and Statistical Manual (DSM-IV-TR). 4th Text Revision.* Arlington, VA: American Psychiatric Association, 2000.

35. **Golembiewski J.** The subcortical confinement hypothesis for schizotypal hallucinations. *Curēus* 2013; **5**: e118.
36. **Le Hunte B, Golembiewski J.** Stories have the power to save us: a neurological framework for the imperative to tell stories. *Arts and Social Sciences Journal* 2014; **5**: 73–77.
37. **Baron-Cohen S, Ring H, Bullmore E, Wheelwright S, Ashwin C, Williams S.** The amygdala theory of autism. *Neuroscience and Biobehavioral Reviews* 2000; **24**: 355–364.
38. **Blanchard DC, Blanchard RJ.** Innate and conditioned reactions to threat in rats with amygdaloid lesions. *Journal of Comparative and Physiological Psychology* 1972; **81**: 281.
39. **Adolphs R, Tranel D.** Preferences for visual stimuli following amygdala damage. *Journal of Cognitive Neuroscience* 1999; **11**: 610–616.
40. **McGilchrist I.** Reciprocal organization of the cerebral hemispheres. *Dialogues in Clinical Neuroscience* 2010; **12**: 503–515.
41. **Chadwick P.** The stepladder to the impossible: a first hand phenomenological account of a schizoaffective psychotic crisis. *Journal of Mental Health* 1993; **2**: 239–250.
42. **Freeman D, Freeman J.** *Paranoia the 21st Century Fear.* Oxford and New York: Oxford University Press, 2008.
43. **Ellett L, Freeman D, Garety P.** The psychological effect of an urban environment on individuals with persecutory delusions: the Camberwell walk study. *Schizophrenia Research* 2008; **99**: 77–84.
44. **Golembiewski J.** All common psychotic symptoms can be explained by the theory of ecological perception. *Medical Hypotheses* 2012; **78**: 7–10.
45. **Ashby FG, Turner BO, Horvitz JC.** Cortical and basal ganglia contributions to habit learning and automaticity. *Trends in Cognitive Sciences* 2010; **14**: 208–215.
46. **Ginovart N, Kapur S.** Dopamine receptors and the treatment of schizophrenia. In: KA Neve (ed.) *The Dopamine Receptors.* New York: Springer, Humana Press, 2010, pp. 431–477.

Chapter 10

The psychogenic city

Francesca Solmi and James B. Kirkbride

Teeming, swarming city, city full of dreams,
Where specters in broad day accost the passer-by!
(*Les Fleurs du mal,* Charles Baudelaire, 1857)

Over half of us globally now live in cities. By 2050 this figure is predicted to rise to a staggering two-thirds of the world's population. This unprecedented change in the organization of human populations—combined with an ever increasingly connected world—will have both positive and negative consequences on a wide variety of social, political, economic, and health-related domains for individuals and society. In this chapter, we will focus on one of the apparent negative consequences of city living; namely, the raised *incidence* rates of some types of psychotic disorders (but, as we shall see, not others) associated with urban living. Regardless of the possible causes of this phenomenon, which we review later in this chapter, it reveals an uncontroversial, largely replicable, and pivotal tenet in the epidemiology of psychotic disorders: schizophrenia and other non-affective psychotic disorders manifest themselves at a higher rate in more urban environments. What is more controversial is the extent to which living in an urban environment *causes* psychosis. The first section of this chapter ('Evidence of association') reviews the epidemiological studies describing the association between urban living and the incidence of psychotic disorders. The extent to which *causality* matters here depends on the perspective from which one approaches the issue. From an epidemiological point of view, understanding whether *urbanicity* is causally related to psychosis risk is central to a complete understanding of the polygenetic and multifactorial aetiology of these disorders. From a public mental health perspective, causality is still a fundamental issue, as prevention strategies will only be successful if removal or prevention of an exposure leads to a corresponding reduction in risk. From a health services research approach, however, causality, arguably, matters to a lesser extent, as resource allocation mainly depends on need, regardless of its determinants. Thus, if the rate of presentation for potential psychotic disorders is twice as high in urban areas than in rural ones, *early intervention in psychosis* services need to be deployed according to this need, regardless of whether it is driven by sociodemographic factors, environmental stressors, or social drift. We will explore the major hypotheses to account for this increased risk in the second section of this chapter ('An overview of the main exploratory hypotheses'). At the outset, it is important to be mindful of the need to appraise carefully the strength of the evidence in terms of the likely causal role the urban environment might play in generating psychotic experiences and disorders. While this caveat should permeate reading of the entirety of this chapter, we pay specific attention to the issue of causality in the third section ('Causal inference in the association between urbanicity and psychosis risk'). We also discuss how a causal association (if true) between urban living and psychosis risk fits with current socio-neurodevelopmental perspectives on psychosis; in other words, how does the urban environment get *under the skin*?

Evidence of association

Early evidence

That rates of psychotic disorders are higher in cities is far from a new observation. The seminal study to first demonstrate this was published by Robert E.L. Faris and H. Warren Dunham, two sociologists from the Chicago School of Sociology who set out to examine variation in hospital admission rates for several psychiatric disorders in the same city in the 1920s. Their methodological rigour—and adherence to several epidemiological principles—means that Faris and Dunham's monograph *Mental disorders in urban Areas* [1] is to social and psychiatric epidemiology what John Snow's *On the Mode of Communication of Cholera* [2] is to epidemiology. Much like Snow's work, Faris and Dunham's careful spatial analysis of the occurrence of episodes of psychotic disorders provided clues to their aetiology. This involved the meticulous investigation of approximately 35,000 hospital admissions in the city of Chicago for a first occurrence of a set of major mental disorders—including schizophrenia, bipolar disorder, alcohol-induced psychoses, and drug-induced disorders. Each case was linked to the census tract in which they resided at the time of hospitalization, allowing Faris and Dunham to estimate and map crude hospitalized admission rates for these disorders. Table 10.1 provides an overview of their main findings. They found that admissions for schizophrenia and substance abuse

Table 10.1 Summary of main findings from Faris and Dunham [1] in relation to psychotic disorders

Condition	Number of cases	Area-level findings	Individual-level findings	Comments and hypotheses raised
Schizophrenia	7253	◆ High rates in and near the centre of the city, lowest rates in the city's periphery ◆ Higher rates in areas inhabited by black ethnic groups and migrant communities ◆ Same pattern observed when the population is stratified by gender and when the time period is extended to 1934	◆ Higher rates in males than females (117 to 100) ◆ Higher rates in younger age groups among men and in older age groups among women ◆ Higher rates of schizophrenia among single men, while, among women, rates were higher in married ones	◆ Gradient in the distribution of schizophrenia in thee areas inhabited almost exclusively by black ethnic communities suggests presence of risk factors other than ethnicity alone ◆ Hypothesized that ethnic fragmentation could be a risk factor for schizophrenia for all ethnic groups, rates are higher in black and white ethnic groups who are living in areas primarily inhabited by people of different ethnicity
Manic depressive psychoses	2311	◆ Small range of cases between areas with low and high rates ◆ No evidence of a geographical variation in the distribution of manic-depressive psychoses, even when stratified by gender and type (manic, depressive)	◆ Higher rates in women than men ◆ The distribution of manic–depressive psychoses did not show variation across public and private hospitals, and ethnic background ◆ Higher rates of manic-depressive psychoses among married individuals ◆ People with manic-depressive psychoses have higher SES than those with schizophrenia	◆ 50% of cases admitted in private hospitals compared to a much smaller proportion of cases of schizophrenia. This could be explained by differential diagnoses between public/private institutions or tendency of people with manic depressive to use private institutions

(continued)

Table 10.1 Continued

Condition	Number of cases	Area-level findings	Individual-level findings	Comments and hypotheses raised
Paranoid schizophrenia	2154	◆ The geographical distribution of paranoid and hebephrenic types of schizophrenia is very similar to the overall patterns seen in schizophrenia ◆ In areas inhabited by black ethnicity communities higher rates near the centre and lower in the south	◆ Higher rates in men than women ◆ Higher rates in older age groups compared to other types of schizophrenia ◆ Among men, higher proportion of cases in younger groups (< 30 years old); among women, higher proportion in older age groups (> 30 years old)	◆ High rates of paranoid and hebephrenic types of schizophrenia (and low rates of the catatonic type) in areas where populations are highly mobile, with little family and neighbouring life ◆ In areas inhabited by Italian immigrants and black communities with low levels of social organization, high rates of paranoid and hebephrenic types of schizophrenia, although lower than in other areas, and high rates of catatonic schizophrenia ◆ Hypothesized link between social organization and rates of schizophrenia
Hebephrenic schizophrenia	3447		◆ Higher rates in men than women ◆ Higher rates in younger age groups ◆ Among people > 30 years of age, rates are higher among women than men	

Catatonic schizophrenia	1360	◆ Higher rates of catatonic schizophrenia areas inhabited by migrant communities, but not near the centre ◆ In areas inhabited by black ethnicity communities, lowest rates near the centre and higher in the south	◆ Higher rates in women than men ◆ Higher rates in younger age groups than the other two groups ◆ Higher rates of catatonic-type than paranoid-type schizophrenia among black ethnic minority groups	◆ As for schizophrenia, it is hypothesized that ethnic fragmentation could be a risk for alcoholic psychoses. Higher rates observed in ethnic groups who are a minority in their area of residence
Alcoholic psychoses	1930	◆ The distribution of alcoholic psychoses is similar to that of schizophrenia with highest rates at the centre of Chicago, in areas inhabited by Black ethnic communities, and in highly mobile areas	◆ Rates of alcoholic psychoses are higher among men than women ◆ Higher rates among older age groups (35–64 years) ◆ Higher rates in low-income groups	
Drug addiction (without psychoses)	772	◆ Similar pattern in the distribution of drug addiction as for alcoholic psychoses and schizophrenia: a general concentration in and near the centre of the city. High rates in the mobile areas, although also high in the apartment areas	◆ Rates of alcoholic psychoses are higher among men than women, and among single than married individuals ◆ The highest rates are in the native-born white groups, and the lowest in the foreign-born white group. Intermediate rates were found in the black ethnic communities	◆ Smaller number of admissions for drug addiction could explain higher variability in estimates ◆ Hypothesized that higher rates of drug addictions are found in mobile areas as these might be less subject to scrutiny

Source data from Faris R.E.L. and Dunham H.W., *Mental disorders in urban areas*. 1939, University of Chicago Press, Chicago, USA. SES, socio-economic status.

disorders followed a distinct spatial gradient, with higher rates concentrated among deprived inner-city regions. In contrast, they did not find comparable evidence with respect to affective psychoses, including manic depressive psychoses and alcoholic psychoses. Faris and Dunham went on to compare the social characteristics of those communities with the highest and lowest rates of schizophrenia and substance abuse disorders. They observed strong negative correlations between degree of social organization and admission rates of these disorders, which led the authors to hypothesize that social isolation and poor social cohesion were likely to increase people's susceptibility to its core symptoms, such as hallucinations and delusions [1, 3] (see the next section for further discussion).

Faris and Dunham's work catalysed a series of epidemiological studies investigating the incidence rates of psychotic disorders in urban areas on both sides of the Atlantic over the next half century, with further important contributions by Edward Hare in Bristol (in the southwest of the UK) [4], John Giggs and John Cooper in Nottingham (central UK) [5–7], Heinz Hafner in Mannheim (in the west of Germany) [8–10], Norbett Mintz and David Schwartz in Boston (Massachusetts, USA) [11], August Hollingshead and Fredrick Redlich in New Haven (Connecticut, USA) [12], and Benjamin Malzberg in New York (New York, USA) [13]. For example, Hare [4] conducted the first methodologically comparable study to that of Faris and Dunham to take place outside of the United States. Using hospitalized admission data for five broad types of mental disorders (including schizophrenia and bipolar disorder) in Bristol between 1949 and 1953, Hare calculated incidence rates for 28 small-area neighbourhoods, using the 1951 Census of Great Britain to estimate the denominator across these areas. Critically, Hare advanced Faris and Dunham's methodology by standardizing incidence rates for age and sex. Following this, he observed that schizophrenia rates were twice as high towards the central parts of Bristol, and were correlated with worse social conditions, including social isolation, population density, and deprivation. Similar findings have since been reported elsewhere. For example, in Nottingham and Mannheim a remarkable series of studies—by Giggs, Cooper [5–7], and Brewin [14] (Nottingham), and Hafner [8–10] (Mannheim)—have demonstrated that patterns of higher incidence of psychotic disorders in urban areas is a stable phenomenon over relatively long time periods (up to 25 years).

In the USA, Mintz and Schwartz [11] examined the incidence of first hospital admissions for schizophrenia and bipolar disorder in the Greater Boston area over 2.5 years, with a particular focus on the role of *ethnic density* effects first observed in Chicago [1]. Here, they investigated whether incidence rates for Italian (born, or by descent) groups varied by both the proportion of Italians in each neighbourhood and its socio-economic profile. They found a strong negative correlation between the proportion of Italian-born people in a given neighbourhood and the incidence of both schizophrenia and bipolar disorder. Moreover, these correlations persisted after adjustment for the median monthly rental cost in each area, a measure of socio-economic deprivation negatively associated with schizophrenia (although not with bipolar disorder).

Non-affective versus affective psychoses

One longstanding observation from the Chicago study was the apparent differential pattern in incidence rates between non-affective psychoses (including schizophrenia) and 'manic depression', now more commonly referred to as bipolar disorder. In their study, the centripetal gradient in incidence observed for schizophrenia-related disorders observed by Faris and Dunham—highest in downtown Chicago—was not apparent for bipolar disorder [1]. Instead, a much more mixed pattern of rates emerged across the Chicago *catchment area*, with the authors concluding that 'manic-depression showed a random pattern—[with] no particular relationship between incidence and the stability of areas' [1: pp. 78–81]. While much of the literature that has followed has supported the observation that non-affective psychoses and bipolar disorder differ with respect to spatial variance, this conclusion was not universally supported. In a re-analysis of Faris and Dunham's data, for example, Mintz and Schwarz [11] suggested that both schizophrenia and bipolar disorder were highly negatively correlated with the degree of neighbourhood stability (reporting correlation coefficients of –0.87 and –0.74, respectively [11; p. 102]), but only for white groups. Although Mintz and Schwarz's [11] re-analysis was itself not without limitations (a sub-group analysis which also discounted an area of Chicago with the highest proportion of African Americans), the extent to which bipolar disorder is not associated with the social environment is deserving of careful attention (see 'Urbanicity and the incidence of affective psychoses'), given its implications for aetiology and mechanistic pathways through which the environment may contribute to psychosis risk, if causal.

Urbanicity and the incidence of non-affective psychoses

Evidence for an association between the urban environment and incidence of psychotic disorders is most robust for non-affective psychoses. In the UK, a series of publications from the Aetiology and Ethnicity in Schizophrenia and Other Psychoses (ÆSOP) study have demonstrated that their incidence varies across small areas within South East London [15], and at a national level [16], with rates (adjusted for age, sex, and ethnicity) 30–40% times higher in urban South East London than more mixed rural, suburban, and urban populations in Nottinghamshire and Bristol. Up to a 61% increase in incidence rates have also been found in urban South East London compared with rural Scotland [17]; however, when the authors restricted these analyses to the majority white ethnic group this difference did not persist. This suggests that some of the differences in rates in this study may have been driven by the underlying ethnic composition of the respective populations, given a large and consistent body of evidence showing that black and minority ethnic groups in the UK (and elsewhere) are at elevated risk of psychosis [18]. Nevertheless, further studies have demonstrated that rural–urban variation in schizophrenia risk persists after adjustment for ethnicity [15, 16, 19, 20]. Furthermore, two of these studies [19, 20] found that spatial variation in incidence persisted after additional adjustment for individual-level socio-economic status. Having controlled for these factors, rates were greater in more densely populated parts of the regions studied. A major systematic review and meta-analysis of all incidence studies of psychotic disorders published in England since 1950 found consistent evidence of an urban gradient in risk across studies of broad and narrow definitions of schizophrenia, but—in keeping with earlier research—no such variation for the affective psychoses [18]. Findings that the incidence of schizophrenia is up to twice as high in urban than rural areas—when measured close to the time of onset—have also been observed in other European settings, including France [21] and Ireland [22], although not in one region of north-east Italy [23] in contrast to an earlier finding [24]. Studies from Spain [25] and the Netherlands [26, 27] have also observed similar urban–rural differences with respect to *prevalence*, although this *measure of disease frequency* may be more prone to issues of *reverse causality*.

Studies utilizing Scandinavian population registers have made important contributions to understanding the incidence of psychotic disorders by place. Uniquely, these studies can address temporal associations between urban exposure and later schizophrenia risk. One early example of this approach was conducted by Lewis et al. [28] using data on conscripts to the Swedish military linked to nationwide population and health registers covering the entire country. The authors found that those (all male) conscripts brought up in more urban areas were also 65% more likely to receive a later diagnosis of schizophrenia than their rural-born counterparts. The importance of this finding—which was independent of possible confounding by age and sex (implicitly, via study design) and family finances, parental divorce, and family history of previous psychiatric admission (via statistical adjustment)—was in the methodological advance this study introduced over studies which came before it (see 'Early evidence'). Here, the study used prospectively recorded data to assess the temporal relationship between urban living and later psychosis risk, ascertained through high-quality linkage of routinely recorded national data. This study was among the first to classify participants based on their exposure to urbanicity further from the time of presentation for psychotic disorder, a major limitation of most studies referenced thus far in this chapter. This significant change thus reduced the likelihood that exposure status was a consequence of the *prodromal phase* of disorder, a form of reverse causality termed *social drift*. This phenomenon is thought to arise when individuals with early signs and symptoms of psychotic disorder move into more deprived, fragmented, or marginal areas (historically, although perhaps no longer, thought of as inner-city urban environments in many high-income countries) because of a decline in socio-economic status or desire for anonymity (a perverse feature of modern, densely populated environments is that they may afford a greater degree of anonymity than smaller rural communities). As found by Hollingshead and Redlich [12], lower socio-economic status at presentation for psychosis is strongly associated with higher incidence, although parental SES seems less so [29], providing some support for the idea of social drift; nonetheless, whether such *social* drift leads to a corresponding level of downward *spatial* drift is an area requiring further investigation.

A series of larger, nationwide longitudinal cohort studies from Denmark and Sweden have added support for an association between greater urbanicity and higher incidence rates of schizophrenia and other non-affective psychoses. In a landmark study published in the *New England Journal of Medicine* in 1999 [30], Preben Bo Mortensen and colleagues reported a dose–response relationship between the degree of urbanicity of birthplace (from rural areas through to provincial towns and cities and suburbs of Copenhagen and the capital city itself) and later incidence of schizophrenia, even after adjustment for several factors, including age, sex, parental age, family history of schizophrenia, and season of birth. Rates were 2.4 times greater for those born in Copenhagen than those born in rural parts of Denmark. Later research from the same group showed that longer time lived in urban areas was associated with increased incidence of schizophrenia in a dose–response fashion [31]. In the Netherlands, Marcelis et al. [32] found that urban birth also predicted increased incidence rates of broadly or narrowly defined schizophrenia (approximately double) later in life. Moreover, their data suggested that this effect was stronger than the effect of the urban environment closer to the time of onset, supporting the idea that early life and cumulative exposure to factors in the urban environment may be associated with schizophrenia risk. Population-based register data from Sweden also support an association between urban birth and higher rates of other non-affective psychoses, although point estimates for schizophrenia were not significantly different for people born in rural versus urban environments

[33]. Nevertheless, urban living at 15 years of age has been associated with schizophrenia incidence in another, more recent study of schizophrenia [34] (although this study calls into question the causality of this relationship, see 'Causal inference in the association between urbanicity and psychosis risk'), and a further Swedish nationwide study has found a strong association between place of residence (time period not specified, although presumed to be at time of onset) and schizophrenia incidence [35]. In Finland, register-linkage studies have suggested that rural–urban differences in the rates of schizophrenia may be less important than regional variation in incidence. While urban birth may be an emerging risk factor for younger cohorts [36], rural areas in the north and east of Finland have particularly pronounced rates of disorder, although this effect may, in part, be driven by genetic isolation [36, 37].

Fewer studies on urban–rural differences in the rate of schizophrenia have been conducted in low-and-middle-income (LAMI) countries. To date, nine studies from LAMI countries have investigated this issue, with mixed evidence of rural–urban differences across heterogeneous settings and study designs. For example, the prevalence of schizophrenia has been reported to be higher in urban Chile [38] and China [39–41], but the opposite was found in India [42] and in the Chinese famine study [43]. Data from a further study in China [44], a study from Tibet [45], and one from Uganda [46] have observed no differences in the prevalence of schizophrenia between rural and urban populations. Incidence studies from LAMI settings investigating rural–urban differences in schizophrenia and other psychotic disorders are largely missing, and would represent a vital area for further research given that rapid urbanization is greatest in such settings. Many (although not all [41, 43]) of these studies had notable methodological limitations, including validity of definitions of urban exposure [38], small sample sizes [46], and limited statistical analysis [42, 45, 47], which will need to be overcome to provide robust evidence on rural–urban differences in psychosis risk in LAMI settings. In general, there is a strong legacy of well-conducted epidemiological studies of schizophrenia in LAMI settings [48–52], and such designs could easily be extended to examine rural–urban differences in the future. Data from LAMI settings on this issue are particularly important given that the composition and risk profiles of rural and urban populations in low-, middle-, and high-income countries may differ considerably.

Overall, the evidence for an association between urban living—whether measured at birth, during upbringing or closer to the time of onset is strong, and largely consistent in high-income countries (see March et al. [53] for a review), with more limited and mixed evidence from LAMI countries (see Solmi et al. [54] for a recent review). The variation in rates between rural and urban areas appears to operate in a dose–response fashion, and does not appear to be confounded by several important factors including individual- and family-based sociodemographic differences, or by family history of psychosis. In the next section we will explore the main hypotheses to explain these differences.

Urbanicity and the incidence of affective psychoses

Unlike the incidence of schizophrenia and other non-affective psychoses (see 'Urbanicity and the incidence of non-affective psychoses'), fewer differences in the incidence of affective psychoses—such as bipolar disorder with psychosis or severe depression with psychosis—seem to exist across urban and rural environments, despite an apparent overlap in genes for both sets of mental health disorders [55, 56]. The absence of a clear spatial patterning of the affective psychoses was first noted by Faris and Dunham [1] and replicated in more recent epidemiological research [15, 20, 57–59], including a nationwide Danish study of 2.2 million people [57], which also failed to show an association between urban factors and later affective psychosis risk. Only three studies have observed higher rates of affective psychoses in urban than in rural areas [16, 21, 60]. However, not only was the magnitude of this association smaller than observed for non-affective psychoses, but these studies only controlled for basic confounders (e.g. age, sex, ethnicity), suggesting further research is required on this issue. One under-researched possibility is that the urban environment acts at the symptom-level rather than at the disorder-level; for example, Oher et al. [61] observed that the urban environment was more strongly associated with positive symptoms (specifically hallucinations) than disorganized or manic symptoms, whereas depressive symptoms were higher in people with *first-episode psychosis* (FEP) in less densely populated areas of South East London. In a non-clinical sample of the population, van Os et al. [62] have also found that positive and negative symptoms of psychosis (i.e. the core non-affective dimensions) were correlated with increased population density.

An overview of the main explanatory hypotheses

Several hypotheses have been proposed to explain the higher rate of non-affective psychotic disorders associated with exposure to urban living (see Table 10.2 for an overview). These include hypotheses relating to social drift (H1, H2), gene-environment interplay (H2, H3), characteristics of the individual (H4) or places in which individuals are exposed to adverse environmental factors (H5, H6), and to detection bias in rural areas (H7).

The idea of social drift represents perhaps the largest threat to validity in demonstrating a causal relationship between urban exposure and later psychosis risk. This phenomenon—falling under the broader epidemiological term

Table 10.2 Main hypotheses proposed to explain urban–rural differences in the incidence of schizophrenia and other non-affective psychoses

	Hypothesis title	Hypothesis description	First proposed by ... (year)	Evidence for	Evidence against	Notes
H1	Individual social drift	After onset/in the prodromal phase of schizophrenia an individual's SES deteriorates leading them to 'migrate' to more deprived neighbourhoods, often located in urban areas	Faris and Dunham (1939) [1]	Consistent with studies employing place of residence at diagnosis (for examples, see [1, 17, 16, 21, 35])	Studies of exposure to urban birth and upbringing (i.e. [28, 30, 31, 33, 60])	
H2	Intergenerational social drift (gene–environment correlation)	Families with characteristics that can act as risk factors for schizophrenia are more likely to migrate to urban areas. Increased schizophrenia risk in children born in urban areas therefore reflects familial genetic liability, with or without an independent effect of environmental exposures	Pedersen and Mortensen (2006) [66]	A Danish study found that a person's schizophrenia risk was associated with older sibling's place of birth. Among children born in rural areas, having a sibling born in urban areas was associated with higher risk of schizophrenia [66]	Control for family history of psychiatric disorder does not remove urban birth effect [30, 31]	Pedersen and Mortensen suggested genetic causes associated with both the parents migrating to the city and subsequent offspring risk of psychosis may exist (gene–environment correlation)

				A Swedish study found the association between population density and neighbourhood deprivation at age 15, and schizophrenia incidence was partially mediated by unobserved familial risk factors [34]		The advent of gXe studies, polygenic risk scores and causal inference methods in epidemiology hold promise to elucidate pathways (i.e. H1, H2, H5)
H3	Gene–environment interactions	Environmental exposures interact with genetic liability to increase risk of psychosis	Van Os et al. (2003) [26]	The effect of urbanicity on psychosis risk was greater for those with identifiable family liability for psychosis than those without in two studies [26, 67]. Statistically, this interaction was more than additive		Statistical interaction depends on the scale used (additive vs multiplicative), and does not necessarily correspond to biological synergy [68]
H4	Sociodemographic characteristic	Sociodemographic and socio-economic differences between areas explain the observed differences	Silver et al. (2002) [90]	In a Dutch study, area-level differences disappeared after adjustment for individual-level SES [111]	Significant effect of area-level characteristics after adjusting for individual-level ones [19, 20, 112–114]	Not all studies adjust for the same individual level characteristics, therefore residual confounding could potentially account for area-level variability observed in some studies
H5	Antenatal and perinatal risk factors	Obstetric complications and infections in early life associated with schizophrenia risk are more common in urban areas	Bleuler (1911) [71] Takei et al. (1992) [73]	Urban birth effect may be stronger among those born in winter, suggestive of an interaction between urban environments and seasonal risk factors [74]	No evidence that obstetric complication mediates the association between urban birth and schizophrenia [33, 59]	Support for this hypothesis comes from one short report [74]

(continued)

Table 10.2 Continued

	Hypothesis title	Hypothesis description	First proposed by ... (year)	Evidence for	Evidence against	Notes
H6	Social stress	Stressors in the urban environment increase schizophrenia risk, including social isolation, low SES, and social threat	Faris and Dunham (1939) [1]; Link and Phelan (1995) [81]	Compatible with: ◆ studies finding higher rates in urban areas (assuming urban areas are more stressful) [16, 21, 28, 30, 31, 33, 35, 60] ◆ studies finding higher rates of psychosis in ethnic minority groups living in low ethnic density areas [115, 116] ◆ - studies finding higher rates of psychosis in areas with low levels of social capital [86, 111, 113, 116]	None	Direct evidence still required
H7	Differences in healthcare provisions between urban and rural areas	The number of people with psychosis in rural areas could have been underestimated owing to lack of contact with mental health care providers.	Schelin et al. (2000) [91]	Consistent with studies employing place of residence at diagnosis (for examples, see [1, 16, 21, 35, 17])	Studies of exposure to urban birth and upbringing (i.e. [28, 30, 31, 33, 60]). No variation in DUP at environmental level [93]. Incidence studies in rural areas show variation by environmental factors [19, 88]	There may be overlap here with H1 and H2 if people with psychosis (or in the prodromal phase) move to more urban environments to be closer to mental health care services

SES, socioeconomic status; gXe, gene–environment interaction; DUP, duration of untreated psychosis.

reverse causality—may take place in two ways. Firstly, an individual in the prodromal phase of disorder—a period that may be marked by cognitive decline and impairment in social functioning—may move into more urban environments as a result of a decline in socio-economic status, income, and increased propensity for social seclusion (H1, Table 10.2). This finding is compatible with all studies that have found an association between urban living close to the time of presentation and psychosis risk (i.e. [1, 16, 17, 21, 35]). It also accords with one of Faris and Dunham's central observations—that higher rates of schizophrenia are found in areas with more social instability, greater isolation, and higher residential turnover [1]. While they ultimately argued for a causal association between such environments and risk, social drift cannot be excluded. Nonetheless, there are both empirical and theoretical arguments against this hypothesis. Empirically, dose–response relationships between urbanicity at birth, and time spent in urban environments during upbringing and later psychosis risk are incompatible with the *individual social drift* hypothesis. From a theoretical perspective, we should also consider the function and role of the modern, urban environment in many high-income countries. While such environments may, indeed, afford more anonymity than rural ones (in which unusual behaviour may be tolerated to a lesser degree), it is unclear whether modern, urban environments still offer the low-rent housing upon which the *individual social drift* hypothesis is partially predicated. While this was undoubtedly true in historic investigations in inner-city Chicago, Boston, and Nottingham, the gentrification of modern-day inner cities calls into question whether the stereotype of the inner city as a space into which social drift is permissible requires careful consideration in future theoretical and empirical research.

At this juncture, it is worth noting that recent research from a Canadian sample of people presenting with psychotic disorder has highlighted the fact that people with psychosis experience both upward and downward mobility following a first diagnosis [63]. This finding underscores the fact that social mobility for people with psychosis is likely to be complex, both in the run up to and following onset of disorder. Social drift is not mutually exclusive with causal aspects of the social environment, as demonstrated in a recent longitudinal study of schizophrenia in Denmark [64]. As we have previously noted [65], the majority of people with FEP experience considerable disadvantage; regardless of whether this is a cause or a consequence of disorder, it is vital for public mental health and mental health services commissioning that services for people with FEP are located in communities proportional to need. This may mean a preponderance of services need to be provided in more urban areas, both as a function of the rate of disorder and population size.

The second hypothesis, which proposes that social drift may explain higher rates of non-affective psychotic disorders in urban areas, suggests that this effect may operate *intergenerationally* (H2, Table 10.2). That is, a set of factors operating on the family confer both a higher likelihood of moving into more urban environments among previous generations (grandparents, parents) and increase the likelihood of developing psychosis in the subsequent (child) generation. Where the factors which influence social drift and psychosis risk are genetic, this is an example of gene–environment correlation. Examples might include risk genes for psychosis (i.e. dopaminergic synthesis genes) or genes for other neuroendophenotypes such as genes that regulate cognitive processes, which are known to be impaired in schizophrenia, and which might result in intergenerational drift into more urban environments. In such an example, impaired cognitive ability in previous generations may limit educational and socio-economic attainment, resulting in a progressive social drift into more urban, or more socially disadvantaged neighbourhoods over generations. Such genes must also increase psychosis liability, which will be phenotypically expressed at the onset of frank psychosis in a given generation, whereupon urban birth would appear to predict later schizophrenia risk. It is possible that the effect of intergenerational drift—if it exists—is augmented by upward social mobility among those without such vulnerability into less socially disadvantaged areas with correspondingly lower rates of psychosis. Evidence for intergenerational drift is growing. Pedersen and Mortensen [66] found that place of birth of the older sibling predicted psychosis risk in the *proband*, implying that some of the exposure to urban risk is transmitted through familial effects. A similar conclusion was drawn in a more recent Swedish study [34], which demonstrated that population density and deprivation at 15 years of age predicted later schizophrenia risk in the general population, but that this effect was diminished and non-significant (respectively), among cousins and siblings discordant for exposure at 15 years of age. Arguments against the intergenerational drift hypothesis include the persistence of an effect of urban birth on psychosis risk after controlling for a family history of psychosis [30, 31]. To date, there are insufficient data to prove or disprove this hypothesis, but novel methods in causal inference, including propensity score matching/adjustment and polygenic risk scores, promise to shed further light on this hypothesis (see the next section).

As with the first hypothesis, the presence of intergeneration drift would not negate the possibility of a causal relationship between the urban environment and psychosis; following drift into urban environments, continued exposure to deleterious environmental stressors may further increase risk. This may be particularly likely for people who have an underlying genetic susceptibility for psychosis, and has led to the formulation of gene–environment interaction as a hypothesis to explain increased psychosis rates seen in urban areas (H3, Table 10.2) [26]. In an initial study [26] and replication [67], van Os et al. found evidence that the effect of urban living (cross-sectionally, close to the time of onset) was more pronounced in people with a family history of psychiatric illness. These effects were observed at the subclinical level (i.e. in the general population) [26] and in a clinical sample [67], respectively. They were observed on an additive statistical scale, meaning that the risk for people exposed to both urban living and family history was greater than the sum of both effects. There is some dispute as to whether a statistical interaction—either on an additive or multiplicative scale—corresponds to biological synergism [68], and the observations from van Os et al. were based on cross-sectional data collected in adulthood; social drift could not be excluded. Nonetheless, the advent of polygenic risk scores in large population-based cohorts [69] and the development of gene–environment interaction studies in psychosis epidemiology [70] hold promise for potential discovery of genetic and environmental interplay in psychosis.

A set of hypotheses proposing that individual- (H4, H5) and area-level risk factors acting on the individual (H6) explain higher rates of schizophrenia in urban environments have also been proposed (Table 10.2). For example, whether higher rates in cities are simply explained by compositional effects of the population is an obvious, although largely disproven possibility (H4, Table 10.2). Cities, after all, typically attract younger populations and have a higher proportion of migrants and ethnic minority groups than more rural communities. Both younger age and ethnic minority status also confer substantially increased psychosis risk [18], making it possible that these factors confound the association between urban exposure and psychosis risk. Nonetheless, the evidence for this is weak. Even the earliest studies conducted by Faris and Dunham [1] and Hare [4] controlled for age and sex. Allardyce et al. [17] suggested that urban–rural differences between urban South East London and rural Scotland might be explained by the higher proportion of ethnic minority groups in the former catchment area, as rates did not differ for the majority white group between these settings. However, similar comparisons between rural and urban environments, having controlled for age, sex, and ethnicity have shown that rural–urban differences in risk still persist [16, 19]. Moreover, urban–rural differences [19] and neighbourhood variation in risk [20] are still apparent after further adjustment for socio-economic status, making confounding by basic sociodemographic factors an unlikely explanation for the differences presented in this chapter.

Eugen Bleuler [71] proposed that prenatal and perinatal risk factors might be important in the genesis of schizophrenia, including infection, malnutrition, and obstetric complications, and a large body of robust evidence supports a role for altered early life neurodevelopment in the aetiology of these psychotic disorders (for a recent overview, see Howes and Murray [72]). Takei et al. extended this hypothesis to suggest that infections may also account for urban–rural differences in schizophrenia risk (H5, Table 10.2) [73]. This possibility is supported by observations of a small excess of schizophrenia associated with winter births [30], and that the risk of schizophrenia associated with urban birth appears to be stronger in this winter-born group [74]. Thus, people born in urban environments may have been exposed—either *in utero* or in early life—to a range of infections that may impinge on typical neurodevelopment, including influenza [75] and herpes simplex virus [76]. The infectivity of such pathogens may be greater in more urban environments, due to higher population densities or overcrowding, although no direct association with schizophrenia has been found with respect to the latter [77]. Torrey and Yolken [78] have gone as far as suggesting that closer proximity to cat faeces contaminated with *Toxoplasmosis gondii* in urban environments may contribute to this effect, although a recent longitudinal study of adolescent psychotic symptoms and early life cat ownership found no such association [79]. With respect to obstetric complications—which increase schizophrenia risk [80]—there is no evidence that they mediate the association with urban birth [33, 59]. Overall, there is presently only limited evidence that the urban excess in schizophrenia is confounded by pre- and perinatal infection or obstetric complications, although there is some evidence that such factors play a direct role in later psychosis risk.

A lot of discussion—although perhaps outweighing current empirical evidence—has focused on the role the urban environment plays as a reservoir for deleterious experiences that causally contribute to the psychogenesis of schizophrenia and other psychotic disorders. The main mechanism through which such factors impinge on psychotic experiences is through the catchall generic label 'social stress' (H6, Table 10.2). This hypothesis was first mooted by Faris and Dunham [1], and extended to encompass social conditions as a risk factor for a wide range of physical and mental health conditions by Link and Phelan in 1995 [81]. Several underlying theories with respect to psychosis have been broadly proposed to link adverse social exposures to psychosis risk. These include Selten's [82, 83] model of *social defeat* and Howes and Murray's [72] *integrated sociodevelopmental-cognitive model*. While such theories differ in prescription and detail, they broadly suggest that exposure to adverse social conditions—which may range from personal traumatic experiences such as parental death or child abuse through to chronic disadvantage from living in a deprived neighbourhood—result in stressful experiences, which subsequently disrupt critical neurodevelopmental or neurocognitive pathways and lead to the onset of psychotic experiences (see the next section). While direct evidence that prolonged exposure to factors in the urban environment lead to psychosis in this way is still lacking, the wider epidemiological literature on this topic is consistent with this possibility. This includes (1) the dose–response relationship between degree of urbanicity, time spent in urban environments and later psychosis risk discussed earlier; (2) higher rates of schizophrenia in areas with greater levels of potential social stressors, including deprivation [19, 20, 34, 84, 85] and inequality [20]; and (3) higher rates in neighbourhoods with the least social support (typically indexed with low social cohesion [86], or high social fragmentation [87, 88] and residential instability [1, 89, 90]). These studies will only support this hypothesis if the implicit assumption that urban communities are more stressful—or lack the social support to mitigate such stress—are shown to be true, and further evidence here is still required.

The final main hypothesis proposed to explain higher rates of psychotic disorder in urban environments surrounds the issue of detection bias (H7, Table 10.2). Schelin et al. [91] proposed that the differences in the provision of mental healthcare services in rural and urban areas—typically harder to access, smaller, and less frequent in rural areas—may lead to under-detection of cases in typical observational studies reliant on contact with mental health care providers as the primary means for case ascertainment. This hypothesis is consistent with studies that have described variation in the incidence of psychotic disorders between rural and urban areas [1, 16, 17, 21, 35]. Moreover, recent studies that have estimated the incidence of psychotic disorders from whole systems registers (rather than solely based on mental health care contacts) have found much higher estimates of psychosis than previously reported [92]. Unfortunately, these studies did not investigate whether this accounted for previously- reported rural–urban differences in schizophrenia rates, but this would be an important future research question with respect to this hypothesis. Nonetheless, this hypothesis is not compatible with the association between urban birth and schizophrenia, and one study (although exclusively in an urban environment) found no evidence of neighbourhood variation in the *duration of untreated psychosis* (DUP) [93]; if geographical variation in healthcare provision did account for some of the variation in incidence between rural and urban regions, one would also expect to observe variation in DUP. Finally, studies conducted in more rural populations still show considerable variation in incidence rates between geographical regions [19, 88].

Causal inference in the association between urbanicity and psychosis risk

In this chapter, we have shown that the incidence of schizophrenia and other psychotic disorders is consistently associated with exposure to urban environments, although evidence for the affective psychoses, including bipolar disorder, is more mixed ('Evidence of assocation'). Various hypotheses to explain these patterns have been proposed ('An overview of the main exploratory hypotheses'), including those that ascribe raised rates of non-affective psychoses to reverse causality (H1, H2), confounding (H4, H5), or bias (H7). The extent to which the patterns of incidence for both non-affective and affective psychoses are causal with respect to the urban environment require careful consideration. Here, we briefly place the currently available evidence—from epidemiology and neuroscience—into context, using the nine *Bradford-Hill criteria* [94] for causation to structure our thinking.

The first Bradford-Hill criterion was in regard to the *strength of association* between exposure and outcome. Thus, larger effect sizes may be more likely to remain after eliminating issues of bias and confounding through careful study design and analysis. The effect size for urban living in relation to non-affective psychotic disorders appears to be in the region of 1.5–2 times greater for people exposed to urban rather than rural environments [16, 28, 30], after adjustment for potential confounders, placing this as a moderate effect size. Effect sizes for the affective psychoses appear to be smaller than this, and even large, well-powered longitudinal studies have failed to find a statistically robust association with urban birth and upbringing [57]. Secondly, *consistency* of findings may indicate a higher likelihood of a causal relationship, and there is good evidence for this in high-income settings with respect to non-affective psychoses (see 'Urbanicity and the incidence of non-affective psychosis'). Further well-designed epidemiological research from LAMI settings would permit further clarification of the consistency of the urbanicity effect on risk. The evidence for affective psychoses is less consistent overall (see 'Urbanicity and the incidence of affective psychoses'), with most [1, 15, 20, 57–59] (although not all [16, 21, 60]) studies failing to identify an association. These differences are not readily explained by sample size with null and positive findings reported in both small and large samples (see previous references).

Bradford-Hill's third criterion was in regard to *specificity*. Here, we interpret the evidence as broadly indicating that exposure to the urban environment is specific to non-affective psychoses. In addition to inconsistent evidence regarding the affective psychoses, there is little consistent evidence that depression or other psychiatric illnesses show a strong urban gradient [54], while suicidal outcomes may show the reverse [54]. This therefore raises the possibility that factors in the urban environment may act specifically on neural mechanisms that lead to the development of psychotic symptomatology. If true, such a hypothesis may be sufficient to account for the mixed findings from studies of affective samples, which have included people with bipolar disorder both with and without psychotic phenomena. Further, previous studies of symptom dimensions in people with FEP have found that psychotic (i.e. positive and negative) rather than affective (i.e. depressive and manic) symptoms were most strongly associated with urban living [61, 62, 95]. This specificity requires further research, and should link to other clinical and social characteristics that distinguish schizophrenia from (non-psychotic) bipolar disorder. One such example is the role of premorbid cognition that appears to be impaired in psychotic-related disorders (including bipolar with psychosis) [96, 97], but not non-psychotic bipolar disorder.

Two further criteria—the *temporality* of association and a *biological gradient*—support a causal role for the urban environment in schizophrenia and other psychotic disorders. As we have shown, studies of urban birth and later schizophrenia risk demonstrate a clear temporal relationship between exposure and outcome, notwithstanding the possible caveats of *gene–environmental correlation* and *intergenerational drift* discussed in 'An overview of the main exploratory hypotheses'. Demonstration of dose–response gradients observed with both the degree of urbanicity [30] and time spent in urban environments [31] are consistent with a biological gradient in the aetiology of schizophrenia.

Bradford-Hill also proposed that the *plausibility* and *coherence* of an association should be consistent with existing knowledge about the disease process. Here, then, we need to consider whether exposure to factors in the urban environment may cause psychosis via a plausible neurobiological mechanism coherent with current theories in psychosis research. While the neurobiology of psychotic disorders is far from definitively established, evidence suggests several pathways are disrupted in psychosis [98, 99], including abnormal dopaminergic, glutamatergic, γ-aminobutyric acid-(GABA)ergic and voltage-gated calcium channel signalling function. Of these, perhaps sensitization of the mesolimbic dopamine system, has garnered the greatest attention to date, given its well-established role in the emergence of hallucinations and delusions. Neuroimaging studies have revealed that people with schizophrenia have altered presynaptic dopamine functioning, including an increased capacity for synthesis and release [72]. Howes and Kapur have suggested that repeated exposure to stressful environmental experiences might lead to sensitization of this dopaminergic system [100], and a series of animal [101, 102] and human studies (see Mizrahi [103] for a recent review) have shown that such experiences are associated with hyperdopaminergic activity (the confluence of animal and human evidence may—speculatively—satisfy Bradford-Hill's ninth criteria). In turn, as dopamine is a critical neurotransmitter involved in reward processing and salience recognition, excess release and synthesis may result in altered perception; that is, reality distortion, manifesting in the positive symptoms typical in schizophrenia [100]. This raises the possibility that cognitive ability—which may also be influenced by dopamine function—is also involved in the attribution of salience to environmental stimuli [72], as impairments in this domain may lead to a higher likelihood to misattribute environmental factors as threatening; here, paranoia is a core delusion in schizophrenia, and may be more common in more urban, deprived environments [61, 104]. Further, people with psychosis show a greater tendency to perform worse on a variety of social cognition tasks [105], including jumping to conclusions and external attribution bias. As cognitive impairments also distinguish schizophrenia and bipolar disorder from non-psychotic affective disorders [96, 97], we suggest that the increased risk of schizophrenia in urban environments may arise as a result of increased exposure to social adversity and threatening experiences, and impairments in processing the salience of such events. There is some empirical epidemiological evidence to support this possibility [95, 106]. By contrast, in non-psychotic bipolar disorder, where typical cognition is preserved, exposure to urban environments is less likely to lead to prediction errors about external environmental stimuli, and may therefore explain the lack of association between urban exposure and later risk of disorder.

The last Bradford-Hill criteria we have yet to discuss is *experiment*. Consistent with modern epidemiological enquiry, experimental studies often provide the gold-standard methodology for establishing causation between exposure and outcome, typically because participants can be randomized to receive the 'active' or 'control' condition so that all observed and unobserved confounders are balanced between the two arms of the study (i.e. in randomized controlled trials). Nonetheless, deliberate randomization to area-level exposures (e.g. urban living) are difficult to achieve both ethically and practically, although examples such as the US 'Moving To Opportunity' study [107] exist (although too small to investigate psychotic outcomes). In the last decade, methods to simulate the randomization achieved in trials have been developed for observation data, including propensity scoring, instrumental variable analysis (including Mendelian randomization), and novel sibling-based designs. While such causal inference methods are still an active area of statistical development, and are not without challenges within social and psychiatric epidemiology, they offer promise as a way of overcoming some of the threats to validity discussed in 'An overview of the main exploratory hypotheses'. For example, Sariaslan et al.

[34] have used a family-based design to show that the risk of schizophrenia associated with urban birth progressively decreases with familial aggregation (i.e. general population, cousins, siblings), suggesting that a degree of the effect of urban exposure (measured at 15 years of age) may be due to shared genetic and environmental familial factors. Beyond randomized designs, experimental studies integrating epidemiology and neuroscience perspectives reveal novel pathways in the aetiology of psychotic disorders. For example, in a health convenience sample in Germany, Andreas Meyer-Lindenberg [108] has demonstrated that those brought up and living in more urban environments showed greater activation of the pregenual anterior cingulate cortex (pACC) and amygdala in response to a stress task than their rural-dwelling counterparts. As with striatal dopamine dysregulation, the amygdala is involved in environmental threat perception, while the pACC is involved in modulating limbic stress regulation and amygdala activity. Similar observations have been made with respect to ethnic minority status [109], suggesting that environmental stressors may have discernible effects on brain function. Extension of these results into clinical populations and—perhaps—in relation to other neural pathways would provide the necessary evidence as to whether our environments were able to modify mental processes potentially relevant to the onset of psychotic symptoms and disorder.

Conclusion

In this chapter we have outlined the epidemiological evidence which shows that exposure to urban living—at birth, during childhood, and into adulthood—is robustly and consistently associated with increased rates of schizophrenia and other non-affective psychotic disorders in those communities. Leaving aetiology aside, this spatial variation should be used to a greater degree than is currently apparent in informing mental health service providers about need for psychosis services (including the provision of Early Intervention Psychosis programmes) across different populations. Examples of how this can be achieved to ensure services reach the populations who most need them exist [110], but more can be done. With respect to aetiology it is premature to conclude that urban living increases risk, but the available evidence satisfies a number of causal criteria here. Most critically, we suggest that future studies investigating the association between exposure to urban environments and psychotic disorders are designed, where possible, with attempts to build in causal inference techniques to examine the extent to which a causal association exists. One particularly notable threat to validity is the possibility of intergenerational drift as an explanation of the overrepresentation of schizophrenia cases in urban areas. In either case, conclusively refuting or demonstrating that such an effect underpins the association between urban living and psychosis risk would inform public mental health by facilitating interventions which aimed to prevent the transition to psychosis in high risk groups, wherever they live.

References

1. **Faris REL, Dunham HW.** *Mental Disorders in Urban Areas.* Chicago, IL: University of Chicago Press, 1939.

2. **Snow J.** *On the Mode of the Communication of Cholera*, 2nd ed. London: John Churchill, 1855 (reprinted 1936: New York).

3. **Cockerham W.** *Social Causes of Health and Disease.* Chicago, IL: Polity, 2007.

4. **Hare EH.** Mental illness and social condition in Bristol. *Journal of Mental Science* 1956; **102**: 349–357.

5. **Giggs JA, Cooper JE.** Ecological structure and the distribution of schizophrenia and affective psychoses in Nottingham. *British Journal of Psychiatry* 1987; **151**: 627–633.

6. **Giggs JA.** Distribution of schizophrenics in Nottingham. *Transactions of the Institute of British Geographers* 1973; **59**: 5–76.

7. **Giggs JA.** Mental disorders and ecological structure in Nottingham. *Social Science & Medicine* 1986; **23**: 945–961.

8. **Maylaih E, Weyerer S, Hafner H.** Spatial concentration of the incidence of treated psychiatric disorders in Mannheim. *Acta Psychiatrica Scandinavica* 1980; **80**: 650–656.

9. **Hafner H, Reimann H.** Spatial distribution of mental disorders in Mannheim, 1965. In: **EH Hare, JK Wing** (eds) *Psychiatric Epidemiology.* London: Oxford University Press, 1970, pp. 341–354.

10. **Loffler W, Hafner H.** Ecological patterns of first admitted schizophrenics to two German cities over 25 years. *Social Science & Medicine* 1999; **49**: 93–108.

11. **Mintz NL, Schwartz DT.** Urban ecology and psychosis: community factors in the incidence of schizophrenia and manic-depression among Italians in Greater Boston. *International Journal of Social Psychiatry* 1964; **10**: 101–118.

12. **Hollingshead AB, Redlich FC.** *Social Class and Mental Illness.* New York: Wiley, 1958.

13. **Malzberg B.** Internal migration and mental disease among the white population of New York state, 1960–1961. *International Journal of Social Psychiatry* 1967; **13**: 184–191.

14. **Brewin JS, Harrison GL, Cantwell R, Dalkin T, Fox R, Glazebrook C, Medley I.** Schizophrenia in Nottingham 1978–1994: secular trends in incidence. *Schizophrenia Research* 1996; **18**: 106.

15. **Kirkbride JB, Fearon P, Morgan C, Dazzan P, Morgan K, Murray RM, Jones PB.** Neighbourhood variation in the incidence of psychotic disorders in Southeast London. *Social Psychiatry and Psychiatric Epidemiology* 2007; **42**: 438–445.

16. **Kirkbride JB, Fearon P, Morgan C, Dazzan P, Morgan K, Tarrant J,** et al. Heterogeneity in incidence rates of schizophrenia and other psychotic syndromes: findings from the 3-center AeSOP study. *Archives of General Psychiatry* 2006; **63**: 250–258.

17. Allardyce J, Boydell J, Van Os J, Morrison G, Castle D, Murray RM, McCreadie RG. Comparison of the incidence of schizophrenia in rural Dumfries and Galloway and urban Camberwell. *British Journal of Psychiatry* 2011; **179**: 335–339.

18. Kirkbride JB, Errazuriz A, Croudace TJ, Morgan C, Jackson D, Boydell J, et al. Incidence of schizophrenia and other psychoses in England, 1950–2009: a systematic review and meta-analyses. *PLoS One* 2012; 7: e31660.

19. Kirkbride JB, Hameed Y, Ankireddypalli G, Ioannidis K, Crane CM, Nasir M, et al. The Epidemiology of First-Episode Psychosis in Early Intervention in Psychosis Services: Findings From the Social Epidemiology of Psychoses in East Anglia [SEPEA] Study. *American Journal of Psychiatry* 2017; **174**: 143–153.

20. Kirkbride JB, Jones PB, Ullrich S, Coid JW. Social deprivation, inequality, and the neighborhood-level incidence of psychotic syndromes in East London. *Schizophrenia Bulletin* 2014; **40**: 169–180.

21. Szöke A, Charpeaud T, Galliot A-M, Vilain J, Richard J-R, Leboyer M, et al. Rural-urban variation in incidence of psychosis in France: a prospective epidemiologic study in two contrasted catchment areas. *BMC Psychiatry* 2014; **14**: 78.

22. Kelly BD, O'Callaghan E, Waddington JL, Feeney L, Browne S, Scully PJ, et al. Schizophrenia and the city: a review of literature and prospective study of psychosis and urbanicity in Ireland. *Schizophrenia Research* 2010; **116**: 75–89.

23. Lasalvia A, Bonetto C, Tosato S, Zanatta G, Cristofalo D, Salazzari D, et al. First-contact incidence of psychosis in north-eastern Italy: influence of age, gender, immigration and socioeconomic deprivation. *British Journal of Psychiatry* 2014; **205**: 127–134.

24. Thornicroft G, Bisoffi G, De Salvia D, Tansella M. Urban-rural differences in the associations between social deprivation and psychiatric service utilization in schizophrenia and all diagnoses: a case-register study in Northern Italy. *Psychological Medicine* 1993; **23**: 487–496.

25. Moreno-Küstner B, Mayoral F, Navas-Campaña D, Garcia-Herrera JM, Angona P, Martin C, Rivas F. Prevalence of schizophrenia and related disorders in Malaga (Spain): results using multiple clinical databases. *Epidemiology and Psychiatric Sciences* 2016; **25**: 38–48.

26. van Os J, Hannssen M, Bak M, Bijl RV, Vollebergh W. Do urbanicity and familial liability coparticipate in causing psychosis? *American Journal of Psychiatry* 2003; **160**: 477–482.

27. van Os J, Hanssen M, Bijl R V, Vollebergh W. Prevalence of psychotic disorder and community level of psychotic symptoms: an urban-rural comparison. *Archives of General Psychiatry* 2011; **58**: 663–668.

28. Lewis G, David A, Andreasson S, Allebeck P. Schizophrenia and city life. *Lancet* 1992; **340**: 137–140.

29. Byrne M, Agerbo E, Eaton WW, Mortensen PB. Parental socio-economic status and risk of first admission with schizophrenia—a Danish national register based study. *Social Psychiatry and Psychiatric Epidemiology* 2004; **39**: 87–96.

30. Mortensen PB, Pedersen CB, Westergaard T, Wohlfarht J, Ewald H, Mors O, et al. Effects of family history and place and season of birth on the risk of schizophrenia. *N Engl J Med* 1999; **340**: 603–608.

31. Pedersen CB, Mortensen PB. Evidence of a dose-response relationship between urbanicity during upbringing and schizophrenia risk. *Archives of General Psychiatry* 2001; **58**: 1039–1046.

32. Marcelis M, Takei N, van Os J. Urbanization and risk for schizophrenia: does the effect operate before or around the time of illness onset? *Psychological Medicine* 1999; **29**: 1197–1203.

33. Harrison G, Fouskakis D, Rasmussen F, Tynelius P, Sipos A, Gunnell D. Association between psychotic disorder and urban place of birth is not mediated by obstetric complications or childhood socio-economic position: a cohort study. *Psychological Medicine* 2003; **33**: 723–731.

34. Sariaslan A, Larsson H, D'Onofrio B, Långström N, Fazel S, Lichtenstein P. Does population density and neighborhood deprivation predict schizophrenia? A nationwide Swedish family-based study of 2.4 million individuals. *Schizophrenia Bulletin* 2015; **41**: 494–502.

35. Sundquist K, Frank G, Sundquist J. Urbanisation and incidence of psychosis and depression: follow-up study of 4.4 million women and men in Sweden. *British Journal of Psychiatry* 2004; **184**: 293–298.

36. Haukka J, Suvisaari J, Varilo T, Lonnqvist J. Regional variation in the incidence of schizophrenia in Finland: a study of birth cohorts born from 1950 to 1969. *Psychological Medicine* 2001; **31**: 1045–1053.

37. Perälä J, Saarni SI, Ostamo A, Pirkola S, Haukka J, Härkänen T, et al. Geographic variation and sociodemographic characteristics of psychotic disorders in Finland. *Schizophrenia Research* 2008; **106**: 337–347.

38. Vicente B, Kohn R, Rioseco P, Saldivia S, Navarrette G, Veloso P, Torres S. Regional differences in psychiatric disorders in Chile. *Social Psychiatry and Psychiatric Epidemiology* 2006; **41**: 935–942.

39. Long J, Huang G, Liang W, Chen Q, Xie J, Jiang J, Su L. The prevalence of schizophrenia in mainland China: evidence from epidemiological surveys. *Acta Psychiatrica Scandinavica* 2014; **130**: 244–256.

40. Chan KY, Zhao F-F, Meng S, Demaio AR, Reed C, Theodoratou E, et al. Prevalence of schizophrenia in China between 1990 and 2010. *Journal of Global Health* 2015; **5**: 10410.

41. Xiang Y-T, Ma X, Cai Z-J, Li SR, Xiang YQ, Guo HL, et al. Prevalence and socio-demographic correlates of schizophrenia in Beijing, China. *Schizophrenia Research* 2008; **102**: 270–277.

42. Ganguli HC. Epidemiological findings on prevalence of mental disorders in India. *Indian Journal of Psychiatry* 2000; **42**: 14–20.

43. Song S, Wang W, Hu P. Famine, death, and madness: schizophrenia in early adulthood after prenatal exposure to the Chinese Great Leap Forward Famine. *Social Science & Medicine* 2009; **68**: 1315–1321.

44. Phillips MR, Zhang J, Shi Q, Song Z, Ding Z, Pang S, et al. Prevalence, treatment, and associated disability of mental disorders in four provinces in China during 2001-05: an epidemiological survey. *Lancet* 2009; **373**: 2041–2053.

45. Wei G, Liu X, Liu S, et al. The first epidemiological study of mental disorders of Tibetans. *World Cultural Psychiatry Research Review* 2008; 1–3.

46. Lundberg P, Cantor-Graae E, Rukundo G, Ashaba S, Östergren P-O. Urbanicity of place of birth and symptoms of psychosis, depression and anxiety in Uganda. *British Journal of Psychiatry* 2009; **195**: 156–162.

47. Chan KY, Zhao F-F, Meng S, Demaio AR, Reed C, Theodoratou E, et al, Urbanization and the prevalence of schizophrenia in China between 1990 and 2010. *World Psychiatry* 2015; **14**: 251–252.

48. Bhugra D, Hilwig M, Hossein B, Marceau H, Neehall J, Leff J, et al. First-contact incidence rates of schizophrenia in Trinidad and one-year follow-up. *British Journal of Psychiatry* 1996; **169**: 587–592.

49. Hickling FW, Rodgers-Johnson P. The incidence of first contact schizophrenia in Jamaica. *British Journal of Psychiatry* 1995; **167**: 193–196.

50. Leff J, Mallett RM, Bhugra D, Mahy GE, Hutchinson G, Takei N. Incidence rates for schizophrenia and migration, another view of the excess risk for schizophrenia among African-Caribbeans in Britain. *Schizophrenia Research* 1998; **29**: 13–14.

51. Menezes PR, Scazufca M, Busatto G, Coutinho LMS, Mcguire PK, Murray RM. Incidence of first-contact psychosis in São Paulo, Brazil. *British Journal of Psychiatry* 2007; **191**: 2–7.

52. Morgan C, John S, Esan O, Hibben M, Patel V, Weiss H, et al. The incidence of psychoses in diverse settings, INTREPID (2): a feasibility study in India, Nigeria, and Trinidad. *Psychological Medicine* 2016; **46**: 1923–1933.

53. March D, Hatch SL, Morgan C, Kirkbride JB, Bresnahan M, Fearon P, Susser E. Psychosis and place. *Epidemiologic Reviews* 2008; **30**: 84–100.

54. Solmi F, Dykxhoorn J, Kirkbride JB. Urban-rural differences in major mental health conditions. In: N Okkels, C Blanner Kristiansen, P. Munk-Jørgensen (eds) *Mental Health and Illness in the City*. Springer, 2017, pp. 27–132.

55. Cross-Disorder Group of the Psychiatric Genomics Consortium, Lee SH, Ripke S, Neale BM, Faraone SV, Purcell SM, et al. Genetic relationship between five psychiatric disorders estimated from genome-wide SNPs. *Nature Genetics* 2013; **45**: 984–994.

56. Neale BM, Sklar P. Genetic analysis of schizophrenia and bipolar disorder reveals polygenicity but also suggests new directions for molecular interrogation. *Current Opinion in Neurobiology* 2015; **30**: 131–138.

57. Pedersen CB, Mortensen PB. Urbanicity during upbringing and bipolar affective disorders in Denmark. *Bipolar Disorders* 2006; **8**: 242–247.

58. Mortensen PB, Pedersen CB, Melbye M, Mors O, Ewald H. Individual and familial risk factors for bipolar affective disorders in Denmark. *Archives of General Psychiatry* 2003; **60**: 1209–1215.

59. Eaton WW, Mortensen PB, Frydenberg M. Obstetric factors, urbanization and psychosis. *Schizophrenia Research* 2000; **43**: 117–123.

60. Marcelis M, Navarro-Mateu F, Murray R, Selten JP, Van Os J. Urbanization and psychosis: a study of 1942–1978 birth cohorts in The Netherlands. *Psychological Medicine* 1998; **28**: 871–879.

61. Oher FJ, Demjaha A, Jackson D, Morgan C, Dazzan P, Morgan K, et al. The effect of the environment on symptom dimensions in the first episode of psychosis: a multilevel study. *Psychological Medicine* 2014; **44**: 2419–2430.

62. **van Os J, Hanssen M, de Graaf R, Vollebergh W.** Does the urban environment independently increase the risk for both negative and positive features of psychosis? *Social Psychiatry and Psychiatric Epidemiology* 2002; **37**: 460–464.

63. **Ngamini Ngui A, Cohen AA, Courteau J, Lesage A, Fleury M-J, Grégoire J-P,** et al. Does elapsed time between first diagnosis of schizophrenia and migration between health territories vary by place of residence? A survival analysis approach. *Health & Place* 2013; **20**: 66–74.

64. **Pedersen CB.** Persons with schizophrenia migrate towards urban areas due to the development of their disorder or its prodromata. *Schizophrenia Research* 2015; **168**: 204–208.

65. **Kirkbride JB.** Hitting the floor: understanding migration patterns following the first episode of psychosis. *Health & Place* 2014; **28**: 150–152.

66. **Pedersen CB, Mortensen PB.** Are the cause(s) responsible for urban-rural differences in schizophrenia risk rooted in families or in individuals? *American Journal of Epidemiology* 2006; **163**: 971–978.

67. **van Os J, Pedersen CB, Mortensen PB.** Confirmation of synergy between urbanicity and familial liability in the causation of psychosis. *American Journal of Psychiatry* 2004; **161**: 2312–2314.

68. **Zammit S, Owen MJ, Lewis G.** Misconceptions about gene-environment interactions in psychiatry. Evidence Based Mental Health. 2010; **13**: 65–68.

69. **Zammit S, Hamshere M, Dwyer S, Georgiva L, Timpson N, Moskvina V,** et al. A population-based study of genetic variation and psychotic experiences in adolescents. *Schizophrenia Bulletin* 2014; **40**: 1254–1262.

70. **van Os J, Rutten BPF, Poulton R.** Gene–environment interactions in schizophrenia: review of epidemiological findings and future directions. *Schizophrenia Bulletin* 2008; **34**: 1066–1082.

71. **Bleuler E.** *Dementia Praecox oder Gruppe der Schizophrenien.* Tubingen: Diskord, 1911.

72. **Howes OD, Murray RM.** Schizophrenia: an integrated sociodevelopmental-cognitive model. *Lancet* 2014; **383**: 1677–1687.

73. **Takei N, Sham PC, O'Callaghan E, Murray RM.** Cities, winter birth, and schizophrenia. *Lancet* 1992; **340**: 558–559.

74. **Takei N, Sham PC, O'Callaghan E, Glover G, Murray RM.** Schizophrenia: increased risk associated with winter and city birth--a case-control study in 12 regions within England and Wales. *Journal of Epidemiology & Community Health* 1995; **49**: 106–107.

75. **Brown AS, Begg MD, Gravenstein S, Schaefer CA, Wyatt RJ, Bresnahan M.** Serologic evidence of prenatal influenza in the etiology of schizophrenia. *Archives of General Psychiatry* 2004; **61**: 774–780.

76. **Buka SL, Cannon TD, Torrey EF, Yolken RH.** Maternal exposure to herpes simplex virus and risk of psychosis among adult offspring. *Biological Psychiatry* 2008; **63**: 809–815.

77. **Agerbo E, Torrey EF, Mortensen PB.** Household crowding in early adulthood and schizophrenia are unrelated in Denmark: a nested case-control study. *Schizophrenia Research* 2001; **47**: 243–246.

78. **Torrey E, Yolken RH.** Could schizophrenia be a viral zoonosis transmitted from house cats? At issue. *Schizophrenia Bulletin* 1995; **21**: 167–171.

79. **Solmi F, Hayes JF, Lewis G, Kirkbride JB.** Curiosity killed the cat: no evidence of an association between cat ownership and psychotic symptoms at ages 13 and 18 years in a UK general population cohort. *Psychological Medicine* 2017; **47**: 1659–1667.

80. **Cannon M, Jones PB, Murray RM.** Obstetric complications and schizophrenia: historical and meta-analytic review. *America Journal of Psychiatry* 2002; **159**: 1080–1092.

81. **Link BG, Phelan J.** Social conditions as fundamental causes of disease. *Journal of Health and Social Behavior* 1995; **35**: 80–94.

82. **Selten JP, Cantor-Graae E.** Social defeat: risk factor for schizophrenia? *British Journal of Psychiatry* 2005; **187**: 101–102.

83. **Selten J-P, van der Ven E, Rutten BPF, Cantor-Graae E.** The social defeat hypothesis of schizophrenia: an update. *Schizophrenia Bulletin* 2013; **39**: 1180–1186. 84. **Croudace TJ, Kayne R, Jones PB, Harrison GL.** Non-linear relationship between an index of social deprivation, psychiatric admission prevalence and the incidence of psychosis. *Psychological Medicine* 2000; **30**: 177–185.

85. **Bhavsar V, Boydell J, Murray R, Power P.** Identifying aspects of neighbourhood deprivation associated with increased incidence of schizophrenia. *Schizophrenia Research* 2014; **156**: 115–121.

86. **Kirkbride JB, Morgan C, Fearon P, Dazzan P, Murray RM, Jones PB.** Neighbourhood-level effects on psychoses: re-examining the role of context. *Psychological Medicine* 2007; **37**: 1413–1425.

87. **Allardyce J, Gilmour H, Atkinson J, Rapson T, Bishop J, McCreadie RG.** Social fragmentation, deprivation and urbanicity: Relation to first-admission rates for psychoses. *British Journal of Psychiatry* 2005; **187**: 401–406.

88. **Omer S, Kirkbride JB, Pringle DG, Russell V, O'Callaghan E, Waddington JL.** Neighbourhood-level socio-environmental factors and incidence of first episode psychosis by place at onset in rural Ireland: the Cavan-Monaghan First Episode Psychosis Study [CAMFEPS]. Schizophrenia Research 2014; **152**: 152–157.

89. **Paksarian D, Eaton WW, Mortensen PB, Pedersen CB.** Childhood residential mobility, schizophrenia, and bipolar disorder: a population-based study in Denmark. *Schizophrenia Bulletin* 2015; **41**: 346–354.

90. **Silver E, Mulvey EP, Swanson JW.** Neighborhood structural characteristics and mental disorder: Faris and Dunham revisited. *Social Science & Medicine* 2002; **55**: 1457–1470.

91. **Schelin EM, Munk-Jorgensen P, Olesen A V, Gerlach J.** Regional differences in schizophrenia incidence in Denmark. *Acta Psychiatrica Scandinavica* 2000; **101**: 293–299.

92. **Hogerzeil SJ, van Hemert AM, Rosendaal FR, Susser E, Hoek HW.** Direct comparison of first-contact versus longitudinal register-based case finding in the same population: early evidence that the incidence of schizophrenia may be three times higher than commonly reported. *Psychological Medicine* 2014; **44**: 3481–3490.

93. **Kirkbride JB, Lunn DJ, Morgan C, Lappin JM, Dazzan P, Morgan K,** et al. Examining evidence for neighbourhood variation in the duration of untreated psychosis. *Health & Place* 2010; **16**: 219–225.

94. **Bradford-Hill A.** The environment and disease: association or causation? *Proceedings of the Royal Society of Medicine* 1965; **58**: 295–300.

95. Kaymaz N, Krabbendam L, de Graaf R, Nolen W, ten Have M, van Os J. Evidence that the urban environment specifically impacts on the psychotic but not the affective dimension of bipolar disorder. *Social Psychiatry and Psychiatric Epidemiology* 2006; **41**: 679–685.

96. Hill SK, Reilly JL, Keefe RS, Gold JM, Bishop JR, Gershon ES, et al. Neuropsychological impairments in schizophrenia and psychotic bipolar disorder: findings from the Bipolar-Schizophrenia Network on Intermediate Phenotypes (B-SNIP) study. *American Journal of Psychiatry* 2013; **170**: 1275–1284.

97. Reichenberg A, Weiser M, Rabinowitz J, Caspi A, Schmeidler J, Mark M, et al. A population-based cohort study of premorbid intellectual, language, and behavioral functioning in patients with schizophrenia, schizoaffective disorder, and nonpsychotic bipolar disorder. *American Journal of Psychiatry* 2002; **159**: 2027–2035.

98. Schizophrenia Working Group of the Psychiatric Genomics Consortium. Biological insights from 108 schizophrenia-associated genetic loci. *Nature* 2014; **511**: 421–427.

99. Kahn RS, Sommer IE. The neurobiology and treatment of first-episode schizophrenia. *Molecular Psychiatry* 2015; **20**: 84–97.

100. Howes OD, Kapur S. The dopamine hypothesis of schizophrenia: version III—the final common pathway. *Schizophrenia Bulletin* 2009; **35**: 549–562.

101. Hall FS, Wilkinson LS, Humby T, Inglis W, Kendall DA, Marsden CA, Robbins TW. Isolation rearing in rats: pre- and postsynaptic changes in striatal dopaminergic systems. *Pharmacology, Biochemistry and Behavior* 1998; **59**: 859–872.

102. Tidey JW, Miczek KA. Social defeat stress selectively alters mesocorticolimbic dopamine release: an in vivo microdialysis study. *Brain Research* 1996; **721**: 140–149.

103. Mizrahi R. Social stress and psychosis risk: common neurochemical substrates? Neuropsychopharmacology 2016; **41**: 666–674.

104. Wickham S, Taylor P, Shevlin M, Bentall RP. The impact of social deprivation on paranoia, hallucinations, mania and depression: the role of discrimination social support, stress and trust. *PLoS One* 2014; **9**: e105140.

105. Green MF, Horan WP, Lee J. Social cognition in schizophrenia. *Nature Reviews Neuroscience* 2015; **16**: 620–631.

106. Weiser M, van Os J, Reichenberg A, Rabinowitz J, Nahon D, Kravitz E, et al. Social and cognitive functioning, urbanicity and risk for schizophrenia. *British Journal of Psychiatry* 2007; **191**: 320–324.

107. Ludwig J, Duncan GJ, Gennetian LA, Katz LF, Kessler RC, Kling JR, et al. Neighborhood effects on the long-term well-being of low-income adults. *Science* 2012; **337**: 1505–1510.

108. Lederbogen F, Kirsch P, Haddad L, Streit F, Tost H, Schuch P, et al. City living and urban upbringing affect neural social stress processing in humans. *Nature* 2011; **474**: 498–501.

109. Akdeniz C, Tost H, Streit F, Haddad L, Wüst S, Schäfer A, et al. Neuroimaging evidence for a role of neural social stress processing in ethnic minority-associated environmental risk. *JAMA Psychiatry* 2014; **71**: 672–680.

110. Kirkbride JB, Jackson D, Perez J, Fowler D, Winton F, Coid JW, et al. A population-level prediction tool for the incidence of first-episode psychosis: translational epidemiology based on cross-sectional data. *BMJ Open* 2013; **3**: 1–14.

111. **Drukker M, Krabbendam L, Driessen G, van Os J.** Social disadvantage and schizophrenia : A combined neighbourhood and individual-level analysis. *Social Psychiatry and Psychiatric Epidemiology* 2006; **41**: 595–604.

112. **Werner S, Malaspina D, Rabinowitz J.** Socioeconomic status at birth is associated with risk of schizophrenia: population-based multilevel study. *Schizophrenia Bulletin* 2007; **33**: 1373–1378.

113. **Lofors J, Sundquist K.** Low-linking social capital as a predictor of mental disorders: a cohort study of 4.5 million Swedes. *Social Science & Medicine* 2007; **64**: 21–34.

114. **van Os J, Driessen G, Gunther N, Delespaul P.** Neighbourhood variation in incidence of schizophrenia. Evidence for person-environment interaction. *British Journal of Psychiatry* 2000; **176**: 243–248.

115. **Veling W, Susser E, van Os J, Mackenbach JP, Selten J-P, Hoek HW.** Ethnic density of neighborhoods and incidence of psychotic disorders among immigrants. *American Journal of Psychiatry* 2008; **165**: 66–73.

116. **Kirkbride JB, Boydell J, Ploubidis GB, Morgan C, Dazzan P, McKenzie K, et al.** Testing the association between the incidence of schizophrenia and social capital in an urban area. *Psychological Medicine* 2008; **38**: 1083–1094.

Chapter 11

Cross-cultural contact: psychosis and the city in modern life

Shuo Zhang, Vishal Bhavsar, and Dinesh Bhugra

Introduction

The city is a focus of modern social, economic, and political life. It has always presented a rich tapestry of interest for sociology, social psychology, anthropology, geography, and urban studies research. It is from this interdisciplinary milieu in the early twentieth century that Faris and Durham produced the first epidemiological description of the socio-spatial distribution of presentations of psychosis across city zones [1]. Since then, the social sciences and social psychiatry have developed on synchronous but divergent paths. Social psychiatry has focused on the mental health impacts of the urban environment through associating, correlating, and classifying factors of interest such as differences in urban density, noise pollution, loss of community, social capital, and social fragmentation [2–8].

In this chapter we outline the importance of culture in urban mental health through historical, sociological, and epidemiological contexts. We argue that the modern multicultural metropolis can be conceptualized as a global hub of migration, a place where individuals encounter the other and boundaries intersect. We propose that the psychological process of acculturation is a useful beginning in terms unpicking the phenomenology of identity formation and cross-cultural contact. The chapter will first trace the historical development of the city in parallel to the literature on psychosis and the city in developed and developing contexts, before critically examining the role of culture in informing our explanatory and interpretive frameworks of psychosis epidemiology.

Growth of the modern city

Defining the city sets the boundaries of this discussion. What is a city? Is it defined by the physical environment or the processes through which the individual engages with its institutions? In the changing conceptualizations of the city from antiquity to modernity, to what extent have sociocultural processes shaped the development and form of the contemporary city?

The idea of the city as a polis, literally defined as 'an ancient Greek city-state' [9], has embedded meanings of citizenship, governance, and politics. Archaeologists define the ancient city in terms of size, population density, complexity, and its interaction with other settlements—a city is 'a community with a significant degree of division of labour that makes it part of a network of cities' [10, 11]. Modelski distinguishes the city from a settlement of farmers that is 'protected […] by a wall, not operating in a system of cities' [10]. The idea of the city therefore combines two components: population size and a particular structure, where the city is a set of social relations that have a global reach.

Since the industrial revolution, cities have been associated with modernity, progress, and industrialization. Cities grew in conjunction with the social, economic, technological, and political changes that shaped the modern world, changes described as 'a widening, deepening and speeding up of worldwide interconnectedness in all aspects of contemporary social life' [12]. Cowgill also emphasizes the importance of individual experience, the 'practices, perceptions, experiences, attitudes, values, calculations and emotions' of the city beyond considerations of size and complexity [11]. Cities did not simply 'happen' out of technological, political, and economic innovations, but were purposely created. The city's infrastructure and institutions act as 'active instruments for shaping behaviour, attitudes and emotions' [11]. Therefore, an understanding of the city should consider size and social relations, as well as individual experience.

This conceptualization of the city as having grown out of social relations offers a particular interpretation of the processes that underlie urbanization. The creation of a global community with division of labour is a key driver for migration both between countries and between the countryside and cities.

The city of London is a good example of how multiple phases of migration changed a Roman town into the diverse neighbourhoods of today. The city grew from the industrialization of eighteenth century into divided neighbourhoods based on class and industry, before expanding to incorporate its peripheral towns and villages. Immigration and emigration expanded rapidly after the fall of the British Empire, with mass migration into London of people from across the former colonies, forming diverse communities and identities. Peckham, one such previous agricultural village, now has a high street populated by micro-businesses run by migrants from all over the world [13].

However, this is not the story across the board. There are significant differences between and within developed and developing countries, in terms of infrastructure, governance, jobs, and population makeup. Global geo-political forces shape cities, as well as individual sociocultural contexts. In regions of Africa, there are lower initial and total levels of urbanization [14]. Equally, cities have different political contexts, for example the creation of Israel reshaping Jerusalem, and different opportunities or the lack thereof in the slums of India. Therefore, the experience of living in a city is not universal, and the mix of social relations is continually being negotiated.

The modern city is presented here to be global and multicultural, with its form, structure, and character specific to its particular contexts. The city is both complex and changeable, and individuals exist simultaneously as family units and also in differing ways as a part of a global community with forces that they cannot control. It is this disjuncture, between the individual's internal cultural identity and the external reality, that is present in everyday city life that will be explored. The city therefore for individuals can offer sociopolitical and economic benefits, and host 'concentrated impoverishment and human hopelessness' [15].

Studying 'mental life in the metropolis'

The beginnings of studying psychosis and the city in terms of the impacts of the wider social environment on mental illness and human well-being ran parallel to the development of the social sciences. It is important to remember that early theorists were important to the development of the disciplines of sociology, psychology, and anthropology, and used both epidemiological and qualitative approaches to understand the individual in their cultural context.

An emerging urban sociology articulated the rapidly changing social structures emergent within cities as people moved between urban and rural settings, and reconciled that with an understanding of how an individual made sense of their social world. George Simmel began a sociological enquiry into the negotiation of individual identity, collective identity, and shifting cultural processes in modern life through an analysis of 'the attempt of the individual to maintain the independence and individuality of his existence against the sovereign powers of society, against the weight of historical heritage and the external culture and technique of life' [16]. Later, in *Suicide* [17], Émile Durkheim used demographic data to study the effects of societal factors on mental illness across urban populations of different countries, which combined interpretive analysis with a more formalized empirical approach. It was the role of the sociologist, Durkheim argued, to look at the social factors of suicide, and of the clinician to look at the individual's psychology. 'Instead of seeing in them separate occurrences, unrelated and separately studied ... it appears that this total is not simply a sum of independent units, a collective total, but is itself a new fact *sui generis*, with its own unity, individuality and consequently its own nature- a nature, furthermore, dominantly social' [17]. Rates of suicide were found not to be constant across societies or throughout time. Through grouping the outward expression of suicide as mental distress into categories of egoistic, altruistic, and anomic [17], Durkheim recognized the importance of social factors in the causation of an individual's distress; the expectations and adjustment of the self to society were not the same across different cultures. However, this approach also led to a sociological tradition that focused on an empirical study of social facts that was set apart from understanding individual phenomenon.

As mentioned in Chapter 2, and further discussed in Chapter 10, Faris and Dunham [1] used epidemiological approaches, and were very much interested in rates of psychosis across different neighbourhoods. They drew heavily on Ernest Burgess's typology of the city [18]—a system of concentric zones with business zones in the centre surrounded by industrial zones, workingmen's homes, and commuter zones. Here, they divided the city into distinct populations with transitional boundaries and compared rates of psychosis. Two 'distinct types of disorganizing factors' were identified: the isolation of an older, foreign-born generation, and the social isolation of the second and third generations 'growing out of … the mental conflict of the person who is in process of transition between two cultures'. This tension of finding order in the disorder was a process Richard Sennett [19] sees as universal to all, and not just to immigrants. The 'purification' of community life is a result of an attempt by the affluent to order their physical materiality. He argues that a solution for the 'emotional poverty' of American cities is 'if multiple points of social contact once characterizing the city can be reawakened … then some channels of experiencing diversity and disorder will again be open to men'. Sennett presents a conceptualization of the social fabric of cities as an overlay of individual cultures [19], with those belonging to the elite as having the greatest control in creating their physical manifestations—homogenous and sanitized streets, which are alienating to others.

We have seen that the study of mental health within cities has been interdisciplinary at its core. This is in opposition to sociology's departure into more empirical approaches, and anthropology into ethnography. Ethnography is now the mode through which the individual's experience of sociopolitical and economic processes, as well as on the cultural meanings of the urban environment, is studied. The city has now moved beyond components to an interest in process. Setha Low argues beyond 'essentialising the city as an institution … through population density, unique physical qualities or appearance, and styles of social interaction' [20]. He does not subscribe to a purely symbolic analysis, but argues that 'urban' should be considered a process rather than a category. We propose that in understanding such processes that led to psychosis within the city, taking into account the social psychological processes of an experience of a city is as just as important as a social epidemiological approach. Therefore, it is important to go back to an interdisciplinary approach that examines city life from different perspectives.

The development of an urban social psychiatry

In social psychiatry the work of Faris and Durham [1] should be seen as the beginning an epidemiological enquiry in associating the city as aetiological factor in the development of psychosis; however, it is only now incorporating some of the richness of an interdisciplinary approach. It has been shown that the city is complex, and that there are multiple conceptualizations that are being continually negotiated. This section reviews the key conclusions from current work and highlights the theoretical and methodological limitations in disaggregating urban and rural differences in isolation of a sociocultural approach.

Developed contexts

For developed contexts, research focuses on either intra-city or urban–rural differences with an aim to characterize the impact of an urban ecology on schizophrenia. Key questions have focused on temporal relation of exposure to an urban environment [21], effect size, and neighbourhood characteristics [3, 7]. Approaches have been limited by the social data available and the confinements of an epidemiological methodology. It has been difficult to characterize which factors of urban life are most influential, and how they interact are still much debated. In examining neighbourhood characteristics there is an emerging recognition that sociocultural processes such as migration and economic deprivation interact with the physical environment to create social stress [22].

Temporal exposure

Debate initially focused around urban drift, where people with psychosis move down in social class to poorer areas or urban shift, where people are left behind by others who can move away. Hollingshead and Redlich [23] proposed that this was partly owing to people with psychosis being both geographically and socially down mobile, or the difference in availability and ability to access services. Environmental characteristics of cities were later found to be independent of social factors. Lewis et al. [8] found that Swedish conscripts who were brought up in cities had a 1.65 higher incidence of schizophrenia, after controlling for cannabis use, parental divorce, and family history of psychiatric disorder. It has been further demonstrated that urbanicity at birth and during upbringing increases risk [24], but urban residence at onset was not significant when controlling for birth [25]. However, service provision does explain some differences in urban–rural incidence [26].

Effect size

It is now widely accepted that populations living in urban areas have greater risk of psychosis [3, 8, 25, 27]. The effect size of urban environments has been difficult to quantify owing to inconsistent methods. Faris and Dunham [1] and Van Os et al. [28] measure psychotic symptomology, whereas others measure schizophrenia incidence [3]. Systematic reviews have reported figures of increased risk such as 1.92 in males and 1.34 in females [29]. For specific contexts, the extent of urban–rural difference has been quantified as a 61% increase in the UK, but was insignificant when corrected for ethnicity [3].

Neighbourhood characteristics

Intra-city differences were first associated with social factors of causation—such as material deprivation, social fragmentation, and other neighbourhood dimensions, such as deprivation, community organizational structure, and ethnic composition [4–6]. Allardyce et al. [4] looked at social fragmentation independently from material deprivation and urban–rural category and identified a dose–response relationship.

Measurement is often inconsistent, and urbanicity has been characterized in different ways according to various social research traditions. For example, urban environments related to descriptions of population density in the Scandinavian literature are similar to the neighbourhood boundaries already predetermined [24, 30], such as electoral wards in the UK. Definitions of urbanicity are also inconsistent: Van Os et al. [28] used a number of single households to indicate that perceived social isolation was indicated by perceived social isolation, whereas Peter Congdon [31] uses the number of privately rented household, single-person households, and number of unmarried persons as an indicator for social fragmentation.

Research interest has now moved on to characterizing particular dimensions of the physical urban environment, such as infrastructure, economic issues, environmental pollutants, and social conditions as a way of structuring the wide range of, and how it causes, social stress [32]. These encompass a diverse range of indicators such as social coherence, density of social networks, rates of employment, working conditions, population density, and access to green space, and has begun to be associated with a neurobiological stress hypothesis through functional neuroimaging [33]. Emphasis has also been placed on a multidimensional approach, whereby neighbourhoods were characterized by a continuum of factors rather than dichotomies such as urban/rural, affluent/non-affluent.

Developing contexts

The research bias towards developed countries applies to epidemiological findings and, in particular, psychiatric epidemiology [34]. Primarily studies in developing countries have focused on health impacts of the urban poor, and emphasized how their disease patterns reflects their existence at the interface between underdevelopment and industrialization. Solvig Ekblad characterizes a triad of these impacts [35]: infectious and gastrointestinal disease; chronic degenerative diseases; and conditions associated with stress precipitated by social isolation, insecurity, dissolution of primary family relations, and cultural conflicts.

Owing to the wide range of development strategies and city-specific contexts, generalizable conclusions from the literature on psychosis in developing countries are elusive. They do act as important points of cross-cultural comparison. Trudy Harpham found little work on intra-city differences [14]. There is more work on urban–rural differences in psychosis incidence. In some studies, the mental health impacts of urban settings are attributed to negative living standards, such as noise, low wages, and high population density, contrasted against a supportive rural ideal [36, 37]. This is not universal. Andrew Cheng found no urban–rural differences in Taiwan [38]; Ekblad attributes this to cultural differences [35]. Xiang et al. [39] recently published a 5926-subject prevalence study of China, drawing attention to the urban and rural heterogeneity in diagnosis and service provision with subsequent public health implications. Lack of social provision is also important in Korea for people with depression [40].

However, research has mainly focused on mental health outcomes and not on psychosis in particular. Findings suggest that there is a wealth of information to be uncovered in specific contexts. Often, even simple prevalence is not known, such as in China where only two national surveys have been done on schizophrenia [41, 42].

Migration: the global city

Saskia Sassen's 'global city', characterized by flows of people, goes beyond physical urban geography [43]. There is still a limited understanding of how these populations encounter each other, but the literature on migration and schizophrenia has been a useful beginning. Ornulv Odegaard first observed that the incidence of schizophrenia was much higher for Norwegian migrants to the USA than for those who had remained in Norway [44]. Similar findings hold for the Irish, Indian, Pakistani, and Black-Caribbean ethnicities in the UK [45].

Dinesh Bhugra stresses that migrants are not homogenous groups, and move between urban and rural settings and between developed and less developed countries for different reasons [46]. Migration increases schizophrenia incidence through direct psychological stress caused by reality-expectation mismatch, acculturation, and cultural bereavement, as well as other confounding factors, such as low socio-economic status, limited access to services, and day-to-day racism [46]. The approach used to analyse the effect of migration on psychosis can also be used for the city. Key themes for both are cultural: stigmatization, social disorganization, lack of social capital, and alienation. However, it is worth remembering that a majority of migrants do not develop psychiatric disorders so it is important to take into account the resilience factors.

Understanding processes: the city as a hub of cross-cultural contact

We have traced the theoretical development of an urban social science, and have argued the case for a more interdisciplinary urban social psychiatry. We now turn our attention to focus on an individual's experience of the city and, in particular, how boundaries are formed and crossed. The underlying process, we propose, can be understood in terms of identity formation, cross-cultural contact and wider social and cultural change.

Experience of the city

The city has already been presented as an interwoven series of encounters, places, and spaces that people move through and between. The city was first seen as a completely different experience to smaller units of social organization such as towns. Simmel first developed the idea of a 'metropolitan individuality' as an 'intensification of emotional life' due to changes in 'external and internal stimuli' [16]. Further, the depersonalization of money economies and expectations of 'punctuality, calculability, and exactness' is associated with a capitalistic social order. There is a contradiction between the anonymity experienced in the city and expected socialization. Embedded within this is an idea of an urban–rural difference in the complexity of societal expectations. People are thrown together, yet are quite separate.

Contemporary ways of understanding the city are more complicated [47]. They think about social relations not only as multiple layers, but also as multiple divisions—the ethnic city, the gendered city, the traditional city, the deindustrialized city, the global city. The divided city is physically manifested by city walls and divisions between neighbourhoods, the contested city between cultural movements. This anthropological approach centres on how meaning is created through the social construction and social production of space. Robert

Rotenberg describes a 'subset of knowledge people gain from their lived experience and value' as a kind of socialization into city life [48]. Taking London as an example, the areas of Islington [48], Peckham [13], and Hackney [49] have been areas of interest for ethnographic study. Each neighbourhood has its particular mix of migrant populations that live or transit through for different reasons. The green civic squares of Islington [48], where people are observed to gravitate to people like themselves, is mirrored by Sarah Lester and Nathan Penlington's description of people with flat caps and macintoshes on bikes, who cross the square in front of Hackney Town Hall [50]. The experience for the middle-class resident who walks down Peckham high street is very much different to the experience of the street vendors who participant in street life.

Between these three places the common theme is physical proximity, yet cultural separation. Sennett describes a new kind of urban isolation from the separation of our disparate yet connected lives [19]; a pattern of living is a product of a capitalist and globalized social order where the powerful can create purified spaces in their own image. This is supported by research into 'gentrification' in racially and socioeconomically diverse neighbourhoods show surface changes do not improve perceptions of disorder [51]. The symbolic formation of communities and creation of shared social spaces is vital for healthy cities, and understanding these processes from the point of view of how they impact the individual is an important beginning.

Cultural contact: acculturation, hybridization, and processes of change

Both social sciences and social psychiatry have shown that the negative impacts of cities are a lack of social capital and social cohesion, and both discuss community level phenomena [14, 52]. We go on to consider the vital role of the individual's experience of the city in terms of complex encounters between different social spaces, identities, and relationships. The city consists of divisions and boundaries, and identities are constructed across class, gender, age, sexuality, ethnicity, and even profession. The individual's experience of the modern city can be seen as an intensification of cross-cultural contact, where the individual continually meets the other. These 'meetings' have already been theorized in the migration and schizophrenia literature as the concept of 'acculturation', used to understand identity formation, socialization, and such processes can cause psychological stress [46].

How does acculturation apply to the city?

'Acculturation' was initially used to describe groups coming into first-hand contact with others and 'subsequent changes in the original culture patterns of either or both groups' [53]. The direction of change was unspecified and called assimilation. Later, reactive, creative, and delayed relationships were operationalized in a meeting of the Social Science Research Council [54]. Anthropologists first saw acculturation as a group process that explains how individuals within the group imbibe culture and react to meeting different cultures. Theodore Graves developed the concept of psychological acculturation [55], 'the degree to which [individuals] participate in these community changes' [56]. Anthropological and psychological acculturation therefore function on both the group and individual level. Both have to negotiate changes in identity, values, and attitudes within wider social, economic, and political trends. In thinking about the city, both concepts of acculturation apply, and are used to explain the interactions of the individual and how they adapt to the expectations of city life.

John Berry developed psychological acculturation to incorporate strategies of integration, separation, and marginalization, as well as assimilation [57]. Figure 11.1 also clearly separates identity from society; in this case, society determines particular social and cultural expectations of a divided city.

The process of acculturation causes psychological stress, through both group level and individual level variables [57]. Figure 11.2 is a good illustration of

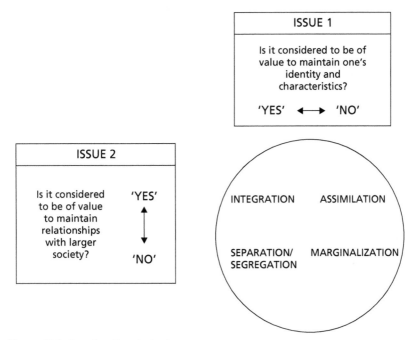

Figure 11.1 Acculturation strategies.
Reproduced from *Applied Psychology*, 46, Berry J. W., Immigration, acculturation, and adaptation, pp. 5–34. Copyright (1997) John Wiley and Sons.

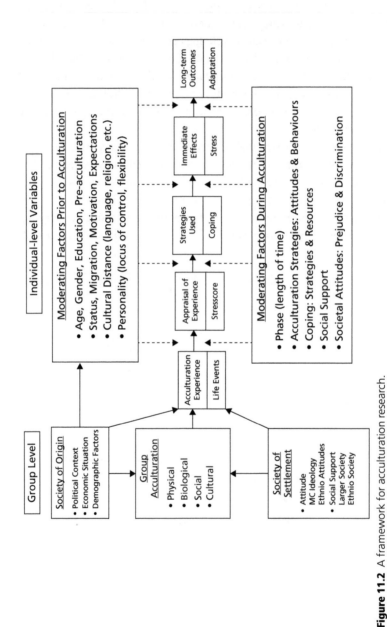

Figure 11.2 A framework for acculturation research.

Reproduced from *Applied Psychology*, 46, Berry J. W., Immigration, acculturation, and adaptation, pp. 5–34. Copyright (1997) John Wiley and Sons.

the modalities of an individual's transition and the protective and detractive moderating factors. Importantly, the time that it takes for the sub-process of cultural shedding, cultural learning, cultural conflict, and, finally, assimilation to occur also determines the timescale of psychological stress. During this process, the individual is aware of the negative attitudes of the other. Supportive relationships with people culturally similar are helpful [58, 59], and experience of prejudice has been shown to be negative [60]. Within the city, the continual buffering between new cultural values to be learnt and assimilated means that the individual is under continual stress. The concept of acculturation is useful in understanding these reactions of the individual.

Challenges

Psychiatrists have taken theories such as acculturation on board as an explanatory framework for epidemiological finding; however, this has been done too uncritically. Thinking of acculturation as a psychological process is too unidirectional, and fails to consider other possibilities when an individual encounters a foreign culture. A useful analogy here might be Erving Goffman's idea of the dialectical self, and the idea of the reciprocal formation of the self [61]. The city has been taken too much as a series of homogenizing forces without a consideration of plurality. The idea of plurality or the possibility of hybridization is a sociological critique of how the individual assimilates new cultural information, and is a reaction against the view that global cultural forces are essentially homogenizing [62]. Local cultures have resistance in their appropriation of Western media [63], and Arjun Appadurai [64] suggests that a 'plurality of imagined communities' can coexist. Acculturation is not a one-way process, but a complex negotiation, moving us beyond simply dichotomized urban–ural, colonizer–colonized, or Eastern–Western cultural relations.

In terms of psychology, Khoa and Van Duesen prescribe different levels of readiness to assimilation according to age [65]. The elderly often show a rejecting pattern, characterized by the unwillingness to adapt to the new cultural reality; the young often show an assimilative pattern, where the new culture is embraced; and others show a bicultural pattern, where values from two cultures are integrated. Approaches to understanding how acculturation causes psychiatric distress using a combined psychiatric and anthropological approach are rare but are extremely valuable. Studies such as Mavreas and Bebbington's [66] investigation of Greek immigrants are key reminders that different cultures acculturate in different ways due to inherent differences in sociocultural values, and how these change. Therefore, within the city these identities are many and complex, and may be too informal or transient to study. Experience of the city can and should be understood in terms of cross-cultural contact; the exact mechanisms are complex and need further investigation.

New approaches: the individual within wider societal change

Cultural identity has been operationalized in terms of religion, rites of passage, language, dietary habits, leisure activities, and so on. When boundaries are crossed in the everyday, 'interactions can be both non-cultural and cultural, and yet the change is cultural' [67]. Both cultural identity in the city on a group level and the psychological process of acculturation are more complex than previously thought. Neither can be reduced to simple processes whereby the individual or 'society may either become fully homogenized or break into smaller more homogenous independent societies' [67]. Further work needs to be done to understand the impact on an individual of (1) the perceived conception of city life; (2) the processes of contact with others; (3) state of having multiple identities; and (4) ways of measuring the objective and subjective levels of change.

Combining two approaches

Psychiatry, anthropology, and the wider social sciences have always shared an intertwined history. Arthur Kleinman cautions, however, that 'for all this cross-disciplinary interest [...] there is little evidence that anthropology exerts any significant influence in psychiatry' [68]. This is really the crux of the problem and Kleineman's observations are, indeed, relevant for the current research landscape of psychosis and the city, where anthropology's more informal and heuristic approach has not been combined with clinical and epidemiological thinking. Kleinman's criticism of anthropology as unsystematic in 'relevant diagnostic, epidemiological or treatment issues' also holds true.

In thinking about psychosis and the city, we draw together both literatures and clarify their theoretical and methodological orientations. We explore the experience of the city through cultural contact theories, and borrow from work on schizophrenia and migration. The social environment of the city reflects the increasingly complex flows of people, economics, and technology in the age of globalization. Yet the social physical environment around us always affects the every day, and ultimately has an impact on our psychologies. In order to understand the city and psychosis, psychiatry has to look beyond sociology, its natural companion within the social sciences, and consider the approaches of social psychology and anthropology. We need to look at both the macrosocial level and the level of individual processes.

Kleinman's critique finishes with four anthropological questions for psychiatry [68]. It is a good starting point for thinking about how the social sciences can inform the ecological study of psychosis and the city in the future. Firstly, to what extent do psychiatric disorders differ in different societies? Secondly, does cross-cultural psychiatry exaggerate biological dimensions of disease and de-emphasize the cultural dimensions of illness? Thirdly, what place does translation have in cross-cultural research? And, finally, does the standard approach to cross-cultural research in psychiatry commit a category fallacy? Although concerns about translation are less relevant to this topic, these questions should be kept in mind when thinking about culture. Further, the cross-cultural validity of epidemiological findings has not been considered, as the work on cities has mainly concentrated on neighbourhood and urban–rural differences within cities. The disaggregation of psychosis to neighbourhood characteristics follows an inherent drive within the discipline of classification, which errs on the side of being too reductionist. Fundamentally, Kleinman is asking us to be aware of interpretation and to make sure that measurement is coupled with understanding.

Conclusion

In this chapter we have attempted to combine approaches from social psychiatry with those from the social sciences that consider the individual. However, there are always limitations in subject boundaries drawn, the remit considered, and the evidence examined. The primary assumption that underlies current work is that the physical environment affects the social landscape, and, in turn, people's psychologies. In the work explored, this is thought to be a significant impact. However, this assumption is limited in negotiating the changing role of the city in the twenty-first century in our global society facilitated by technological advancements. Media theorists explore the contraction of the sense of place and space, and understand society in terms of cultural flows [64]. New technology has transformed cultural contact into an everyday event, cultures are losing physical separation, and there is constant re-negotiation of power dynamics between transmission and reception of culture [69]. The Internet, in particular, has transformed the way in which the individual engages, connects with, and contacts others. Individuals can now interact across a number of levels, and form a variety of non-traditional communities and identities [70, 71]. The challenge for understanding the social and cultural aspects of mental health is to be able to account for multilevel and multidimensional analysis of changing social forces. Although understanding psychosis and the city is just one lens through which to view such entanglements, it is an important beginning.

References

1. **Faris REL, Dunham HW.** *Mental Disorders in Urban Areas.* Chicago, IL: University of Chicago Press, 1939.

2. **Van Os J, Driessen G, Gunther N, Delespaul P.** Neighbourhood variation in incidence of schizophrenia. Evidence for person-environment interaction. *British Journal of Psychiatry* 2000; **176**: 243–248.

3. **Allardyce J, Boydell J.** Environment and schizophrenia: review: the wider social environment and schizophrenia. *Schizophrenia Bulletin* 2006; **32**: 592–598.

4. **Allardyce J, Boydell J, Van Os J, Morrison G, Castle DJ, Murray RM, Mccreadie RG.** Comparison of the incidence of schizophrenia in rural Dumfries and Galloway and urban Camberwell. *British Journal of Psychiatry* 2001; **179**: 335–339.

5. **Allardyce J, Gilmour H, Atkinson J, Rapson T, Bishop J, Mccreadie RG.** Social fragmentation, deprivation and urbanicity: relation to first-admission rates for psychoses. *British Journal of Psychiatry* 2005; **187**: 401–406.

6. **Boydell J, Van Os J, Mckenzie K, Allardyce J, Goel R, Mccreadie RG, Murray RM.** Incidence of schizophrenia in ethnic minorities in London: ecological study into interactions with environment. *British Medical Journal.* 2001; **323**: 1336.

7. **Kirkbride JB, Fearon P, Morgan C, Dazzan P, Morgan K, Murray RM, Jones PB.** Neighbourhood variation in the incidence of psychotic disorders in Southeast London. *Social Psychiatry and Psychiatric Epidemiology* 2007; **42**: 438–445.

8. **Lewis G, David A, Andréasson S, Allebeck P.** Schizophrenia and city life. *The Lancet* 1992; **340**: 137–140.

9. Collins English Dictionary. 11th edition. New York: Collins Press, 2011.

10. **Modelski G.** Ancient world cities 4000–1000 BC: Centre/Hinterland in the World System. *Global Society* 1999; **13**: 382–392.

11. **Cowgill GL.** Origins and development of urbanism: archaeological perspectives. *Annual Review of Anthropology* 2004; **33**: 525–549.

12. **Held D, McGrew A, Goldblatt D, Perraton J.** *Global Transformations: Politics, Economics, and Culture.* Stanford, CA: Stanford University Press, 1999.

13. **Hall SM.** Super-diverse street: a 'trans-ethnography' across migrant localities. *Ethnic and Racial Studies* 2015; **38**: 22–37.

14. **Harpham T.** Urbanization and mental disorder. In: **D Bhugra, J Leff** (eds) *Principles of Social Psychiatry.* London: Blackwell, 1993, pp. 346–354.

15. **Harvey D.** The city in a globalizing world. In: **C Lemert** (ed.) *Social Theory: The multicultural and classic reading.* Boulder, Colorado: Westview Press, 2009, pp. 616–620.

16. **Simmel G.** The metropolis and mental life. In: **G Bridge, S Watson** (eds) *The Blackwell City Reader.* Malden, MA: Wiley-Blackwell, 2010 [1903], pp. 103–110.

17. **Durkheim E.** *Suicide: A Study in Sociology.* Glencoe, IL: The Free Press, 1951.

18. **Burgess EW.** The cultural approach to the study of the personality. *Mental Hygiene* 1930; **16**: 307–325.

19. **Sennett R.** *The Uses of Disorder: Personal Identity and City Life.* New York: W.W. Norton, 1992.

20. **Low SM.** The anthropology of cities: imagining and theorizing the city. *Annual Review of Anthropology* 1996; **25**: 383–409.

21. **McGrath JJ.** Variations in the incidence of schizophrenia: data versus dogma. *Schizophrenia Bulletin* 2006; **32**: 195–197.

22. **Freeman H.** Schizophrenia and city residence. *British Journal of Psychiatry Supplement* 1994; (23): 39–50.

23. **Hollingshead AB, Redlich FC.** Social stratification and schizophrenia. *American Sociological Review* 1954; **19**: 302–306.

24. **Pedersen CB, Mortensen PB.** Evidence of a dose-response relationship between urbanicity during upbringing and schizophrenia risk. *Archives of General Psychiatry* 2001; **58**: 1039.

25. **Marcelis M, Navarro-Mateu F, Murray R, Selten J, Van Os J.** Urbanization and psychosis: a study of 1942-1978 birth cohorts in The Netherlands. *Psychological Medicine* 1998; **28**: 871–879.

26. **Mccreadie R, Leese M, Tilak-Singh D, Loftus L, Macewan T, Thornicroft G.** Nithsdale, Nunhead and Norwood: similarities and differences in prevalence of schizophrenia and utilisation of services in rural and urban areas. *British Journal of Psychiatry* 1997; **170**: 31–36.

27. **Mortensen PB, Pedersen CB, Westergaard T, Wohlfahrt J, Ewald H, Mors O,** et al. Effects of family history and place and season of birth on the risk of schizophrenia. *New England Journal of Medicine* 1999; **340**: 603–608.

28. **Van Os J, Hanssen M, Bijl R V, Vollebergh W.** Prevalence of psychotic disorder and community level of psychotic symptoms: an urban-rural comparison. *Archives of General Psychiatry* 2001; **58**: 663.

29. **Kelly BD, O'Callaghan E, Waddington JL, Feeney L, Browne S, Scully PJ,** et al. Schizophrenia and the city: A review of literature and prospective study of psychosis and urbanicity in Ireland. *Schizophrenia Research* 2010; **116**: 75–89.

30. **Peen J, Schoevers R, Beekman A, Dekker J.** The current status of urban-rural differences in psychiatric disorders. *Acta Psychiatrica Scandinavica* 2010; **121**: 84–93.

31. **Congdon P.** Suicide and parasuicide in London: a small-area study. *Urban Studies* 1996; **33**: 137–158.

32. **Lederbogen F, Kirsch P, Haddad L, Streit F, Tost H, Schuch P,** et al. City living and urban upbringing affect neural social stress processing in humans. *Nature* 2011; **474**: 498–501.

33. **Abbott A.** Urban decay. *Nature* 2012; **490**: 162.

34. **Patel V, Boyce N, Collins PY, Saxena S, Horton R.** A renewed agenda for global mental health. *The Lancet* 2011; **378**: 1441–1442.

35. **Ekblad S.** Family stress and mental health during rapid urbanization: the vulnerability of children in growing Third World cities. In: **E Nordberg, D Finer** (eds) *Society, Environment and Health in Low-income Countries.* Stockholm: Karolinska Institute, 1990, pp. 113–128.

36. **Fromm E.** *The Anatomy of Human Destructiveness.* New York: Holt, Reinhart, and Winston, 1973.

37. **Greenblatt M.** The troubled mind in the troubled city. *Comprehensive Psychiatry* 1970; **11**: 8–17.

38. **Cheng TA.** Urbanisation and minor psychiatric morbidity. *Social Psychiatry and Psychiatric Epidemiology* 1989; **24**: 309–316.

39. **Xiang YT, Ma X, Cai ZJ, Li SR, Xiang YQ, Guo HL**, et al. Prevalence and socio-demographic correlates of schizophrenia in Beijing, China. *Schizophrenia Research* 2008; **102**: 270–277.

40. **Kim JM, Stewart R, Shin IS, Yoon JS, Lee HY**. Lifetime urban/rural residence, social support and late life depression in Korea. *International Journal of Geriatric Psychiatry* 2004; **19**: 843–851.

41. **Twelve-Region Psychiatric Epidemiological Study Work Group**. A national 12-region psychiatric epidemiological study: methodology and results. *Chinese Journal of Neurology and Psychiatry* 1986; **19**: 65–69.

42. **Chen C, Shen Y, Zhang W**. Epidemiological survey on schizophrenia in 7 areas of China (in Chinese). *Chinese Journal of Psychiatry* 1998; **31**: 72–74.

43. **Sassen S**. The global city: introducing a concept. *Brown Journal of World Affairs* 2004; **11**: 27.

44. **Odegaard O**. Emigration and insanity: a study of mental disease among the Norwegian-born population of Minnesota. *Acta Psychiatrica Scandinavica* 1932; **7**: 1–206.

45. **Cochrane R**. Mental illness in immigrants to England and Wales: an analysis of mental hospital admissions. *Social Psychiatry and Psychiatric Epidemiology* 1977; **12**: 25–35.

46. **Bhugra D**. Migration and schizophrenia. *Acta Psychiatrica Scandinavica* 2002; **102**: 68–73.

47. **Low SM**. The anthropology of cities: imagining and theorizing the city. *Annual Review of Anthropology* 1996; **25**: 383–409.

48. **Rotenberg R**. *Time and Order in Metropolitan Vienna*. Washington, DC: Smithsonian Institutional Press, 1992.

49. **Butler T**. Living in the bubble: gentrification and its' others' in North London. *Urban Studies* 2003; **40**: 2469–2486.

50. **Lester S, Penlington N**. *An Attempt at Exhausting a Place in London*. Portishead: Burning Eye Books, 2015.

51. **Sullivan DM, Bachmeier JD**. Racial differences in perceived disorder in three gentrifying neighbourhoods. *Advances in Applied Sociology* 2012; **2**: 229–236.

52. **Sampson RJ, Raudenbush SW, Earls F**. Neighbourhoods and violent crime: a multilevel study of collective efficacy. *Science* 1997; **277**: 918–924.

53. **Redfield R, Linton R, Herskovits MJ**. Memorandum for the study of acculturation. *American Anthropologist* 1936; **38**: 149–152.

54. **Social Science Research Council**. Acculturation: an exploratory formulation. *American Anthropologist* 1954; **56**: 973–1000.

55. **Graves TD**. Psychological acculturation in a tri-ethnic community. *Southwestern Journal of Anthropology* 1967; **23**: 337–350.

56. **Berry JW**. Marginality, stress and ethnic identification in an acculturated Aboriginal community. *Journal of Cross-Cultural Psychology* 1970; **1**: 239–252.

57. **Berry JW**. Immigration, acculturation, and adaptation. *Applied Psychology* 1997; **46**: 5–34.

58. **Berry JW**. Understanding and managing multiculturalism. *Psychology & Developing Societies* 1991; **3**: 17–49.

59. **Berry J, Kostovcik N.** Psychological adaptation of Malaysian students in Canada. Third Asian Regional Conference of the International Association for Cross-Cultural Psychology, University of Malaysia, Bangi, Malaysia, 1983.

60. **Halpern D.** Minorities and mental health. *Social Science & Medicine* 1993; **36**: 597–607.

61. **Goffman E.** *The Presentation of Self in Everday Life.* New York: Doubleday, 1959.

62. **Pieterse JN.** Globalisation as hybridisation. *International Sociology* 1994; **9**: 161–184.

63. **Madianou M.** Contested communicative spaces: rethinking identities, boundaries and the role of the media among Turkish speakers in Greece. *Journal of Ethnic and Migration Studies* 2005; **31**: 521–541.

64. **Appadurai A.** Disjuncture and difference in the global cultural economy. In: M Featherstone (ed.) *Global Culture: Nationalism, Globalization and Modernity.* London: Sage Publications, 1990.

65. **Khoa LX, Vandeusen J.** Social and cultural customs: their contribution to resettlement. *Journal of Refugee Resettlement* 1981; **1**: 48–51.

66. **Mavreas V, Bebbington P.** Acculturation and psychiatric disorder: a study of Greek Cypriot immigrants. *Psychological Medicine* 1990; **20**: 941–951.

67. **Bhugra D, Bhui K, Mallett R, Desai M, Singh J, Leff J.** Cultural identity and its measurement: a questionnaire for Asians. *International Review of Psychiatry* 1999; **11**: 244–249.

68. **Kleinman A.** Anthropology and psychiatry. The role of culture in cross-cultural research on illness. *British Journal of Psychiatry* 1987; **151**: 447–454.

69. **Sullivan DM.** The Media and Modernity. London: Blackwell, 2012.

70. **Rheingold H.** *The Virtual Community.* London: Secker and Warburg, 1997.

71. **Turkel S.** *Life on the Screen: Identity in the Age of the Internet.* London: Orion Publishing.

Chapter 12

Research challenges

Todd Litman

Introduction

Does urban living threaten our mental health and happiness? Popular culture is rife with stories suggesting that urban environments, apartment living, and public transit travel cause emotional stress and unhappiness. Some scientific studies also find higher mental illness and depression rates in urban areas. Are these claims credible? What are their implications? How can communities and individuals maximize urban mental health and happiness? These are important and timely questions. The human experience is increasingly urban; the world's population is currently transitioning from being approximately 80% rural in 1920 to 80% urban in 2060. Many people whose grandparents lived in traditional villages have children who will live in large, industrial cities. Decision-makers and individuals need practical guidance on how to maximize sanity and happiness when planning cities and choosing where to live.

Abundant empirical evidence indicates that people can benefit overall from city living. Many people migrate from rural to urban areas to achieve healthier, wealthier, and more satisfying lives. Public policies to discourage urbanization, such as China's *hukou* registration system, which limits rural-to-urban migrations, and restrictions on building density and height common in many cities, are often unsuccessful, indicating that many people prefer city living overall.

Of course, migrating itself can be stressful, and urban living can impose certain physical and emotional stresses. However, as humans are adaptable beings, most migrants eventually adapt successfully to their new communities. Rural and urban environments each offer advantages and disadvantages, and some people are more suited to one or the other, but there is little evidence that most people cannot adapt to urban conditions.

This type of analysis is challenging. Much research concerning urban mental health impacts is incomplete and biased, focusing on specific impacts or groups, and most guidance for improving urban mental health and happiness is vague and unrealistic. There are many possible ways to define and measure mental health and urban conditions, and various factors to consider when evaluating these impacts, making quantification difficult.

This chapter investigates these issues. It examines scientific evidence concerning the mental health risks of urban living, identifies specific mechanisms that explain these impacts, and describes practical strategies that communities and individuals can use to improve urban mental health and happiness. This research should be useful to local officials, public health professionals, planners, and individual households.

Evaluating the mental health impact of urban living is challenging for the reasons discussed below.

Firstly, these are emotional and political issues, so many sources provide incomplete and biased information. For example, Adam Okulicz-Kozaryn's, book *Happiness and Place: Why Life is Better Outside of the City* [1] and Tony Recsei's 2013 blog, Health, Happiness, and Density [2], assume that most experts are irrationally biased *in favour* of cities, which they attempt to correct by describing urban social problems, while James Howard Kunstler's 1994 book, *The Geography of Nowhere* [3], and Edward Glaeser's 2011 book, *The Triumph of the City* [4], argue that policies are irrationally biased *against* cities, which they attempt to challenge by providing information on urban social and economic benefits. As a result, it is important to consult diverse information sources and critically evaluate evidence to obtain comprehensive and objective information [5].

Secondly, mental health and urbanity are difficult to quantify. Studies can measure incidents or rates of mental illnesses such as schizophrenia, suicide rates (which can be considered an indication of mental illness and unhappiness), and self-reported happiness. Similarly, urbanity can be measured by neighbourhood type (downtown, urban neighbourhood, inner or outer suburb, and exurban), density (people and jobs per acre/hectare), crowding (people per square foot/metre in a home), or multifaceted indices [6]. Many reported urban mental health impacts only apply to a subset of conditions, such as distressed neighbourhoods, high-rise buildings, or crowded residences, and so should not be generalized to all city living.

Another challenge is that, because they offer superior economic opportunities and services, cities tend to attract people with elevated mental illness risks, including poverty, homelessness, disability, addiction, and social alienation, so *associations* between urban living and mental illness do not necessarily indicate *causation*. Although these groups may have high rates of mental illness and unhappiness, they are often better off in cities than in smaller communities with fewer opportunities and services. Despite extensive research showing associations between urbanity and some mental illnesses, the mechanisms that explain this have not been identified or measured, so it is possible that these associations reflect confounding factors that affect the types of people who live in cities [7, 8].

These omissions and biases emphasize the importance of properly defining and measuring these effects. For example, a widely cited *Scientific American* article, 'Population density and social pathology' [9] described how rats in extremely crowded colonies demonstrated sexual deviation, cannibalism, child abandonment, frenetic overactivity and pathological withdrawal, which the author claimed demonstrates human urban mental health risks. Critics point out that *crowding* is very different from *density*, the degree of crowding in the study was many times greater than what is commonly associated with urban living, and humans respond to problems differently than rats [10]. More appropriate research finds little or no correlation between urban densities and mental health problems [11, 12]. Research on crowding may be useful for evaluating prison, submarine, and space travel conditions, but has little relevance to common urban planning issues.

Understanding causation

A key issue in this analysis is the degree that urban living actually *causes* mental illness and unhappiness, and therefore harms people who move to cities, in contrast to cities attracting people with elevated risks of mental illness and unhappiness. To explore this, risk factors are categorized in three ways:

1. *Self-selection* factors reflect the types of people who live in urban areas. People experiencing poverty, disability, mental illness, addiction, immigrant status, alienation, and personal crises often locate in cities owing to their better services and opportunities. These conditions tend to increase mental illness and unhappiness, regardless of where people live; in fact, people with these risks are often saner and happier living in cities than in smaller communities with fewer opportunities and services.

2. *Economic and social factors* reflect geographic variations in how people work, interact, and live. As mentioned earlier, people with elevated mental illness risk factors often concentrate in cities. For example, many cities have neighbourhoods where poverty and associated social problems are concentrated and tolerated. Living in such neighbourhoods can increase mental illness and unhappiness, but those factors often apply only to certain neighbourhoods and change over time.

3. *Environmental factors* reflect inherent urban factors such as more interactions with unfamiliar people, more cultural diversity, increased noise and air pollution exposure, and reduced interactions with nature. These

Table 12.1 Factors affecting urban mental health

Self-selection	Economic and social	Environmental factors
Differences in the types of people who locate in different community types. Does not reflect causation.	Differences in how people live and interact. May reflect causation but often changes over time.	Factors innate to urban locations. These do reflect causation but can change over time.
◆ Poverty and income ◆ Age and life stage ◆ Mobility (duration of residency) ◆ Family and community connections	◆ Higher income disparities ◆ Higher costs of living ◆ More subcultures ◆ Higher crime rates	◆ More interactions with strangers · More racial and cultural diversity ◆ Noise and air pollution ◆ Less interaction with nature

This table categorizes factors that affect urban mental health. Most factors are associations; only a few may actually cause cities to increase mental illness and unhappiness.

Reproduced from Todd Litman (2017), Urban Sanity: Understanding Urban Mental Health Impacts and How to Create Saner, Happier Cities, Victoria Transport Policy Institute (www.vtpi.org); at www.vtpi.org/urban-sanity.pdf. Todd Alexander Litman © 2016–2018

mechanisms can be considered to actually *cause* mental illness and unhappiness, although they can change. For example, new technologies and management practices can reduce urban noise and air pollution, and planning changes can increase urban residents' access to nature.

Table 12.1 summarizes these categories.

Although many urban mental health studies try to account for confounding factors, it is not feasible to consider them all [13, 14]. For example, people often move from rural to urban areas following a family break-up, job loss, or disability, which tend to increase stress and unhappiness, regardless of location, yet few studies can incorporate all of these factors in their analysis. This suggests that many studies exaggerate the degree that urban living actually causes mental illness and unhappiness, and results may only apply to certain conditions or people. For example, it would be wrong to apply research findings from distressed neighbourhoods to affluent and stable urban areas.

Summary of previous research

This section summarizes research concerning urban impacts on mental health and happiness.

Overview

The American Psychological Association report, *Toward an Urban Psychology* [15], offers guidance on urban mental health issues for practitioners and policymakers. In this context, *urban* refers primarily to poor and minority communities, so the report mainly explores the effects of poverty and minority status, and associated conditions such as neighbourhood decay, disorder, and gentrification, but provides little guidance on how to plan saner and happier cities.

Urbanity and mental illness

Various chapters in this volume provide epidemiological data on the prevalence of psychiatric disorders in urban settings. Some studies suggest that urban living increases mental illness [16]. Stanley Milgram describes specific ways that urban living may affect residents' daily experiences, social relationships, and mental health, and suggests that cognitive overload and excessive social interactions and fear often leads to defensive behaviours such as unfriendliness and distrust [17]. One meta-analysis concluded that city living increases anxiety disorders by approximately 21%, mood disorders by 39%, and roughly doubles schizophrenia rates [18]. Another found a 2.37 times higher psychosis risk in the most urban-rated areas versus rural rated areas [19]. Such studies measure how reported rates of mental illness or substance abuse treatments, or self-reported depression incidents vary by geographical location, adjusting for demographic factors such as age, income, and relationship status (single, married, divorced, widowed, etc.).

Critics argue that these studies cannot account for all significant confounding factors, such as the tendency of poor and mentally ill people to concentrate in urban areas, and the possibility that cities have better mental illness reporting, which would exaggerate these effects [14, 20]. A critical review of ten studies concerning built environment mental health impacts concluded that there is evidence of *associations* between urban environment and psychological distress, but all studies were cross-sectional and so could not indicate the direction of causation; that is, whether this may reflect the tendency of urban environments to attract higher-risk residents [21].

Brain scan studies suggested that growing up in a city increases psychotic conditions such as schizophrenia [22, 23], but these studies were small (magnetic resonance brain scans are expensive), other researchers challenge their methods [24, 25], and no further such studies have been published, which suggests that subsequent results are less conclusive. A study of British twins (which allows researchers to separate genetic from environmental factors), found that children in deprived urban neighbourhoods were ~80% more likely to experience psychotic symptoms than those in non-urban neighbourhoods, but this primarily reflected increased social disorder and crime risk in deprived neighbourhoods, and so does not apply to affluent urban areas [26].

Some studies identify urban environment mental health benefits. A detailed survey of 6630 Chinese people over 60 years of age found that the urban elderly had better mental health and fewer psychological disorders than the rural elderly [27]. An Ontario College of Family Physician's study concludes that sprawled, automobile-dependent development can harm mental health by eroding social capital, creating unhealthy lifestyles, increasing commuting stress, and degrading natural environments [28].

Overall, the evidence that urban living *causes* mental illness is inconclusive and biased by self-selection, that is, the tendency of people with elevated mental health risks to live in urban neighbourhoods owing to their greater economic and social opportunities. As a result, these studies almost certainly exaggerate the effect that urban living has on mental illness.

Urbanity and self-reported happiness

Studies [29–31] indicate that self-reported happiness (or *life satisfaction*) tends to increase with:

1. Financial situation (incomes relative to living costs and peers' incomes).
2. Family status (being in a stable family).
3. Work status (having a secure and satisfying job).
4. Health (being healthy and physically active).
5. Community connections and close friends (also called *community cohesion* or *social capital*).
6. Social inclusiveness (being a visible minority tends to reduce happiness).
7. Personal freedom and security (having civil rights and security).
8. Positive attitudes and belief in a higher power.

Some studies consider how geographical factors affect happiness [32]. When people move to cities from poor rural areas, they generally gain mental health and happiness. In his book, *Triumph of the City: How Our Greatest Invention Makes Us Richer, Smarter, Greener, Healthier, and Happier*, Glaeser states that [33]:

> Across countries, reported life satisfaction rises with the share of the population that lives in cities, even when controlling for the countries' income and education ... Cities and urbanization are not only associated with greater material prosperity. In poorer countries, people in cities also say that they are happier. Throughout a sample of twenty-five poorer countries, where per capita GDP [gross domestic product] levels are below $10,000, where I had access to self-reported happiness surveys for urban and non-urban populations, I found that the share of urban people saying that they were very happy was higher in eighteen countries and lower in seven. The share of people

saying that they were not at all happy was higher in the non-urban areas in sixteen countries and lower in nine.[1]

Okulicz-Kozaryn counters [34]:

> People are happier in more urbanized countries than in less urbanized countries, but it does not mean that people are happier in cities than in smaller areas. More urbanized countries are simply richer, healthier, better governed, etc., than less urbanized countries. This is one of the most agreed upon findings in happiness literature: In a cross-section of countries, people are happier in more developed areas. Urbanization leads to economic growth, but economic growth does not lead to much happiness over time, especially in developed countries.[2]

Data from the Quality of Life Survey, which asked residents in ten major cities (New York, London, Paris, Stockholm, Toronto, Milan, Berlin, Seoul, Beijing, and Tokyo) to rate their happiness, indicate that happiness tends to increase if cities have efficient public transport; convenient access to cultural and leisure amenities; are considered affordable, safe, clean, and attractive; and foster social connections [35]. A study that examined how location effects on happiness concluded that in the US [36],

> there is no reason to see urbanization as lowering economic welfare, undermining arguments for policies to disperse the population to mitigate negative urban externalities ... that most QOL [quality of life] differences are explained by natural amenities suggests that policy-makers should also consider ways to help households move to places with greater sun, mountains, coastal proximity, or temperate seasons. For instance, they could consider relaxing restrictions to residential development on lands well-endowed by nature, as higher densities are unlikely to reduce, and may even improve, local QOL.[3]

Analysis of World Values Survey data, controlling for personal characteristics such as income, family status, and age, and geographical factors, such as regional income levels, found that life satisfaction depends primarily on personal characteristics, with little variation between rural and city locations in much of the world, excepting in rapidly urbanizing Asia, where dissatisfaction (unhappiness) is *lower* in big cities, and in higher-income countries of Anglo-Saxon heritage, where dissatisfaction is *higher* in large cities [37].

---

[1] Edward L. Glaeser (2011), Triumph of the City: How Our Greatest Invention Makes Us Richer, Smarter, Greener, Healthier, and Happier, Penguin Press.

[2] Adam Okulicz-Kozaryn, Unhappy Metropolis (When American City Is Too Big), Cities, 61, pp. 144–155, 2017.

[3] David Albouy, Are Big Cities Bad Places to Live? Estimating Quality of Life across Metropolitan Areas, University of Michigan and NBER, 2012. Todd Alexander Litman © 2016–2021.

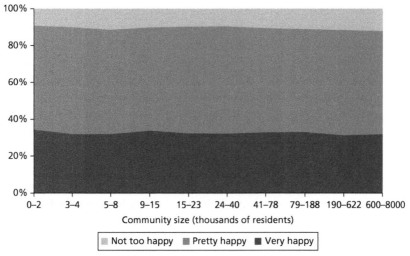

Figure 12.1 City size versus self-reported happiness.
City size has little effect on self-reported happiness. Other demographic and economic factors are more significant, so these results may reflect confounding factors rather than unique North American urban conditions.
Adapted from Todd Litman (2017), Urban Sanity: Understanding Urban Mental Health Impacts and How to Create Saner, Happier Cities, Victoria Transport Policy Institute (www.vtpi.org); at www.vtpi.org/urban-sanity.pdf.

Analysis of US Behavioral Risk Factor Surveillance System data, controlling for various demographic factors, found that urbanization lowers self-reported life satisfaction, with as much as 2.6 percentage points lower ratings for residents in the largest and densest metropolitan areas [38]. Similarly, analysis of US General Social Survey data, which asked respondents whether they feel 'Very Happy', 'Pretty Happy', or 'Not Too Happy', found that in the USA unhappiness peaks at 5000–8000 residents (small towns) and above 250,000 (medium and large cities) [34, 39]. Figure 12.1 presents the results. The variations are small, indicating that community size has little effect. For example, the portion of residents who consider themselves 'not too happy' increases from 9.2% in rural areas to 12.2% in the largest cities, which can be described either as a seemingly large 33% increase or a seemingly small 3.0 percentage point change. The researchers found that poverty and crime significantly affect urban happiness, but overlook other potentially significant factors, so they are wrong to claim that their analysis proves that large cities *make* people unhappy; their results may actually reflect unmeasured differences in the types of people who locate in cities.

Researchers find that human capital (education attainment) has a significant and large positive effect on regional happiness in the US [40]. They suggest that this occurs because increased education provides higher incomes, increased sense of control over life, stable and supportive relationships, more occupational opportunities, plus more stimulating and satisfying work. In addition, the higher incomes and increased incomes it provides allow residents to live in more costly communities with more amenities. They also find that several factors thought to affect community-level happiness, such as density and commute time, do not appear to have a statistically significant effect on happiness when normalized for income. They find that happiness tends to *increase* with housing prices, which probably reflects a combination of increased productivity and therefore economic opportunities, and improved liveability in higher-priced areas. In these regions, individuals can afford and benefit from neighbourhood-related amenities, which, in turn, increases happiness.

As education and wages tend to increase with city size and happiness tends to increase with income, normalizing for income (comparing happiness for people with the same incomes) exaggerates rural happiness and urban unhappiness [41]. Workers who move from impoverished rural areas to cities with better economic opportunities can gain happiness overall because their income gains more than offsets any happiness reduced by city living [37]. Okulicz-Kozaryn argues that people are poor judges of such trade-offs, stating [1]: 'Cities, like capitalism which they embody, lure us by exploiting our passions. Cities promise or even provide momentary enjoyment and pleasure (just like shopping), but not life satisfaction or happiness.' This claim is speculative, while the evidence that happiness tends to increase with incomes, particularly from low-to-moderate incomes, is credible, which suggests that Okulicz-Kozaryn's analysis significantly exaggerates large-city unhappiness.

Canadian Community Health Survey data indicate that self-reported life satisfaction tends to increase with [32]:

♦ *Mental health*. A one-unit increase in perceived mental health, measured on a five-point scale, increases the portion of people who consider themselves very satisfied with life by 17.5 points.

♦ *Perceived health*. A one-unit increase in health status increases the proportion of people very satisfied with life by 8.8 percentage points.

♦ *Marital and immigration status*. Married persons are happier than people who have never been married and recent immigrants are less happy than non-immigrants.

♦ *Lower stress levels*. A one-unit decrease in stress increases *very satisfied* rates by 7.9 percentage points.

♦ *Community belonging*. A one-unit increase in sense of belonging increases the proportion of individuals that are very satisfied with life by 6.5 percentage points.

♦ *Employment and income*. Household income alone has modest impacts: a 10% increase only raises *very satisfied* people by 0.6 percentage points, and, at the community level, average household income is *negatively* associated with individual happiness: a 10% increase in a region's average household income (holding individual income constant) decreases *very satisfied* individuals by 1.1 points, suggesting that relative income is more important than absolute income.[4]

Economic psychology suggests that people tend to overestimate the happiness they gain from the larger and more prestigious housing typically found at the urban fringe, which tends to decline over time, and underestimate the unhappiness caused by their longer commutes and social isolation, which tend to be durable [42]. In his book, *Happy Cities*, Charles Montgomery argues that people *can* be happy in cities provided that they are designed to meet residents' emotional and social, as well as physical, needs [43].

Most of these studies reflect specific times and locations. Urban unhappiness appears to be particularly high in the US, where city living tends to be stigmatized, and receives less policy support (e.g. favourable tax policies and investments in public transport) than in most peer countries [44]. It is therefore possible that high rates of urban unhappiness reflect specific conditions and cannot be considered universal.

Dementia and rates of Alzheimer disease

Rates of dementia and Alzheimer disease tend to be higher in rural areas than cities, particularly for people who grew up in rural areas [45]. A meta-analysis concludes that rural living increases dementia risk by more than 10%, and growing up in a rural area approximately doubles the risk of Alzheimer disease [46]. This may occur because commonly recognized dementia risk factors, including physical and cognitive inactivity, low education, smoking, obesity, depression, diabetes, and high blood pressure, tend to be greater in rural areas. As people are living longer, rates of dementia and Alzheimer disease are likely to increase. In addition, with increased longevity the complex comorbidities are also likely to increase.

Alcohol and drug abuse rates

Drug and alcohol abuse rates vary by geography (Figure 12.2).

Urban areas tend to have more cocaine and heroin addiction, whereas rural areas tend to have more alcohol, prescription drug, and methamphetamine

---

[4] Juan Pablo Chauvin, et al. (2016), "What is Different about Urbanization in Rich and Poor Countries? Cities in Brazil, China, India and the United States," *Journal of Urban Economics*, (doi:10.1016/j.jue.2016.05.003); summary at www.sciencedirect.com/science/article/pii/S0094119016300067.

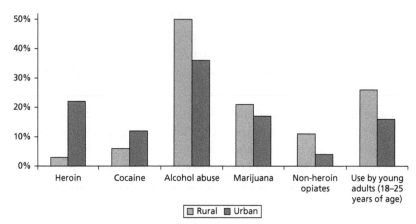

Figure 12.2 Rural versus urban drug abuse.
Heroin and cocaine use is more common in urban areas, while alcohol abuse, marijuana and non-heroin opiate use are higher in rural areas. As alcohol and marijuana abuse is more common than heroin and cocaine addiction, total substance abuse rates tend to be higher in rural areas.
Source data from: SAMHSA (2013), "Drug Abuse Warning Network, 2011: National Estimates of Drug-Related Emergency Department Visits," SAMHSA (2011), "Results from the 2011 National Survey on Drug Use and Health: Mental Health Findings," SAMHSA (2012), "The TEDS Report: A Comparison of Rural and Urban Substance Abuse Treatment Admissions"

abuse [47]. Rural young people are significantly more likely to abuse prescription drugs and alcohol (drinking more than four drinks on a single occasion), than suburban and urban youths [48, 49]. As alcohol and prescription drug abuse are more common than cocaine and heroin addiction, rural areas tend to have more total substance abuse.

Suicide rates

Suicide rates tend to be much higher in rural than in urban areas (Figure 12.3).

In the US, rural male young people had 19.9 suicides per 100,000, versus 10.3 in urban areas, and rural female young people had 4.40 suicides per 100,000 versus 2.39 in urban areas [50]. Suicide rates are particularly high for men working in rural industries such as farming, fishing, and forestry (84.5 per 100,000), which researchers attribute to social isolation and income insecurity [51]. These patterns occur worldwide: suicide rates are much lower in cities in China and India [52], causing national suicide rates decline with urbanization [53, 54].

Conclusions

This analysis suggests that urban living has both positive and negative mental health effects. Studies cited in this chapter indicate that psychosis (e.g. schizophrenia) and mood disorder (e.g. stress and depression) increase with

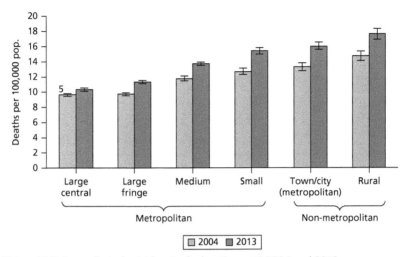

Figure 12.3 Age-adjusted suicide rates by location—US 2004 and 2013.
Suicide rates are lowest in large central cities and increase as community size declines. These rates increased significantly during the last decade. This suggests that mental health and happiness are greater in cities than rural areas.
Source data from CDC (2015), "Age-Adjusted Rates for Suicide, by Urbanization of County of Residence — United States, 2004 and 2013," Morbidity and Mortality Weekly Report (www.cdc.gov/mmwr), U.S. Center of Disease Control

urbanization, but none account for all possible confounding factors, such as the tendency of poor, mentally ill and socially alienated people to move to cities in order to access better services, and economic and social opportunities. In addition, urban areas may have better mental illness reporting. As a result, urban environments probably increase mental illness much less than these studies suggest.

Evidence that cities make people unhappy is also incomplete and biased. In many countries, self-reported happiness tends to be *higher* in cities than rural areas, and even in the US, geography has a small effect, with only three percentage points between the highest and lowest ratings. These differences may reflect other demographic factors and self-selection, so there is little basis to conclude that city living necessarily makes people unhappy.

Urban and rural areas both have significant but different substance abuse problems. Cocaine and heroin addiction rates are higher in large cities, whereas alcohol and methamphetamine abuse rates are higher in rural areas. As alcohol abuse is more common than cocaine and heroin addiction, rural areas probably have higher overall abuse substance rates. Throughout the world, rural areas tend to have higher rates of dementia, particularly Alzheimer disease, and about twice the suicide rates, as in urban areas.

Table 12.2 Urbanization mental health impacts

Increased risk	Reduced risks
◆ Psychosis (e.g. schizophrenia) and mood disorders (e.g. stress and depression) ◆ Self-reported unhappiness (in affluent countries) ◆ Cocaine and heroin addiction	◆ Self-reported unhappiness (in poor countries) ◆ Dementia and Alzheimer disease ◆ Alcohol and methamphetamine abuse ◆ Suicide rates

Urbanization tends to increase some and reduce other mental illness risks.

Table 12.2 summarizes how urban living tends to affect various mental health risks.

Many studies on these issues are limited in scope, and do not account for potentially significant confounding factors, so their results may reflect self-selection and cannot be considered universal. Few studies identify the specific mechanisms by which urban living affects mental health or happiness, and so provides little practical guidance for increasing urban sanity and happiness. Section 2 explores these issues in more detail. It examines possible mechanisms by which urban living may affect mental health, and possible strategies that communities and individuals can apply to help achieve mental health goals.

References

1. **Okulicz-Kozaryn A.** *Happiness and Place: Why Life is Better Outside of the City.* Basingstoke: Palgrave Macmillan, 2015.
2. **Recsei T.** Health, happiness, and density. *New Geography*, 2013. Available at: http://www.newgeography.com/content/003945-health-happiness-and-density (accessed 19 November 2018).
3. **Kunstler JH.** *Geography Of Nowhere: The Rise And Decline of America's Man-Made Landscape.* New York: Simon & Schuster, 1994.
4. **Glaeser EL.** *Triumph of the City: How Our Greatest Invention Makes Us Richer, Smarter, Greener, Healthier, and Happier.* London: Penguin Press, 2011.
5. **Meyer W.B.** Book Review: Happiness and Place: Why Life is Better Outside of the City by Adam Okulicz-Kozaryn. Available at: http://bit.ly/2btYJhW (accessed 19 November 2018).
6. **Ewing R, Hamidi S.** Measuring Urban Sprawl and Validating Sprawl Measures. Available at: https://gis.cancer.gov/tools/urban-sprawl (accessed 20 November 2018).
7. **Golembiewski J.** Architecture, the urban environment and severe psychosis: aetiology. *Journal of Urban Design and Mental Health* 2017; 2: 1.

8. **Gruebner O, Rapp MA, Adli M, Kluge U, Galea S, Heinz A.** Cities and mental Health. *Deutsches Ärzteblatt International* 2017; **114**: 121–127.

9. **Calhoun JB.** Population density and social pathology. *Scientific American* 1962; **306**: 139–148.

10. **1000 Friends.** The Debate over Density: Do Four-Plexes Cause Cannibalism? Available at: www.vtpi.org/1k_density.pdf (accessed 19 November 2018).

11. **Ramsden E.** The urban animal: population density and social pathology in rodents and humans. *Bulletin of the World Health Organization* 2009; **87**, 82–82.

12. **Schmitt RC, Zane LY, Nishi S.** Density, health, and social disorganization revisited. *Journal of the American Institute of Planners* 1978; **44**/2: 209–211.

13. **Bell V.** The Mystery of Urban Psychosis: why are paranoia and schizophrenia more common in cities? Available at: www.theatlantic.com/health/archive/2016/07/the-enigma-of-urban-psychosis/491141 (accessed 19 November 2018).

14. **Sariaslan A, Fazel S, D'Onofrio BM, Långström N, Larsson H, Bergen SE,** et al. Schizophrenia and subsequent neighborhood deprivation: revisiting the social drift hypothesis using population, twin and molecular genetic data. *Translational Psychiatry* 2016; **6**: 796.

15. **American Psychological Association.** Report of the Task Force on Urban Psychology. Toward an Urban Psychology: Research, Action, and Policy. Available at: www.apa.org/pi/ses/resources/publications/urban-taskforce.pdf (accessed 19 November 2018).

16. **Kwon D.** Does City Life Pose a Risk to Mental Health?. *Scientific American*. Available at: www.scientificamerican.com/article/does-city-life-pose-a-risk-to-mental-health (accessed 19 November 2018).

17. **Milgram S.** The experience of living in cities: adaptations to urban overload create characteristic qualities of city life that can be measured. *Science* 1970; **167**: 1461–1468.

18. **Peen J, Schoevers RA, Beekman AT, Dekker J.** The current status of urban-rural differences in psychiatric disorders. *Acta Psychiatrica Scandinavica* 2010; **121**: 84–93.

19. **Vassos E, Pedersen CB, Murray RM, Collier DA, Lewis CM.** Meta-analysis of the association of urbanicity with schizophrenia. *Schizophrenia Bulletin* 2012; **38**: 1118–1123.

20. **Bell V.** The Mystery of Urban Psychosis: Why are paranoia and schizophrenia more common in cities? *The Atlantic*. Available at: www.theatlantic.com/health/archive/2016/07/the-enigma-of-urban-psychosis/491141 (accessed 19 November 2018).

21. **Gong Y, Palmer S, Gallacher J, Marsden T, Fone D.** A systematic review of the relationship between objective measurements of the urban environment and psychological distress. *Environment International* 2016; **96**: 48–57.

22. **Abbott A.** Stress and the city: urban decay. *Nature* 2012; **490**: 162–164.

23. **Lederbogen F, Kirsch P, Haddad L, Streit F, Tost H, Schuch P,** et al. City living and urban upbringing affect neural social stress processing in humans. *Nature* 2012; **474**: 498–501.

24. **Eklund A, Nichols TE, Knutsson H.** Cluster failure: why fMRI inferences for spatial extent have inflated false-positive rates. *Proceedings of the National Academy of Sciences of the United States of America* 2016; **113**: 7900–7905.

25. **Scicurious.** City Living and Your Mental Health: Is city living driving you crazy? *Scientific American*. Available at: http://bit.ly/2c4Aolp (accessed 19 November 2018).

26. **Newbury J, et al.** Why are children in urban neighborhoods at increased risk for psychotic symptoms? Findings from a UK longitudinal cohort study. *Schizophrenia Bulletin* 2016; **42**: 1372–1383.

27. **Tian T, et al.** Effect of air pollution and rural-urban difference on mental health of the elderly in China. *Iran Journal of Public Health* 2015; **8**: 1084–1094.

28. **Ontario College of Family Physicians.** The Health Impacts Of Urban Sprawl Information Series: Volume Four Social & Mental Health. Available at: http://bit.ly/2m5mXpR (accessed 19 November 2018).

29. **Helliwell J, Layard R, Sachs J.** World Happiness Report. Available at: http://worldhappiness.report (accessed 20 November 2018_.

30. **Shekhar S, Joshi S, Sanwal S.** A review: urbanization and life satisfaction. *International Journal on Recent and Innovation Trends in Computing and Communication* 2014; **2**: 12.

31. **Sharpe S, Ghanghro A, Johnson E, Kidwai A.** Does Money Matter? Determining the Happiness of Canadians. Available at: www.csls.ca/reports/csls2010-09.pdf (accessed 19 November 2018).

32. **Chauvin JP, et al.** What is different about urbanization in rich and poor countries? Cities in Brazil, China, India and the United States. *Journal of Urban Economics* 2017; **98**: 17–49.

33. **Glaeser EL.** *Triumph of the City: How Our Greatest Invention Makes Us Richer, Smarter, Greener, Healthier, and Happier.* London: Penguin Press.

34. **Okulicz-Kozaryn A.** Unhappy metropolis (when American city is too big. *Cities* 2017; **61**: 144–155.

35. **Leyden KM, Goldberg A, Michelbach P.** Understanding the pursuit of happiness in ten major cities. *Urban Affairs Review* 2011; **47**: 861–888.

36. **Albouy A.** Are Big Cities Bad Places to Live? Estimating Quality of Life across Metropolitan Areas. Available at: http://davidalbouy.net/improvingqol.pdf (accessed 19 November 2018).

37. **Berry BJL, Okulicz-Kozaryn A.** Dissatisfaction with city life: a new look at some old questions. *Cities* 2009; **26**: 117–124.

38. **Winters J, Li Y.** Urbanisation, Natural Amenities and Subjective Well-being: Evidence from US Counties. Available at: http://blogs.lse.ac.uk/usappblog/2016/05/12/the-bigger-and-denser-the-city-you-live-in-the-more-unhappy-youre-likely-to-be (accessed 19 November 2018).

39. **Okulicz-Kozaryn A.** *Happiness and Place: Why Life is Better Outside of the City.* Basingstoke: Palgrave Macmillan, 2015.

40. **Florida R, Mellander C, Rentfrow PJ.** The happiness of cities. *Regional Studies* 2013; **47**: 613–627.

41. **Jaffe E.** The Great Urban-Rural Happiness Debate. Available at: www.citylab.com/design/2011/10/urban-rural-happiness-debate/290 (accessed 19 November 2018).

42. **Dolan P, Metcalfe R.** Movin' On Up: Happiness and Urban Economics. Available at:https://lsecities.net/media/objects/articles/movin-on-up-happiness-and-urban-economics/en-gb (accessed 19 November 2018).

43. **Montgomery C.** *Happy City: Transforming Our Lives Through Urban Design.* New York: Farrar, Straus & Giroux, 2013.

44. **Hirt S.** *Zoned in the USA: The Origins and Implications of American Land Use Regulation.* New York: Cornell Press.

45. **Nunes B,** et al. Prevalence and pattern of cognitive impairment in rural and urban populations from northern Portugal. *BMC Neurology* 2010; **10**: 42.

46. **Russ T,** et al. Geographical variation in dementia: systematic review with meta-analysis. *International Journal of Epidemiology* 2012; **41**: 1012–1032.

47. **Substance Abuse and Mental Health Services Administration.** A Comparison of Rural and Urban Substance Abuse Treatment Admissions. Available at: www.samhsa.gov/sites/default/files/teds-short-report043-urban-rural-admissions-2012.pdf (accessed 19 November 2018).

48. **Monnat SM, Rigg KK.** Rural Adolescents Are More Likely Than Their Urban Peers to Abuse Prescription Painkillers. Available at: https://carsey.unh.edu/publication/prescription-painkiller-abuse (accessed 19 November 2018).

49. **McInnis OA,** et al. Urban and Rural Student Substance Use. Available at: www.ccsa.ca/Resource%20Library/CCSA-Urban-Rural-Student-Substance-Use-Report-2015-en.pdf (accessed 19 November 2018).

50. **Fontanella CA, Hiance-Steelesmith DL, Phillips GS, Bridge JA, Lester N, Sweeney HA, Campo JV.** Widening rural-urban disparities in youth suicides, United States, 1996–2010. *JAMA* 2015; **169**: 466–473.

51. **McIntosh WL, Spies E, Stone DM, Lokey CN, Trudeau A-RT, Bartholow B.** Suicide rates by occupational group—17 states, 2012,' *Morbidity and Mortality Weekly Report (MMWR)* 2016; **65**: 641–645.

52. **Nolen S.** Suicide Among India's Young Adults at 'Crisis' Levels. Available at: https://www.theglobeandmail.com/news/world/suicide-among-indias-young-adults-at-crisis-levels/article4362016/ (accessed 19 November 2018).

53. **The Economist.** A Dramatic Decline in Suicides: Back from the Edge. Available at:www.economist.com/node/21605942?fsrc=nlw%7Chig%7C27-06-2014%7C5356c195899249e1ccab4314%7C (accessed 19 November 2018).

54. **Wang L, Xu Y, Di Z,** Roehner BM. How are mortality rates affected by population density? Available at: http://arxiv.org/pdf/1306.5179v1.pdf (accessed 19 November 2018).

Mental ill health in cities

Chapter 13

Urban design for adolescent mental health

Jenny Roe and Alice Roe

Introduction

Adolescent mental health

Young people today face unprecedented social, economic, and cultural changes, resulting from globalization and rapid rates of urbanization. Adolescent health and well-being is at risk from global health trends such as obesity, sedentary living, reduced family stability, environmental degradation, armed conflict, and mass migration. There is much debate about whether today's young people are more stressed, depressed, and anxious than previous generations [1, 2]; however, there is no doubt that poor mental health and well-being affects a significant proportion of adolescents.

Issues with data—including differing well-being measures and inconsistent age ranges—make it challenging to grasp a snapshot of young people's mental health across the world; however, evidence suggests that at least one in four or five young people experience at least one mental disorder in any given year globally [3]. In Europe, recent research suggests that adolescent well-being is worsening: a UNICEF study of adolescent well-being has shown that the number of young people living with mental health problems is rising, with one in four adolescents experiencing two or more psychological symptoms more than once a week [4]; in the UK, a study of subjective well-being found that young people's happiness is at its lowest levels since 2010 [5]. There are distinct gender differences in young people's experience of mental health, with almost twice as many girls reporting mental health symptoms than boys aged 13–15 in Europe [4–6]. Moreover, the transition from childhood to adolescence corresponds to worsening mental health, especially for girls: in the UK, results from the Millennium Cohort Study—a longitudinal study following approximately 19,000 children born in 2000 and 2001—showed that between the ages of 11 and 14 the number of girls suffering from emotional problems increased from 12% to 18%, as reported by parents [6], with the most serious mental disorders commonly emerging in the 15–19 year age group [7].

There is therefore a growing need to prioritize mental health care for adolescents. Three-quarters of mental health problems in adults start before their early 20s [8], and many problems in adolescence persist into adulthood [7]. Adolescence is characterized by dynamic brain development in which the interaction with the social environment shapes the capabilities an individual takes forward into adult life; promoting positive well-being in adolescence lays the foundations for positive well-being in adult life. As the Lancet Commission into adolescent health and wellbeing summarized, investing in young people can bring a triple dividend of benefits now, into adult life, and for the next generation of children [7].

Until recently, adolescent health and well-being has been overlooked in global health and policy; however, with a new Lancet Commission on Adolescent Health and Wellbeing [7], together with the United Nation's (UN) Global Strategy for Women's, Children's and Adolescent's Health [9], there is global momentum to drive investment, interventions, research, and evaluation on adolescent health and well-being. The new research vista, however, pays little attention to the built environment and, in particular, the potential of high-quality environments to nurture positive and more equal health and well-being among young people. The role of the built environment in promoting well-being among the adult population is increasingly recognized [10] and can, we posit, significantly advance the health and well-being of young people to build foundations for resilience in later life.

This chapter offers a review of the evidence showing the potential for the built environment to promote health and well-being among young people. We focus on the way that urban outdoor public spaces can promote positive well-being among young people. Firstly, we review the evidence in the general adolescent population—focusing on restorative niches, design for active living, and the playable city—and, secondly, explore the potential of urban design for managing the symptoms of specific adolescent mental health illnesses. Finally, we reflect on how urban design for adolescent mental health is central to a sustainable future for everyone.

Terms of reference: the age span under which adolescent mental health is explored varies. The World Health Organization (WHO) defines 'adolescence' as between the ages of 10 and 19 [11], the age group and term that is used in this chapter.

Defining adolescent mental health and well-being

The WHO defines *mental health* as a state in which an individual 'realizes his or her own potential, can cope with normal stresses of life, can work productively and fruitfully, and is able to make a contribution to her or his community' [12]. Conceived in this way, mental health encompasses both the absence of mental illness and the presence of psychological well-being. Increasingly, mental health is also defined in relation to *resilience* or capacity to cope with life stressors [13], which is particularly important in relation to adolescent mental health and sustaining healthy future adult lives. Adolescence is a period defined by transitions—from childhood to adulthood, education to work, family dependence to autonomy [14]; good mental health in adolescence therefore provides young people with the tools to cope and promotes resilience in adult life [7].

Mental illness refers to the occurrence of cognitive, affective, and behavioural disorders [15]. In adolescence these include highly prevalent conditions such as depression, anxiety, eating disorders, and substance use disorders, as well as autism, attention deficit–hyperactivity disorder (ADHD), and post-traumatic stress disorder. We will explore in the section 'Urban design for specific mental health problems in adolescence' how urban design can ameliorate the symptoms of specific mental health disorders in young people.

Psychological well-being, among the adult population, comprises multiple affective and cognitive components, including *evaluative* well-being (fulfilment), *hedonic* well-being (feelings of happiness, sadness, anger, stress, and pain), and *eudemonic* well-being (sense of purpose and meaning in life) [16]. Additional endeavours critical to human flourishing include the need to achieve (accomplishments), healthy relationships, and engagement in life [17].

For children and young people, however, well-being is a poorly defined concept that fails to encompass the dynamic course of adolescence and transition to adulthood [18].

Measures of adolescent well-being tend to be quantitative, indicator-based (e.g. economic circumstance, education, civic rights), objective (e.g. The Global Youth Wellbeing Index [19] includes only one subjective measure of well-being, on perceived stress), and generally apply adult well-being metrics. Data tends to come from school surveys, meaning marginalized young people (i.e. those not at school, those in juvenile centres) or those in employment are missed. Increasingly, more attention is being paid to children's subjective well-being; for example, The Good Childhood Index, developed in the UK, is one of the most comprehensive studies of children's subjective well-being globally [20]. The index includes ten domains that were identified by children and young people (aged 8–17 years) as most important to their well-being, including appearance and domains associated with autonomy, including time use, choice, and the future.

Restorative niches for adolescents

In this section, we argue that the availability of restorative niches (RNs) in the everyday immediate environment is vital for adolescent psychological well-being. Firstly, we define what an RN is, the importance of RNs for young people's well-being, and give examples of the most effective RNs for adolescent psychological well-being. An RN is defined as a place where you can act as 'your true self' [21]. The concept is related to restorative environments (REs), defined as any setting that offers psychological restoration and recovery from a depleted resource, including cognitive fatigue, stress, or low mood [22]. Typically, an RE offers four attributes [23]: (1) a sense of fascination, promoting intrigue and curiosity; (2) the ability to promote a sense of being away/escape from the everyday; (3) extent (the sense of a 'whole other world'); and (4) compatibility (i.e. it offers a good fit between an individual's goals and the setting).

REs that offer widespread psychological restoration across the general population [24] typically include natural environments (e.g. urban parks, pocket green spaces, urban woodlands). Nature, it is posited, provides the four attributes above, and demands our attention effortlessly, allowing scope for reflection. The restorative properties of natural environments are often assumed to be universal, but the evidence is not substantiated in adolescents. While some studies have found that urban nature exposure in adolescents can assist in stress and anger management [25] and specific behavioural problems (see the section 'Urban design for specific mental health problems in adolescence'), others have suggested that natural settings can have negative health effects in teenagers, fostering experiences of fear, disgust, and discomfort [26].

We suggest that RNs may be a more helpful concept in considering how urban cities can best support adolescent mental health. An RN is one that speaks to our unique character, or our 'fixed personality traits' [21]. An extrovert, for example, might find a party restorative; an introvert, by comparison, might retreat to the woods. Brian Little argues that the availability of RNs becomes particularly important when we 'act out of character', that is, acting in a way that is contrary to our natural disposition to achieve a certain goal, drawing on our 'dynamic personality traits' [21]. For example, an introvert might act out of character by organizing a party for someone they care about and want to please. But prolonged periods of 'acting out of character' exacts a price for health and can cause burnout unless you have an RN where you can indulge your true self [21]. An RN, therefore, is unique and personal, and, we argue, especially important to adolescent well-being for reasons outlined in the following.

Adolescent development is in a steady state of flux, undergoing physical, social, emotional, cognitive growth, and change. Teenagers are continually acting 'out of character', testing out new identities, and exploring ways in which they can 'fit-in' and relate to peer groupings. Adolescents are continually exploring new and novel situations that might require behaving in a manner at odds with their true nature. Such situations can cause social anxiety and exacerbate mental health problems in adolescents. An RN offers young people a place where they can restore emotional balance and actively cope with moods and emotions.

Places that support emotional regulation in adolescents have largely been studied from the perspective of favourite places: Korpela et al. [27] have shown almost half of young adolescents (aged 12–13 years) consciously use an everyday favourite place for emotion regulation in response to challenging events (emotional or cognitive); sport settings, residential areas, natural settings, community facilities (e.g. libraries), and retail facilities were equally used to support emotional self-regulation. Korpela's earlier study [28] on older adolescents (aged 17–18 years) showed the most frequently mentioned favourite places for relieving negative emotion were private homes (39%), natural settings (15%), and retail settings (15%).

Other research on teenagers' place preferences have shown strong preferences for vibrant, urban environments, such as shopping districts and sports centres, offering affordances for social interaction [29]. As social interaction is critical for the well-being of adolescents, it is not surprising they should seek these places out. But—we argue—places to escape peer pressure in the form of RNs—and be oneself—are equally as important.

Research exploring RNs within the context of adolescent goal systems (as a unit of well-being) has shown that the most important RN is most frequently an adolescent's own home, a place associated with more meaningful activities (e.g. intra- and interpersonal goals) but not a place associated with strongest positive affect [30]. This study identified that adolescent RNs are, in fact, spread far and wide across a wide variety of places, including city-centre locations and far-away places offering adventure. RNs have varying qualities and attributes that contribute to adolescent well-being; city-centre locations, for example, were associated with positive affect and autonomy, but with less meaningful and important activities; further afield places were associated with new experiences and adventures, with testing out new identities, and were highly associated with positive affect and self-identity but less meaningful activities [30].

An accompanying qualitative study (n = 45) supported the above findings [31], showing the home environment as the most important RN for emotional self-regulation, particularly for managing negative emotion (e.g. stress, anger, and regret/feeling sorry about something) and/or confiding in someone. Teenage bedrooms were the preferred spaces within the home for mood regulation, followed by the local outdoors with adolescents capitalizing on any available nature space for mood regulation (e.g. by building private dens and treehouses), and including local parks, urban fringe woodland, and recreational playing fields. Describing their favourite RN, almost 75% of respondents referred to the natural outdoors as their ideal RN, providing the freedom to roam, explore, and escape. By far the most significant place for positive mood regulation (e.g. having fun, prolonging positive mood) were city-centre places (e.g. the high street, squares, cafés) providing visual stimulation and opportunities for social interaction. Within the city centre, cafés were the most important RN for young people to relax and interact with their peers, providing comfort, warmth, security, and sensory appeal (nice smells, etc.). Further afield places (e.g. national parks, beaches) offered opportunities for adventure and taking risks.

However, not many adolescents can move freely and independently about a city to access RNs: safety, social, and cultural norms, parental restrictions, and the availability of free and accessible public transportation are all mediating factors. Likewise, the home cannot be assumed to a universal RN for all adolescents; for many young people the home may be a source of conflict and tension. Our research in adolescents from deprived urban backgrounds suggests that— while being inventive at sourcing refuge spaces in their wider local environs— the local youth club provides a vital resource as an 'escape' place, as well as facilitating access to further away RNs that allow young people to explore new activities under safe supervision [30].

In summary, there is very little research on RNs in adolescents. The evidence points to the provision of RNs that are safe, private, comfortable, and offer opportunities for freedom, control, and escape from social pressures. City planning needs to invest in the provision—and maintenance—of attractive, comfortable, and safe spaces that allow for mood regulation in adolescence, particularly for those who lack access to privacy and safety at home.

Design for active living

There is increasing concern about adolescent 'lifestyles' in high-income countries, particularly poor-quality diet and sedentary behaviours. Engagement with social media tends to keep adolescents indoors, often alone—although interacting socially via technology—and exposed to the risks of cyber bullying. The health problems associated with sedentary lifestyles (e.g. obesity) are compounded by late-night use of cell phones and computers in adolescents, causing sleep problems from over exposure to blue light at the wrong time of the day and changes in circadian entrainment and metabolism. Increasingly, urban planning and public health practitioners are turning to the design of the built environment to help promote active travel in young people. Levels of physical activity and health outcomes in adolescents (including lower obesity risk) are closely related to neighbourhood design including residential density, mixed land use, street connectivity, the walkability of the neighbourhood and school environs, the aesthetic of the street, availability of safe crossings, and nearby green space [32, 33]. A recent systematic review of interventions designed to promote active living in adolescents found the most effective interventions were road safety measures (e.g. reducing traffic speed, traffic calming) and providing safe routes to school (e.g. accessible pavements) [34]. Socio-economic factors also impact on active living: poorer teenagers tend to be less active, less likely to participate in team sports, and more likely to engage in sedentary pastimes at home (e.g. watching TV) and therefore at higher risk of obesity [35]. However, it is important to note the patterns between socio-economic status and active living vary based on geography. A large body of the evidence has been generated from the USA, Canada, Australia, New Zealand, and the UK [34]; it is possible in other cultures that low socio-economic status neighbourhoods promote greater walkability in adolescents, owing to better connectivity with destinations and/or less income available for public/private transportation.

The lack of tolerance in our cities for adolescents is a consistent barrier that curtails their mobility, and, in turn, their health and well-being. Public attitudes that cast young people as a problem and threat contribute to their marginalization and social exclusion. Young people hanging around on city streets or urban fringe woodland is perceived as antisocial behaviour. The use of anti-loitering devices, designed to disperse and repel young people from our city centres—including devices like the 'Mosquito'—an audio device that targets young ears only—have been debated under human rights conventions. Inclusive and diverse cities are a worldwide goal (UN 2015 Sustainable Development Goal 11) [36]; sharing our urban space with adolescents and recognizing young people's vital contribution to the life of a city is essential in achieving this goal. Cities need to cater for—and tolerate—'free range teenagers' [37]. This might include the allocation of 'flexible' spaces (e.g. vacant lots) that provide multiple opportunities for adolescents (e.g. 'pop-ups' and creative place-making activities). Cities need to maintain and invest in active living infrastructure for young people (e.g. accessible pavements, cycle lanes, traffic calming) and tolerate unusual forms of mobility (e.g. skateboards, scooters). Understanding where—and how best—to intervene in the city requires multidisciplinary collaborations between researchers, policymakers, planners, and public health—as well as with young people themselves.

The playable city

The right of a child (aged 0–18 years) to play is endorsed in the UN Declaration of the Rights of the Child in 1959, according play equal importance to nutrition, housing, health care, and education in healthy child development [38]. The suitability of a child's local environment is of great importance in promoting play and even more so for young people, where outdoor play becomes a vital opportunity to test independence and to learn to function in the wider local environment.

Play in outdoor environments can make a positive contribution to the well-being of all; its benefits include providing an individual with a sense of autonomy, freedom, control, competence, satisfaction and social connection; opportunities to test and develop self-identity; and a sense of the right to public space [39]. Developmentally, the importance of play in early childhood is well understood [40]. Similarly, the importance of play for adults and older adults is also an emerging area of research, and evidence suggests play has several benefits to adult mental and physical health, adaptability, creativity, and leads to increased social capital—all factors that promote positive well-being [39, 41]. The continued importance of play and unstructured leisure time for young people—and opportunities to encourage this—appear to receive less attention. Yet leisure occupies approximately 50% of adolescents' waking hours, a proportion higher than that of school and work combined [42].

Adolescent leisure activity has been shown to be associated with better psychological well-being [43], life outcomes, and academic performance, and a clear sense of identity [44]. For young people, play provides vital opportunities to test new identities, develop social relationships, and navigate transitional situations that bridge the gap between childhood and adulthood [44]. Play and playfulness have also been shown to have a buffering role against perceptions of stress and its effects on well-being [45].

As the previous two sections have identified, urban green space has multiple mental health benefits for young people and public parks are vital places for young people to engage in play. However, a study of 10–11 year old's play time in the UK illustrated that only 2% of time was spent in green spaces, with the majority of children's time outdoors spent on built surfaces, including streets [46]. The potential of urban areas to promote play among young people is currently under-utilized. Urban play provides adolescents with vital opportunities to experiment with their local environment and to interact with diverse groups of people, crucial to identify formation and well-being [47]; urban areas and public spaces, therefore, are key sites for adolescent development.

Initiatives aimed at promoting outdoor play include the 'Play Streets' initiative introduced in cities across the US, Chile, and the UK. 'Play Streets' are car-free streets that provide children with safe places to play. Evaluations of these schemes suggest they promote social connectedness and well-being among children and their carers but fail to engage older children and adolescents [46, 48]. This shows the need for targeted, inclusive interventions to engage young people that understand their needs as distinct and varied from those of younger children. In addition, 'The Playable City' initiative, developed by Watershed in Bristol, UK, is a global project to reposition everyday urban areas to promote play, sensory awareness and social connectedness, and improve the experience of travelling around a city. Projects include a street game played on bikes, dancing across pedestrian crossings and interactive projections of animals to encourage passersby to play with them. While the initiative is not aimed at young people specifically, it shows the potential of creative ways to reimagine urban play (https://www.playablecity.com).

There is little evidence about the kind of urban outdoor places young people *like* to play in. Graham Bradley [49] found that skate parks—one of the most popular outdoor places for adolescent leisure—promote personal integration, self-esteem, and social bonding in adolescent users in Australia. This evidence counteracts dominant narratives about predominantly adolescent (and male) spaces, such as skate parks, promoting delinquency, substance abuse, and other antisocial behaviours [49].

In addition, the success of 'Pokemon, Go!' in the summer of 2016 suggests the potential of technology and augmented reality (AR) gaming to promote active engagement in our cities, especially among young people. Research suggests that AR gaming can lead to a greater sense of engagement with the environment—i.e. discovering new features in the environment—and prompt excitement and curiosity among users [18, 50, 51]. Curiosity is an integral part of mental well-being linked with motivation and meaning in life; learning to see places differently and 'taking notice' can help promote mental well-being [52]. More research is needed to better understand the potential of AR to promote positive well-being and physical activity among adolescents, in particular to better understand how patterns of use differ according to age, gender, and so on, as well as how initial hype can translate into long-term behaviour change. Early research, however, suggests the potential for such innovative, creative ways to engage young people in urban environments.

The opportunities available for young people to play in urban public spaces are currently limited as a result of design features (see the 'Design for active living' section), parents' perceptions of safety [46]—as well as those of young people themselves [5]—and negative societal perceptions of young people (i.e.

in skate parks), restricting their ability to occupy public spaces. More effort must be made to make our urban streets more inclusive and playful for young people.

Urban design for specific mental health problems in adolescence

There is some evidence to suggest that access to urban green spaces in cities can help ameliorate the symptoms of specific mental health problems [53]. Among adolescents, ADHD is one of the most common psychiatric disorders, and affects between 2% and 7% of children and adolescents worldwide [54]. Symptoms of ADHD include poor attention span, impulsivity, hyperactivity, poor social interaction with peers, poorer school performance, and higher rates of drop-out in high school education [55–57].

Research has consistently demonstrated that access to urban green space (e.g. parks, gardens, school playgrounds) can reduce the symptom severity of ADHD in children [58–63]. It has been suggested that a regular 'dose' of daily nature might serve as a safe, inexpensive, and easily accessible tool for managing ADHD [64]. However, there are very few studies in adolescents. In Scotland, a study in young people (aged 11–13 years) with a range of behavioural problems (which included ADHD) found that 'forest school' (delivering a school curriculum outdoors) delivered positive benefits to mood, anger, and stress, learning outcomes, and that the rate of well-being gain—in the short term—was greater among the young people with behavioural problems than their peers with no identified behavioural problem [25].

Research on autism and the built environment is in its early infancy. Autism is a complex, lifelong condition, often referred to as autism spectrum disorder (ASD), and is characterized by difficulties in social communication (i.e. verbal and non-verbal language), social skills (i.e. understanding and relating to other people), and social imagination (i.e. understanding and predicting other people's behaviour) [65], alongside difficulties in navigating the world owing to sensitivities in sound, touch, taste, light, and colour. Over the past three decades, the rate of autism has increased dramatically worldwide. In the UK the number of school children diagnosed with ASD has increased by over 50% in the last 5 years (2011 UK census data), although it is important to note that this does not mean the condition has become more widespread, simply that it is more easily detected [66].

Current evidence, although very limited, suggests that there is a positive relationship between the amount of urban green space in a neighbourhood and reduced incidence of childhood autism. A recent study found that a higher quantity of green space in urban school districts (i.e. forest, grassland, tree canopy, and near-road tree canopy) was associated with a decrease in autism prevalence, whereas less green space quantity and higher road density in an urban school district were positively associated with an increased prevalence of autism [67]. But further study is needed to explore pathways linking attributes of the built environment (e.g. road density, air quality, traffic noise, urban green space) and autism.

Conclusions

The Lancet Commission on Adolescent Health [7] highlighted the multiple health challenges that face 1.8 billion adolescents worldwide (representing 25% of the population), including obesity and mental health issues such as self-harm. While it is recognized that collaborative and diverse inter-disciplinary and inter-sectoral effort is needed to address these health challenges—including engagement with adolescents themselves—the potential of the urban environment to support adolescent mental health has been completely overlooked to date. Our review found a weak evidence base, both in terms of understanding the nuances of adolescent mental health (and developmental transitions during adolescence) and in how urban design can help. It is imperative that this research is advanced worldwide, with a focus on health equity and those adolescents most disadvantaged. Health urbanism needs to prioritize the most vulnerable as the evidence shows that adolescents in care, ethnic minorities, and those of lower socio-economic status are at higher risk of experiencing mental health problems, exposing them to greater risks of mental illness in their future adult lives. Investing in high-quality urban design—green infrastructure; good community neighbourhood design with safe, walkable streets; smart and connected public transport systems; and promoting ownership of city space by participatory design processes with adolescents—offers a myriad of health benefits that will build assets and resources for resilience in future adult life. This investment is essential in order to support adolescent mental health now and is critical to our sustainable future.

References

1. **Collishaw S, Maughan B, Goodman R, Pickles A.** Time trends in adolescent mental health. *Journal of Child Psychology and Psychiatry* 2004; **45**: 1350–1362.
2. **Hagell A.** *Changing Adolescence: Social Trends and Mental Health.* Bristol: Policy Press, 2012.
3. **Patel V, Flisher AJ, Hetrick S, McGorry P.** Mental health of young people: a global public-health challenge. *Lancet* 2007; **369**: 1302–1312.

4. **Bruckauf Z.** Adolescents' Mental Health: Out of the shadows. Available at: https://www.unicef-irc.org/publications/pdf/IRB_2017_12.pdf (accessed 20 June 2017).

5. **The Children's Society.** The Good Childhood Report 2017. Available at: https://www.childrenssociety.org.uk/the-good-childhood-report-2017 (accessed 1 October 2017).

6. **Patalay P, Fitzsimons E.** *Mental Ill-health Among Children of the New Century: Trends Across Childhood with a Focus on Age 14.* London: Centre for Longitudinal Studies, 2017.

7. **Patton GC, Sawyer SM, Santelli JS, Ross DA, Afifi R, Allen NB,** et al. Our future: a Lancet commission on adolescent health and wellbeing. *The Lancet* 2016; **387**: 2423–2478.

8. **Kessler RC, Amminger GP, Aguilar-Gaxiola S, Alonso J, Lee S, Ustan TB.** Age of onset of mental disorders: a review of recent literature. *Current Opinion in Psychiatry* 2007; **20**: 359–364.

9. **United Nations Secretary General.** The Global Strategy for Women's, Children's and Adolescents Health (2016–2030). Available at: http://www.who.int/life-course/partners/global-strategy/global-strategy-2016-2030/en/ (accessed 16 June 2017).

10. **Giles-Corti B, Vernez-Moudon A, Reis R, Turrell G, Dannenberg AL, Badland H,** et al. City planning and population health: a global challenge. *The Lancet* 2016; **388**: 2912–2924.

11. **World Health Organization.** Definition of key terms. Available at: http://www.who.int/hiv/pub/guidelines/arv2013/intro/keyterms/en/ (accessed 16 June 2017).

12. **World Health Organization (WHO).** *Strengthening Mental Health Promotion (Fact sheet no 220).* Geneva: WHO, 2001.

13. **Huber M, Knottnerus JA, Green L, van der Horst H, Jadad AR, Kromhout D, Leonard B,** et al. How should we define health? *BMJ* 2011; **343**: 4163.

14. **World Bank.** *World Development Report 2007: Development and the Next Generation.* Washington, DC: World Bank, 2007.

15. **Bhugra D, Ventriglio A, Bhui KS.** What's in a name? Reclaiming mental illness. *The Lancet Psychiatry* 2016; **3**: 1100–1101.

16. **Steptoe A, Deaton A, Stone AA.** Subjective wellbeing, health, and ageing. *The Lancet* 2015; **385**: 640–648.

17. **Seligman M.** Flourish: positive psychology and positive interventions. The Tanner Lectures on Human Values. Available at: https://tannerlectures.utah.edu/_documents/a-to-z/s/Seligman_10.pdf (accessed 20 November 2018).

18. **Knöll M, Roe J.** Ten questions concerning a new adolescent health urbansim. *Building and Environment* 2017; **126**: 495–506.

19. **Goldin N, Patel P, Perry K.** Global Youth Wellbeing Index. Available at: https://csis-prod.s3.amazonaws.com/s3fs-public/legacy_files/files/publication/140401_Goldin_GlobalYouthWellbeingIndex_WEB.pdf (accessed 20 November 2018).

20. **Rees G, Goswami H, Bradshaw J.** Developing an index of children's subjective wellbeing in England. Available at: https://www.childrenssociety.org.uk/sites/default/files/tcs/research_docs/Developing%20an%20Index%20of%20Children%27s%20Subjective%20Well-being%20in%20England.pdf (accessed 5 October 2017).

21. **Little BR.** Well-doing: personal projects and the quality of lives. *Theory and Research in Education* 2014; **12**: 329–346.

22. **Hartig T.** Three steps to understanding restorative environments as health resources. In: **CW Thompson, P Travlou** (eds) *Open Spaces, People Space*. Abingdon: Taylor and Francis, 2007, pp. 163–180.

23. **Kaplan R, Kaplan S.** *The Experience of Nature: A Psychological Perspective.* New York: Cambridge University Press, 1989.

24. **Douglas O, Lennon M, Scott M.** Green space benefits for health and well-being: a life-course approach for urban planning, design and management. *Cities* 2017; **66**: 53–62.

25. **Roe J, Aspinall PA.** The restorative outcomes of forest versus indoor settings in young people with varying behaviour states. *Urban Forestry and Urban Greening* 2011; **10**: 205–212.

26. **Milligan C, Bingley A.** Restorative places or scary spaces? The impact of woodland on the mental health of young adults. *Health & Place* 2008; **13**: 799–811.

27. **Korpela K, Kyttä M, Hartig T.** Children's favorite places. Restorative experience, self-regulation, and children's place preferences. *Journal of Environmental Psychology* 2002; **22**: 387–398.

28. **Korpela KM.** Adolescents' favourite places. *Journal of Environmental Psychology* 1992; **12**: 249–258.

29. **Clark C, Uzzell D.** The socio-environmental affordances of adolescents' environments. In: **C Spencer** and **M Blades** (eds) *Children and Their Environments: Learning, Using and Designing Spaces.* Cambridge: Cambridge University Press, 2006.

30. **Roe JJ, Aspinall PA.** Teenager's everyday 'doings' and the restorative niches that support them. *International Journal of Environmental Research and Public Health* 2012; Special Issue: Nature & Health.

31. **Roe, J.,** The restorative power of natural and built environments. Doctoral dissertation. Edinburgh: School of Built Environment, Heriot-Watt University. Available from: http://www.ros.hw.ac.uk/bitstream/handle/10399/2250/RoeJ_0908_sbe.pdf (accessed 20 November 2018).

32. **Ding D, Sallis JF, Kerr J, Lee S, Rosenberg DE.** Neighborhood environment and physical activity among youth a review. *American Journal of Preventative Medicine* 2011; **41**: 442–455.

33. **Carlson JA, Saelens BE, Kerr J, Schipperijn J, Conway TL, Frank LD,** et al. Association between neighborhood walkability and GPS-measured walking, bicycling and vehicle time in adolescents. *Health Place* 2015; **32**: 1–7.

34. **Audrey S, Batista-Ferrer H.** Healthy urban environments for children and young people: a systematic review of intervention studies. *Health & Place* 2015; **36**: 97–117.

35. **Molina-García J, Queralt A, Adams MA, Conway TL, Sallis JF.** Neighborhood built environment and socio-economic status in relation to multiple health outcomes in adolescents. *Prev Med* 2017; **105**: 88–94.

36. **United Nations.** Sustainable Development Goal 11. Available at: https://sustainabledevelopment.un.org/sdg11 (accessed 23 October 2017).

37. **Thompson CW, Roe J, Travlou P.** Free range teenagers: the role of wild adventure space in young people's lives. *Countryside Recreation* 2007; **15**: 12–15.

38. **United Nations General Assembly.** Declaration of the rights of the child. United Nations Treaty Series Volume **1386**, 1959.

39. **Mahdjoubi L, Spencer B.** Healthy play of all ages in public open spaces. In: **H Barton, S Thompson, S Burgess, M Grant** (eds) *The Routledge Handbook of Planning for Health and Well-Being*. London: Routledge, 2015, pp. 136–149.

40. **Ginsburg KR.** The importance of play in promoting healthy child development and maintaining strong parent-child bonds. *Pediatrics* 2007; **119**: 182–191.

41. **Proyer RT.** A new structural model for the study of adult playfulness and exploration of an understudied individual variable. *Personality and Individual Differences* 2017; **108**: 113–122.

42. **Larson RW.** Toward a psychology of positive youth development. *American Psychologist* 2000; **55**: 170–183.

43. **Bartko WT, Eccles JS.** Adolescent participation in structured and unstructured activities: a person-oriented analysis. *Journal of Youth and Adolescence* 2003; **32**: 233–241.

44. **Trainor S, Delfabbro P, Anderson S, Winefield A.** Leisure activities and adolescent psychological well-being. *Journal of Adolescence* 2010; **33**: 173–186.

45. **Staempfli MB.** Adolescent playfulness, stress perception, coping and well being. *Journal of Leisure Research* 2007; **39**: 393–412.

46. **Play England.** Why temporary street closures make sense for public health. Available at: http://www.playengland.org.uk/wp-content/uploads/2017/07/StreetPlayReport1web-4.pdf (accessed 10 October 2017).

47. **Gleeson B, Sipe N.** *Creating Child Friendly Cities: New Perspectives and Prospects.* New York: Routledge, 2006.

48. **Zieff SG, Chaudhuri A, Musselman E.** Creating neighborhood recreational space for youth and children in the urban environment: play(ing in the) streets in San Francisco' *Children and Youth Services Review* 2016; **70**: 95–101.

49. **Bradley GL.** Skate parks as a context for adolescent development. *Journal of Adolescent Research* 2010; **25**: 288–323.

50. **Knöll M.** Bewertung von Aufenthaltsqualität durch Location-Based-Games - Altersspezifische Anforderungen in der Studie "Stadtflucht" in **Frankfurt am Main.' Herausgeber: Gesine Marquardt**. *MATI Mensch - Architektur - Technik - Interaktion für demografische Nachhaltigkeit*. Dresden: Fraunhofer IRB, 2016.

51. **Halblaub, M.M. and Knöll, M.** Stadtflucht—Learning about healthy places with a location-based game. Available at: http://dokumentix.ub.uni-siegen.de/opus/volltexte/2016/1004/pdf/Navigationen_Playin_the_city.pdf (last accessed 20 November 2018).

52. **Aker J, Marks N, Cordon C, Thompson S.** Five Ways to Wellbeing. London: New Economics Foundation, 2008.

53. **Roe J.** Cities, green Space, and Mental Wellbeing. *Oxford Research Encyclopedia of Environmental Science*. Available at: http://environmentalscience.oxfordre.com/view/10.1093/acrefore/9780199389414.001.0001/acrefore-9780199389414-e-93 (accessed 20 November 2018).

54. **Bruchmüller K, Margraf J, Schneider S.** Is ADHD diagnosed in accord with diagnostic criteria? Over diagnosis and influence of client gender on diagnosis. *Journal of Consulting and Clinical Psychology* 2002; **80**: 128–138.

55. **Barkley RA, Fischer M, Smallish L, Fletcher K.** The persistence of attention- deficit/hyperactivity disorder into young adulthood as a function of reporting source and definition of disorder. *Journal of Abnormal Psychology* 2002; **111**: 279–289.

56. **Loe IM, Feldman HM.** Academic and educational outcomes of children with ADHD. *Journal of Pediatric Psychology* 2007; **32**: 643–654.

57. **Nijmeijer JS, Minderaa RB, Buitelaar JK, Mulligan A, Hartman CA, Hoekstra PJ.** Attention-deficit/hyperactivity disorder and social dysfunctioning. *Clinical Psychology Review* 2008; **28**: 692–708.

58. **Amoly EE, Dadvand P, Forns J, López-Vicente M, Basagaña X, Julvez J, et al.** Green and blue spaces and behavioral development in Barcelona. *Environmental Health Perspectives* 2014; **122**: 1351–1358.

59. **Flouri E, Midouhas E, Joshi H.** The role of urban neighbourhood green space in children's emotional and behavioural resilience. *Journal of Environmental Psychology* 2014; **40**: 179–186.

60. **Faber Taylor A, Kuo FE, Sullivan W.** Coping with ADD: the surprising connection to green play settings. *Environment and Behavior* 2001; **33**: 54–77

61. **Kuo FE, Faber Taylor A.** A potential natural treatment for attention-deficit/hyperactivity disorder: evidence from a national study. *American Journal of Public Health* 2004; **94**: 1580–1586.

62. **Markevych I, Tiesler CM, Fuertes E, Romanos M, Dadvand P, Nieuwenhuijsen MJ, et al.** Access to urban green spaces and behavioural problems in children: results from the GINIplus and LISAplus studies. *Environment International* 2014; **71**: 29–35.

63. **Van den Berg AE, Van Den Berg CG.** A comparison of children with ADHD in a natural and built setting. *Child: Care, Health and Development* 2010; **37**: 430–439.

64. **Faber Taylor A, Kuo FE.** Children with attention deficits concentrate better after walk in the park. *Journal of Attention Disorders* 2009; **12**: 402–409.

65. **Delahaye J, Kovacs E, Sikora D, Hall TA, Orlich F, Clemons T. E.** The relationship between Health-Related Quality of Life and sleep problems in children with Autism Spectrum Disorders. *Research in Autism Spectrum Disorders* 2014; **8**: 202–303.

66. **Gotham K, Risi S, Pickles A, Lord C.** The Autism Diagnostic Observation Schedule: revised algorithms for improved diagnostic validity. *Journal of Autism and Developmental Disorders* 2007; **37**: 613–627.

67. **Wu J, Jackson L.** Inverse relationship between urban green space and childhood autism in California elementary school districts. *Environment International* 2017; **107**: 140–146.

Chapter 14

What has changed in children's behavioural problems reported in Mexico City over a 13-year period?

Jorge Javier Caraveo-Anduaga,
Nora Angélica Martínez Vélez,
and José Erazo Pérez

Antecedents

If diagnostic criteria and assessment procedures are held constant over time, temporal trends in child and adolescent mental health can be determined. To our knowledge, there has only been one trend study in Latin America and one in middle-income countries that have shown an increase in psychological problems, particularly behavioural ones, among preschool children over an 11-year period [1, 2].

In 1995 in Mexico City an epidemiological psychiatric study obtaining information across three generations showed that the prevalence of child and adolescent psychological problems was estimated to be 16%, with 3% considered to be highly symptomatic (reporting nine or more symptoms on a 27-item screening instrument). Familial risk for developing psychopathological problems in the third generation was moderate if psychiatric antecedents were present only in grandparents or in one parent, but a twofold increase was found when antecedents were present in both previous generations [3]. Along with familial risk for developing psychopathology, psychosocial correlates—tension over work and less perceived support from family not living at the same household—were both found to contribute highly, as shown by the percentage of population-attributable risk [4]. Two other studies carried out in 1995, using the same screening instrument to detect probable psychopathology in children—one in rural communities of central Mexico with high and low migration rates [5] and the other one in a fisherman's community with high social adversity

[6]—showed that prevalence was higher in the community with more social adversity [7].

Further studies carried out between 2005 and 2008 in a general medical practice setting [8], as well as in primary schools using the same screening instrument, showed a notable increase in the report of psychological problems in children.

Results from these studies, considering different cut-off points for the screening instrument, are shown in Figure 14.1. In the first investigations on urban and rural general populations, children with a high number of symptoms represented a minority (2–6%), whereas in more recent studies on general practice and primary schools, a considerable increase can be appreciated, from 10% to 32% in the most symptomatic children and from 25% to 34% for the middle symptomatic group.

Moreover, an epidemiological study on a young Mexican population in the Mexico City metropolitan area found that almost 40% of adolescents reported a 12-month disorder, and the difference between these results and the 25% median prevalence estimate in developed regions was discussed in terms of the accelerated rate of social change and social adversity [9]. Authors found that 68% of the adolescents had been exposed during infancy to at least one chronic adversity being adverse economic condition the most frequent [10].

The objective of this chapter is to identify what has changed in the frequency of reported behavioural symptoms and syndromes in children aged 4–12 years,

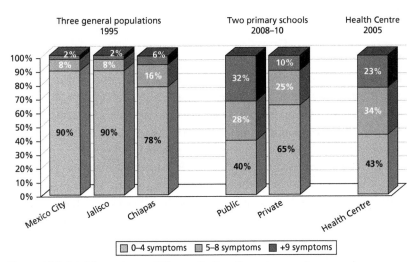

Figure 14.1 Brief Screening and Diagnostic Questionnaire symptom prevalence on children aged 4–12 years.

comparing estimates from the 1995 population study in Mexico City and data from further studies using the same screening instrument over a 13-year period.

Methods

Studies samples

The Mexico City study was designed as a household survey on a representative sample of the adult population aged 18–65 years. The response rate was 60.4%. The total sample size was 1932 adults; 925 respondents with children aged 4–16 years living in the same household were interviewed providing data on 1685 children and adolescents using a standardized screening questionnaire for assessing psychopathology, the Brief Screening and Diagnostic Questionnaire ('CBTD', for its initials in Spanish). The mean age of the children was 9.7 years (SD 3.62), and the distribution by age group was as follows: 4–5 years, 16.3%, 6–8 years, 25.5%, 9–12 years, 30.9%, and 13–16 years, 27.4%. For this chapter, only children aged 4–12 were included (n = 1222) [11].

Further studies were carried out in two different areas of Mexico City and in a close municipality in the metropolitan area. The health centre study included a cohort of consecutive children and adolescents who attended during a 6-month period in 2005; patients already in treatment at the mental health service were excluded [8] and 669 children aged 4–12 years were included for this report. In the study at a public primary school, information on 191 pupils was obtained during 2008 and 2009. At a male primary private school, information on almost all pupils was obtained during 2008; 390 children aged 6–12 years were included in this paper.

Social context

The family has been considered as the nuclear unit of societies, playing a role as a risk or protective factor in children's mental health development. In Mexico, family structure and dynamics have experienced several rapid changes in response to critical economic demands since 1995; even before that they showed an impact on mental health problems across generations [4].

For the 1995 Mexico City study, estimated household income was divided into five levels: 26.04% were at the bottom, 27.35%, 26.09%, and 16.94% at subsequent levels, and only 3.6% at the top. For the other studies, household income was neither estimated nor asked about. However, presumably, families in these other studies corresponded to the first three income levels at the most.

Information about social backward indicators and delictive rates for 2010 in the geographical areas from where the studies samples were obtained, showed that:

1. Poverty represented 31.3% of the total population in the area served by the health centre; 25.5% and 33.8% where the public and private primary schools are located, respectively [12].

2. Many households had a woman as the principal head of the household: 29.4% in the health centre area, and 33% and 22.9% in the schools' geographical areas, respectively [13].

3. In all three geographical areas broadly 50% of the population did not have access to social security [12].

4. Delictive rates (number of denounced delicts/10,000 inhabitants) for each geographical area were 167.5, 208.8, and 169.9, respectively. However, it is known that many transgressions to law are not denounced [14].

Instrument

The CBTD is a 27-item questionnaire answered by a child's parents or care-givers. It explores behavioural symptoms frequently reported as motives for seeking attention at outpatient mental health services. The presence of a symptom requires that each item has to be reported as 'frequently' presented in the last 12-month period. The internal consistency of the questionnaire showed a Cronbach's alpha of 0.81 (range 0.76–0.85). Caseness was defined based on the questionnaire score for those at the ninth decile reporting five or more symptoms [15]. Concurrent validity with any *Diagnostic and Statistical Manual of Mental Disorders*, 4th Edition (DSM-IV) diagnosis using the E-MiniKid standardized interview showed a positive predictive value of 88% (95% confidence interval (CI) 83.7–91.5) and the area under the curve obtained by receiver-operating characteristic curve analysis was 0.78 (95% CI 75–81%) [8].

Syndrome algorithms in order to define probable DSM-IV disorders in children were created based on data from the epidemiological study in Mexico City [16]. Concurrent validity was between good and fair for most of the syndromes [8]. The different behavioural syndromes that derive from the CBTD, mutually exclusive among them, are grouped in the following manner [16]:

Syndromes of externalization: attention deficit and hyperactivity, oppositional behaviour, conduct problems, and explosive conduct.

Syndromes of internalization: depressive syndromes, anxiety, and eating/weight problems.

Other syndromes: language problems, probable manifestations of epilepsy, explosive behaviour with probable brain injury and enuresis.

Mixed type-1: when there is a combination of externalization and internalization syndromes.

Mixed type-2: when there is a combination of externalization and/or internalization syndromes, *and* the group of other syndromes.

Functional impairment was only measured in recent studies, using the Brief Impairment Scale (BIS) [17], which is a 23-item questionnaire exploring interpersonal relationships, work/school performance, and self-attitudes. Each question is answered by parents or caregivers on a Likert scale with four options: 0 (never or no problem); 1 (some problems); 2 (several problems); 3 (serious problems). The internal consistency of the BIS in our population showed a Cronbach's alpha of 0.87.

Analysis

Results from the 1995 population study in Mexico City were used for comparative purposes against the pooled data obtained from the other studies. A chi-square test was used to test for statistical differences between the prevalence of each symptom and behavioural syndrome according to age group (4–5 years, 6–8 years, and 9–12 years), as well as for three different cut-off-point groups in the screening questionnaire: 0–4, 5–8, and ≥ 9 symptoms.

The BIS was not used in the 1995 survey, and as this measurement was introduced during the follow-up of the cohort attended at the health centre, not all of the children initially evaluated also had this assessment; this information was obtained for all children from both school studies. A t-test was used to compare the mean scores on the BIS as related to the three cut-off point groups in the CBTD using the pooled data from the more recent studies.

Results

Comparisons according to sex and age groups between the 1995 population study and the pooled data from recent studies show that for preschool children there is no difference on sex distribution. However, for school-age children, boys are over-represented in the pooled data, as one of the schools is a boys-only one (Table 14.1).

As the requirement of functional impairment for defining caseness and diagnosis has been identified as a major issue on prevalence estimates variability, we tested whether higher scores in the CBTD are associated with higher functional impairment.

Comparisons of the mean total score on the BIS as related to score groups in the CBTD show that there are significant differences between groups, so that children with a higher number of reported symptoms in the CBTD also have higher mean impairment scores (Table 14.2).

Table 14.1 Sex and age groups

	4–5 years					6–8 years					9–12 years				
	Pooled data (n = 179)	Mexico City (n = 273)	Total (n = 452)	χ^2	F	Pooled data (n = 434)	Mexico City (n = 430)	Total (n = 864)	χ^2	F	Pooled data (n = 637)	Mexico City (n = 519)	Total (n = 1156)	χ^2	F
Boys	52.2%	51.5%	51.8%	.024	.477	70.0%	53.5%	61.8%	25.085	.000	63.3%	50.3%	57.4	19.698	.000
Girls	47.8%	48.5%	48.2%			30.0%	53.5%	38.2%			36.7%	49.7%	42.6		

Table 14.2 Comparative Brief Impairement Scale (BIS) and Brief Screening and Diagnostic Questionnaire scores

No. symptoms	0–4	5–8	≥ 9	T	F
Mean BIS score					
	X = 6.86	X = 11.36		33.395	.000
	X = 6.86		X = 15.11	54.389	.000
		X = 11.36	X = 15.11	4.386	.000

Are there differences in the reported prevalence of symptoms according to different cut-off points in the screening questionnaire between the 1995 data and the pooled, more recent data?

When different cut-off points in the questionnaire are considered, most significant differences between the 1995 study and the pooled data from subsequent studies are for those children with fewer reported symptoms, that is, for the probable non-cases (Table 14.3). Across all age groups, nervousness, restlessness, inattentiveness, irritability, and explosiveness show significant reported increases. Sadness, aloofness, physical complaints, disobedience, frequent lying, and not working at school show an increase for school-age children.

For children with a CBTD score of between 5 and 8 symptoms, only a couple of symptoms show a significant increase versus the 1995 results: irritability and explosiveness in late school age, while poor school performance diminishes, as does enuresis in late and early school-age children (Table 14.4).

For children with higher CBTD scores, several symptoms across age groups were absent in the 1995 survey. Notably, frequent lying, aloofness, running away from home, stealing, and restlessness were not reported for the more symptomatic pre-school-age children in 1995 versus recent studies; also, use of alcohol or drugs in older school-age children was absent in 1995. It is important to note that a significant decrease in the report of convulsions and low weight in older school-age children and poor school performance in the younger group, is evident in recent studies versus 1995 data (Table 14.5).

Are there differences in the prevalence of the CBTD syndromes between the results from the 1995 population study and the pooled data from the recent studies across age groups?

Comparison of prevalence of the CBTD syndromes by age group between results from the 1995 survey study and the pooled data from subsequent studies (Table 14.6) shows that there has been a considerable increase in almost all syndromes and across the different age groups.

Table 14.3 Comparative symptom prevalence on low Brief Screening and Diagnostic Questionnaire score (0–4) by age group

Age group	4–5 years				6–8 years				9–12 years			
	Pooled data	Mexico City	χ^2	F	Pooled data	Mexico City	χ^2	F	Pooled data	Mexico City	χ^2	F
Abnormal language	9.9	5.7	1.869	.221	6.2	3.6	2.231	.150	1.3	0.4	1.679	.232
Sleep problems	3.3	0.4	4.756	.061	2.4	1.8	.257	.761	1.9	0.7	2.528	.170
Headaches	2.2	–	5.461	.072	8.1	1.0	20.461	.000	4.7	3.3	1.100	.344
Running away	–	0.4	.370	1.000	–	–	–	–	0.9	0.4	.770	.403
Steals	–	0.4	.370	1.00	1.0	1.0	.006	1.000	0.9	0.4	.770	.403
Nervous	26.4	8.9	17.256	.000	16.7	9.9	5.837	.019	16.5	10.7	5.517	.022
Backward	3.3	1.6	.922	.392	6.7	1.8	9.716	.004	4.4	4.4	.002	1.000
Aloof	3.3	1.2	1.653	.349	4.8	1.3	6.901	.012	2.5	0.4	6.455	.019
Enuresis	3.3	3.2	.001	1.000	5.2	4.6	.134	.694	3.5	2.2	1.204	.368
Dependent	15.4	6.9	5.770	.031	12.4	4.3	1.479	.000	9.5	6.3	2.683	.129
Afraid of school	4.4	1.6	2.218	.218	1.4	0.8	.620	.424	–	0.7	2.073	.275
Restless	38.5	21.9	9.448	.003	33.8	16.8	22.729	.000	19.3	12.0	7.882	.006
Inattentive	16.5	6.1	8.911	.005	22.9	8.9	22.567	.000	16.5	7.2	16.456	.000
Irritable	19.8	3.6	23.559	.000	14.3	6.3	10.436	.002	27.2	11.5	31.216	.000
Sad, depressed	3.3	0.4	4.756	.061	3.8	0.8	7.118	.020	4.7	1.1	9.956	.002
Physical complaints	7.7	2.8	3.953	.063	5.2	1.5	6.913	.017	4.1	1.1	7.547	.007

(continued)

Table 14.3 Continued

Age group	4–5 years				6–8 years				9–12 years			
	Pooled data	Mexico City	χ^2	F	Pooled data	Mexico City	χ^2	F	Pooled data	Mexico City	χ^2	F
Nightmares	5.5	1.2	**5.271**	.035	3.3	2.0	.960	.411	1.9	1.3	.430	.562
Low weight	14.3	8.1	2.891	.100	6.2	4.8	.511	.568	2.8	3.7	.423	.551
Overweight	5.5	0.8	**7.196**	.017	8.6	4.1	**5.246**	.026	11.4	8.5	1.795	.216
Disobedient	13.2	7.3	2.861	.129	13.8	5.8	**11.065**	.001	11.1	6.1	**6.204**	.016
Frequent lies	–	1.2	1.115	.567	6.7	1.0	**15.132**	.000	7.3	1.3	**18.527**	.000
Not working at school	2.2	0.4	2.430	.178	6.2	1.8	**8.336**	.007	3.5	1.3	**4.122**	.048
Explosive	9.9	3.2	**6.159**	.022	6.1	3.3	**6.675**	.017	11.1	4.8	**10.842**	.001
Convulsions	1.1	–	2.722	.269	1.4	1.8	.102	1.000	0.9	0.9	.013	1.000
Staring at emptiness	1.1	0.4	.545	.467	0.5	0.8	.169	1.000	2.2	0.7	3.583	.100
Gathers with problematic children	4.4	1.2	3.318	.087	3.8	1.3	**4.198**	.072	3.2	0.9	**5.548**	.026
Alcohol or drugs	–	–	–	–	–	–	–	–	–	–	–	–

Table 14.4 Comparative symptom prevalence on middle Brief Screening and Diagnostic Questionnaire score (5–8) by age group

Age group	4–5 years				6–8 years				9–12 years			
	Pooled data	Mexico City	χ^2	F	Pooled data	Mexico City	χ^2	F	Pooled data	Mexico City	χ^2	F
Abnormal language	26.3	13.6	1.451	.370	19.3	15.4	.220	.788	13.7	13.0	.015	1.000
Sleep problems	8.8	18.2	1.392	.255	8.6	–	2.402	.217	15.9	6.5	2.696	.152
Headaches	8.8	–	2.060	.315	15.0	3.8	2.373	.205	18.1	21.7	.312	.673
Running away	3.5	4.5	.047	1.000	1.4	–	.376	1.000	1.1	–	.510	1.000
Steals	3.5	–	.792	1.000	5.7	7.7	.152	.657	4.4	2.2	.478	.691
Nervous	52.6	50.0	.044	1.000	52.1	61.5	.778	.401	53.3	41.3	2.113	.187
Backward	17.5	13.6	.176	1.000	20.7	26.9	.498	.450	20.9	37.0	5.185	.033
Aloof	7.0	–	1.626	.572	13.6	11.5	.079	1.000	17.6	13.0	.545	.658
Enuresis	22.8	18.2	.201	.767	17.9	38.5	5.595	.033	9.3	17.4	2.438	.121
Dependent	43.9	54.5	.728	.456	35.0	38.5	.115	.824	30.8	28.3	.109	.858
Afraid of school	10.5	9.1	.036	1.000	4.3	7.7	.555	.612	1.1	–	.510	1.000
Restless	78.9	63.6	1.968	.247	71.4	80.8	.968	.471	47.8	52.2	.281	.624
Inattentive	61.4	54.5	.310	.616	68.6	65.4	.102	.820	56.6	56.5	.000	1.000
Irritable	50.9	72.7	3.091	.127	48.6	42.3	.345	.670	70.3	52.2	5.447	.023
Sad, depressed	21.1	27.3	.349	.561	19.3	19.2	.000	1.000	33.0	28.3	.374	.599

(continued)

Table 14.4 Continued

Age group	4–5 years				6–8 years				9–12 years			
	Pooled data	Mexico City	χ^2	F	Pooled data	Mexico City	χ^2	F	Pooled data	Mexico City	χ^2	F
Physical complaints	21.1	22.7	.026	1.000	22.1	15.4	.602	.602	15.9	13.0	.236	.819
Nightmares	5.3	4.5	.017	1.000	12.9	15.4	.122	.754	13.7	13.0	.015	1.000
Low weight	24.6	31.8	.428	.574	14.3	11.5	.139	1.000	11.0	13.0	.153	.795
Overweight	3.5	9.1	1.029	.309	15.0	7.7	.981	.536	19.2	30.4	2.732	.110
Disobedient	57.9	63.6	.217	.799	50.7	46.2	.182	.831	46.7	54.3	.859	.410
Frequent lies	10.5	27.3	3.456	.083	22.9	15.4	.721	.604	30.8	41.3	1.846	.219
Not working at school	14.0	–	3.436	.098	22.1	19.2	.109	1.000	22.5	30.4	1.254	.334
Explosive	45.6	31.8	1.242	.316	37.1	34.6	.060	1.000	57.1	37.0	6.008	.020
Convulsions	5.3	4.5	.017	1.000	5.0	7.7	.310	.633	1.6	–	.768	1.000
Staring at emptiness	8.8	4.5	.404	1.000	11.4	19.2	1.208	.332	11.0	13.0	.153	.795
Gathers with problematic children	14.0	4.5	1.416	.432	15.0	3.8	2.373	.205	13.2	19.5	1.207	.347
Alcohol or drugs	–	–	–	–	–	–	–	–	–	–	–	–

Table 14.5 Comparative symptom prevalence on high Brief Screening and Diagnostic Questionnaire score (≥ 9) by age group

Age group	4–5 years				6–8 years				9–12 years			
	Pooled data	Mexico City	χ^2	F	Pooled data	Mexico City	χ^2	F	Pooled data	Mexico City	χ^2	F
Abnormal language	39.4	75.0	1.843	.296	33.3	30.0	.045	1.000	25.2	14.3	.823	.520
Sleep problems	39.4	50.0	.166	1.000	33.3	20.0	.731	.494	37.4	21.4	1.411	.381
Headaches	24.2	50.0	1.200	.291	31.0	20.0	.513	.718	38.8	42.9	.086	.781
Running away	15.2	–	.701	1.000	2.4	10.0	1.679	.289	5.0	–	.739	1.000
Steals	9.1	–	.396	1.000	13.1	–	1.483	.600	21.6	14.3	.409	.735
Nervous	81.8	100	.868	1.000	82.1	40.0	9.148	.007	79.1	78.5	.002	1.000
Backward	39.4	25.0	.314	1.000	45.2	80.0	4.321	.048	52.5	35.7	1.437	.271
Aloof	27.3	–	1.442	.554	21.4	10.0	.724	.681	25.9	21.4	.134	1.000
Enuresis	24.2	25.0	.001	1.000	22.6	–	2.835	.204	15.8	21.4	.292	.703
Dependent	81.8	50.0	2.131	.198	61.9	50.0	.531	.508	51.8	42.9	.407	.584
Afraid of school	18.2	25.0	.108	1.000	20.2	20.0	.000	1.000	11.5	14.3	.094	.671
Restless	15.2	–	.701	1.000	77.4	90.0	.850	.683	77.0	92.9	1.896	.304
Inattentive	87.9	50.0	3.768	.115	85.7	90.0	.138	1.000	84.2	100	2.588	.223
Irritable	90.9	100	.396	1.000	86.9	70.0	2.015	.167	87.1	92.9	.394	1.000
Sad, depressed	42.4	75.0	1.524	.315	51.2	60.0	.278	.742	64.0	64.3	.000	1.00
Physical complaints	51.5	50.0	.003	1.000	35.7	20.0	.983	.486	42.9	50.0	.296	.587

(continued)

Table 14.5 Continued

Age group	4–5 years				6–8 years				9–12 years			
	Pooled data	Mexico City	x^2	F	Pooled data	Mexico City	x^2	F	Pooled data	Mexico City	x^2	F
Nightmares	27.3	25.0	.009	1.000	31.0	10.0	1.916	.272	32.4	21.4	.708	.550
Low weight	48.5	50.0	.003	1.000	33.3	40.0	.177	.730	19.4	50.0	6.879	.016
Overweight	3.0	25.0	3.368	.207	21.4	30.0	.378	.688	33.8	50.0	1.459	.250
Disobedient	84.8	75.0	.255	.524	86.9	80.0	.358	.625	73.4	50.0	3.394	.116
Frequent lies	54.5	–	4.249	.105	52.4	40.0	.548	.519	66.9	64.3	.039	1.000
Not working at school	24.2	50.0	1.200	.291	54.8	80.0	2.328	.181	52.5	57.1	.109	.786
Explosive	84.8	50.0	2.824	.155	82.1	100	2.125	.356	77.0	85.7	.562	.736
Convulsions	–	–	–	–	2.4	20.0	6.809	.055	2.9	28.6	16.945	.003
Staring at emptiness	24.2	25.0	.001	1.000	33.3	50.0	1.090	.313	28.8	21.4	.340	.758
Gathers with problematic children	21.2	25.0	.030	1.000	32.1	20.0	.618	.719	32.4	28.6	.084	1.000
Alcohol or drugs	–	–	–	–	–	–	–	–	1.4	–	.204	1.000

Table 14.6 Comparative prevalence of Brief Screening and Diagnostic Questionnaire syndromes by age groups

Age group	4–5 years				6–8 years				9–12 years			
	Pooled data (n = 179)	Mexico City (n = 273)	x^2	F	Pooled data (n = 434)	Mexico City (n = 430)	x^2	F	Pooled data (n = 637)	Mexico City (n = 519)	x^2	F
Externalized												
ADHD-combined	15.4	2.6	25.403	.000	16.1	3.0	41.724	.000	17.6	2.7	65.245	.000
ADHD-inatenttive severe	3.3	1.1	2.740	.096	8.3	0.7	28.925	.000	6.1	1.0	20.790	.000
ADHD-inatenttive mild	5.5	1.1	7.643	.007	4.1	0.9	9.010	.002	3.9	0.6	13.552	.000
ADHD-hyperactive-impulsive	12.1	4.4	9.417	.002	9.2	1.9	22.276	.000	6.4	2.1	12.406	.000
Oppositional behaviour	25.8	5.8	36.682	.000	25.3	3.3	85.744	.000	20.9	3.9	72.190	.000
Conduct problem: severe	6.0	0.4	13.765	.000	8.3	1.2	24.307	.000	8.9	1.0	35.924	.000
Conduct problem: mild	4.4	0.7	6.851	.011	3.7	1.4	4.570	.026	8.0	2.1	19.526	.000
Explosive conduct	14.3	1.8	26.800	.000	16.1	1.6	55.951	.000	17.5	2.5	63.717	.000
Feeding/ weight												
Low weight mild	1.7	2.9	.716	.538	3.7	1.4	4.570	.050	4.7	3.3	1.508	.234
Low weight severe	10.4	0.0	29.848	.000	5.1	0.9	12.677	.000	2.8	0.2	12.265	.000
Overweight mild	6.1	1.8	5.892	.019	6.2	1.9	10.567	.002	6.6	3.1	7.396	.007
Overweight severe	0.5	0.4	.085	.639	3.5	0.0	15.124	.000	5.7	0.8	20.395	.000

(continued)

Table 14.6 Continued

Age group	4–5 years				6–8 years				9–12 years			
	Pooled data (n = 179)	Mexico City (n = 273)	χ^2	F	Pooled data (n = 434)	Mexico City (n = 430)	χ^2	F	Pooled data (n = 637)	Mexico City (n = 519)	χ^2	F
Internalized												
Generalized anxiety	24.2	6.6	28.857	.000	20.5	3.7	57.008	.000	22.4	3.7	83.778	.000
Anxiety with inhibition	17.6	5.8	16.012	.000	18.2	3.3	50.239	.000	14.3	2.9	44.590	.000
Depression-2 severe	8.8	2.6	8.881	.003	11.5	1.9	32.188	.000	16.9	2.1	67.223	.000
Depression-2 mild	1.1	1.1	.000	.663	0.7	0.7	.000	.652	3.0	0.8	7.176	.005
Depression-1 severe	18.7	3.3	30.354	.000	17.3	3.5	44.034	.000	18.2	3.7	58.695	.000
Depression-1 mild	8.8	3.6	5.377	0.18	7.1	1.2	19.344	.000	7.1	3.3	8.088	.003
Other												
Language, severe	10.4	2.2	14.363	.000	8.5	0.9	27.565	.000	7.1	0.2	35.344	.000
Language, mild	6.6	2.9	3.519	.052	3.5	1.9	2.123	.106	2.5	0.8	5.099	.018
Enuresis	0.4	–	–	–	0.7	–	–	–	0.6	–	–	–
Epilepsy	6.0	0.7	11.150	.001	6.5	1.4	14.607	.000	6.4	1.2	20.444	.000
Epilepsy probable	2.2	0.7	1.815	.176	2.3	0.9	2.588	.091	2.5	0.2	10.615	.001
Explosive conduct, organic	3.3	1.5	1.720	.162	3.2	0.2	11.344	.000	6.9	0.8	27.061	.000

ADHD, attention deficit–hyperactivity disorder.

Among the externalized syndromes is noteworthy that along with the increase in the combined attention deficit–hyperactivity disorder (ADHD), oppositional, and conduct problems, there is also a significant and steady increase in the report of explosive behaviour for all age groups.

Among internalizing manifestations both anxiety syndromes show a significant increase with variations across age groups in a similar manner to that observed in the 1995 study.

Depressive syndrome with both irritable and depressed mood as cardinal symptoms shows an increasing prevalence from preschool to late childhood, whereas depressive syndrome with only one cardinal symptom, predominantly irritable mood, shows a consistent increase across all age groups.

Among the other syndrome groups, those with higher threshold definitions show a significant increase in all age groups versus those with less stringent criteria. Explosiveness, possibly associated with brain damage, shows a significant increase, most notably for older school-age children.

Among the feeding/weight-related syndromes, severe low weight and mild overweight show a higher prevalence across all age groups versus 1995 data, whereas severe overweight shows higher prevalence among school-age children in recent studies.

Whenever symptoms were reported as present in the CBTD, the respondent was asked if he/she had considered the need of mental health services for the child. Results are presented in Table 14.7 and show notable differences to results from the 1995 study and an increasing need for attention as related to children's age, similar to 1995.

Groups of CBTD syndromes are also presented in Table 14.7. Externalized, as well as both mixed-type syndromes, are more frequent in recent studies and across all age groups, whereas internalized syndromes are only more frequent in late school-age children.

Discussion

Our study has several limitations. Firstly, The pooled sample from the recent studies do not represent the whole population, and for school-age children boys are over-represented versus the 1995 epidemiological data, so that any generalizations should be made with caution. Secondly, comparisons are limited to the CBTD symptom and syndrome prevalence for the whole 1995 study sample and the pooled data from recent studies, not distinguishing between boys and girls. Therefore, possible differences by sex are not considered. Thirdly, CBTD syndromes are only indicative of probable clinical conditions—they do not represent mental disorders as defined by International Classification of Diseases

Table 14.7 Need of mental health services and syndromes' groups prevalence by age

Age group	4–5 years				6–8 years				9–12 years			
	Pooled data (n = 179)	CdMX (n = 273)	χ^2	F	Pooled data (n = 434)	CdMX (n = 430)	χ^2	F	Pooled data (n = 637)	CdMX (n = 519)	χ^2	F
Needing attention	40.1	10.9	367.343	.000	50.9	11.2	702.267	.000	56.8	15.4	891.159	.000
Externalized	6.6	0.7	12.634	.000	6.0	0.9	16.504	.000	4.2	0.8	13.179	.000
Internalized	2.7	2.9	.012	.578	5.3	2.3	5.200	0.17	4.7	1.7	7.767	.004
Other	1.6	0.0	4.546	.063	0.5	0.2	.325	.503	0.5	0.2	.642	.392
Mixed type1	19.9	4.7	25.778	.000	20.3	2.8	64.528	.000	20.3	4.2	64.65	.000
Mixed type2	18.7	3.6	28.343	.000	18.9	3.3	53.483	.000	19.6	2.5	79.720	.000

CdMX, Mexico City.

(ICD) or DSM diagnostic categories. Finally, although information about familial income was not estimated for the pooled sample, the population served by the health centre and both schools broadly correspond to low- and medium-to-low-income families, which represent 60% of the total population.

The strengths of this study are firstly, the same screening instrument and criteria were used in the different studies across time, so that confounding due to changes in reporting is somehow limited. Secondly, children with a higher number of reported symptoms also show higher impairment scores. Moreover, the mean score found on the BIS, 15 points, in children with ≥ 9 symptoms reported on the CBTD, is almost the same as the cut-off point of 14 proposed by the authors in order to define probable cases [17], thus variability on prevalence estimates is also limited.

The main goal for this chapter was to find out what has changed in the reporting of behavioural symptoms and syndromes in Mexican children living in different areas of Mexico City.

Across all age groups, nervousness, restlessness, inattentiveness, irritability, and explosiveness show significant reported increases in children not considered as probable 'cases' based on the cut-off point, with fewer reported symptoms in the screening questionnaire. Notably, in preschool-age children, the differential ratio for irritability between prevalence in the pooled data and results from 1995 show a fivefold increase, which is higher than that observed for the other symptoms. However, this ratio diminishes and becomes practically the same as for these other behaviours in school-age children.

Could the observed increase, especially for irritability and explosive behaviours in preschoolers, be the result of different sources of tension in the familial and social envirinment as a whole? Have these behaviours become accepted as 'normal'?

Notably, for children with a CBTD score of 5–8 symptoms, but not for the group with the highest score, irritability and explosiveness in late school-age are the only two symptoms with a significant increase compared with 1995 data.

Lastly, and of great concern, is the fact that frequent lying, aloofness, running away from home, stealing, and restlessness were not reported for the more symptomatic preschool-age children in 1995 versus recent studies, as well as the reporting of alcohol or drugs use in older school-age children, suggesting that there have been considerable changes negatively affecting the mental health status of children living in areas with more economic and social disadvantage conditions.

A study investigating the prevalence of psychiatric disorders in junior high students found that prevalence was higher, especially major depressive disorder, in students from public schools than in private schools [18].

Independently of any causal explanations, these findings suggest that in terms of symptoms, irritability and explosiveness are core behaviours that should be considered for surveillance and study starting from early-age stages. Moreover, in exploring pooled data and information from clinical samples, not included for this chapter, in more depth we have identified a strong association between the early report of explosive and irritable behaviour, not evident in 1995 data, that is currently under study. Moreover, Dougherty et al. [19, 20] have presented results from longitudinal studies showing that preschool irritability predicted increases in anxiety, depressive, and disruptive behaviour disorder symptoms at the ages of 6 and 9 years.

Taking into account the diferential ratios between the prevalence of syndromes in the pooled data and the 1995 study, explosiveness clearly becomes an issue. Explosiveness as an exacerbated conduct syndrome is 7.9, 10, and 7 times more frequent for each age group, respectively, in recent studies versus prevalence in 1995. The more symptomatic definition of explosiveness in the CBTD, suggesting probable organic damage, has been shown to be less prevalent in both the pooled data and in the 1995 study; however, the results show a significant 16- and 8.6-fold increase, respectively, for school-age children's groups, while for preschoolers a non-significant 2.2-fold increase was found. Is this because explosiveness has become normatively frequent and expected until it clearly interferes at school age?

The differential ratios for explosiveness are important when compared with other frequent and clinically relevant externalized and internalized syndromes. For example, ADHD is 5.9, 5.3, and 6.5 times more frequent in each age group in recent studies; general anxiety syndrome is 3.6, 5.5, and 6 times more frequent for each age group, respectively, in the pooled data versus 1995.

As a non-specific behavioural syndrome explosiveness has bio-social roots. Both are of special interest for psychosocial researchers, as well as for clinicians and epidemiologists.

Explosiveness may be a component associated with different medical conditions, including neuropsychiatric and neurodevelopmental problems, but can also be the outcome of nurtural deficiencies. Both CBTD screening syndromes (probable organic and as a noticeable conduct) showed a high positive predictive power as indicators of any psychiatric diagnosis in the general practice [8] Results from the health centre study have found explosiveness to be associated with depressive syndromes, mainly when irritable mood is the cardinal symptom, and with ADHD-impulsive syndrome in highly symptomatic children [21].

In sum, explosiveness seems to be a relevant issue for surveillance and study as an emerging indicator of actual or eventual psychopathology. Our findings replicate, somehow, results presented by Matijasevich et al. [1] about the increase in externalizing problems and aggressive behaviour in Brazilian preschoolers, and extend suggestive evidence on the same path into school-age Mexican children.

Lastly, parents' perceived need for mental health advice for their children is considerably higher in recent studies versus 1995. Data on the use of psychiatric services in Mexico City during 2010 showed that 43.5% of the total consultations corresponded to child psychiatrists. ICD-10 diagnostic categories for children attending the outpatient service of the Child Psychiatric Hospital were as follows: behaviour disorders (F90-F98) 39.6%; affective disorders (F30-F39) 30%; neurotic and somatoform disorders (F40-F49) 8%; psychological developmental disorders (F80-F89) 4.4% [22].

A study reviewing 100 clinical files of children attending medical services provided by the Popular Security System in a northern state of Mexico between January 2011 and December 2013 showed that 78% were sent by the schools. The most frequent motives were conduct problems, restlessness, bothering other children, aggressiveness, not completing school work, disobediency, having troubles with other children, and biting other children [23].

As a whole, the results suggest that there has been an increase in the prevalence of almost all of the CBTD behavioural syndromes from the pooled data from recent studies versus results from the epidemiological survey carried out in 1995 in Mexico City, and that mixed-type clinical manifestations are more frequently presented than just externalized or internalized problems across all age groups, following the same path as previously observed in 1995.

Our estimate of 20.7% of children with ≥ 9 symptoms is higher than the estimated 12.3% worldwide pooled prevalence for any mental disorder in children aged 6–11 years reported in a recent thorough meta-analysis [24]. Also, the severe and early behaviour problems that were absent in the most symptomatic preschoolers in 1995, possibly associated with different types of disadvantages, as shown by the social contexts from where data for recent studies were obtained, are a matter of public mental health concern as childhood psychological problems tend to be chronic and have a long-lasting impact on later life [25–27]. An example, is the report of alchol consumption in older school-age children, which is another behaviour clearly indicating considerable mental health problems.

Efforts toward research, prevention, early detection, and attention of the different mental health problems in children should be a public health priority. However, the magnitude is high above the available mental health services so that educators, general practitioners, and paediatricians should be involved, capable, and willing to deal with these emerging needs.

References

1. Matijasevich A, Murray E, Stein A, Anselmi L, Menezes AM, Santos IS, et al. Increase in child behavior problems among urban Brazilian 4 year olds: 1993 and 2004 Pelotas birth cohorts. *Journal of Child Psychology and Psychiatry* 2014; **55**: 1125–1134.

2. Collinshaw S. Secular trends in child and adolescent mental health. *Journal of Child Psychology and Psychiatry* 2015; **56**: 370–393.

3. Caraveo-Anduaga J, Nicolini SH, Villa RA, Wagner EF. Psicopatología en familiares de tres generaciones: un estudio epidemiológico en la Ciudad de México. *Salud Pública De México* 2005; **47**: 20–26.

4. Caraveo JJ. Familial risk across three generations and psychosocial correlates for developing psychopathology in a changing world. *Journal of Child Adolescent Behavior* 2014; **2**: 131.

5. Salgado de Synder VN, Díaz-Pérez MJ. Los trastornos afectivos en la población rural. *Salud Mental* 1999; **22**: 68–74.

6. Sarmiento AR. *Detección de Problemas de Salud Mental en una Población Rural.* Puebla: Universidad Popular Autónoma del Estado de Puebla, 2000.

7. Caraveo-Anduaga JJ. Adversidad social y el reporte de conducta en niños y adolescentes. *Fromm, Humanismo y Psicoanálisis* 2010; **3**: 14–24.

8. Caraveo-Anduaga JJ, López-Jiménez JL, Soriano-Rodríguez A, López-Hernández JC, Contreras-Garza A, Reyes-Mejía A. Contreras G. Eficiencia y validez concurrente del CBTD para la vigilancia de la salud mental de niños y adolescentes en un centro de atención primaria de México. *Revista De Investigación Clínica* 2011; **63**: 590–600.

9. Benjet C, Borges G, Medina-Mora M, Zambrano J, Aguilar-Gaxiola S. Youth mental health in a populous city of the developing world: results from the Mexican adolescent mental health survey. *Journal of Child Psychology and Psychiatry* 2009; **50**: 386–395.

10. Benjet C, Borges G, Medina-Mora ME, Zambrano J, Cruz C, Méndez E. Descriptive epidemiology of chronic childhood adversity in Mexican adolescents. *Journal of Adolescent Health* 2009; **45**: 483–489.

11. Caraveo AJ, Martínez N, Rivera E. Un modelo para estudios epidemiológicos sobre la salud mental y la morbilidad psiquiátrica. *Salud Mental* 1998; **21**: 48–57.

12. CONEVAL. Indice de rezago social 2010 a nivel municipal y por localidad. Available at: http://www.coneval.org.mx/Medicion/IRS/Paginas/%C3%8Dndice-de-Rezago-social-2010.aspx (accessed 23 October 2016).

13. INEGI. Censo de Población y Vivienda 2010, México. Available at: http://www.inegi.org.mx/est/contenidos/proyectos/ccpv/cpv2010/ (accessed 10 February 2016).

14. PGJDF. Informe Estadístico Delicitivo en el Distrito Federal, en el 2010, México. Available at: http://www.pgjdf.gob.mx/index.php/procuraduria/estadisticas (accessed 23 October 2016).

15. Caraveo-Anduaga J. Cuestionario Breve de tamizaje y diagnóstico de problemas de salud mental en niños y adolescentes, CBTD: confiabilidad, estandarización y validez de construcción. *Salud Mental* 2006; **29**: 65–72.

16. Caraveo-Anduaga J. Cuestionario Breve de tamizaje y diagnóstico de problemas de salud mental en niños y adolescentes: algoritmos para síndromes y su prevalencia en la Ciudad de México. *Salud Mental* 2007; **30**: 48–55.

17. **Bird HR, Canino GJ, Davies M, Ramírez R, Chávez L, Duarte C**, et al. The brief impairment scale (BIS): A multidimensional scale of functional impairment for children and adolescents. *Journal of the American Academy of Child & Adolescent Psychiatry* 2005; **44**: 699–707.

18. **De la Peña F, Gómez C, Heinze G, Palacios L**. Social adversity and psychiatric disorders: comparative study among junior high-school students in public and private schools. *Salud Mental* 2014; **37**: 483–489.

19. **Dougherty LR, Smith VC, Bufferd SJ, Kessel E, Carlson GA, Klein DN**. Preschool irritability predicts child psychopathology, functional impairment, and service use at age nine. *Journal of Child Psychology and Psychiatry* 2015; **56**: 999–1007.

20. **Dougherty LR, Smith VC Bufferd SJ, Stringaris A, Leibenluft E, Carlson GA, Klein DN**. Preschool irritability: longitudinal associations with psychiatric disorders at age 6 and parental psychopathology. *Journal of the American Academy of Child & Adolescent Psychiatry* 2013; **52**: 1304–1313.

21. **Caraveo-Anduaga JJ**. *Vigilando la Salud Mental Infantil en Atención Primaria.* Saarbrüchen: Editorial Académica Española, 2016.

22. **SAP**. Anuario estadístico 2010, México, Secretaría de Salud. Available at: http://www.sap.salud.gob.mx/principales/estad%C3%ADsticas/anuario-estad%C3%ADstico.aspx (accessed 21 November 2016).

23. **Figueroa A, Campbell C**. Health's social determinants: their relevance for children's mental health. *Boletín Clínico Del Hospital Infantil Del Estado De Sonora* 2014; **31**: 66–76.

24. **Polanczyk GV, Salum GA, Sugaya LS, Caye A, Rodhe LA**. A meta-analysis of the worldwide prevalence of mental disorders in children and adolescents. *Journal of Child Psychology and Psychiatry* 2015; **56**: 345–365.

25. **Fergusson DM, Horwood LJ**. The Christchurch Health and Development Study: Review of findings on child and adolescent mental health. *Australian & New Zealand Journal of Psychiatry* 2001; **35**: 287–296.

26. **Copeland WE, Adair CE, Smetanin P, Stiff D, Briante C ,Colman I**, et al. Diagnostic transitions from childhood to adolescence to early adulthood. *Journal of Child Psychology and Psychiatry* 2013; **54**: 791–799.

27. **Costello J, Copeland W, Angold A**. Trends in psychopathology across adolescent years: what changes when children become adolescents, and when adolescents become adults? *Journal of Child Psychology and Psychiatry* 2011; **52**: 1015–1025.

Chapter 15

Common mental disorders in cities

Santosh K. Chaturvedi
and Narayana Manjunatha

Introduction

Common mental disorders (CMDs) are noted and reported globally. These have are particularly common in primary care, which also means rural dwellings. With rapid urbanization and industrialization, cities have sprouted unabated. There are even many types of cities—metropolis, cosmopolitan, those with urban slums, and so on. In 2007, the the urban population exceeded the rural population. This trend of urbanization is now a global phenomenon, causing a rapid rise in populations living in urban areas worldwide. This trend is expected to grow, with six out of ten of people living in towns and cities by 2030, and being four times faster in developing countries than in developed countries. On the bright side, this urbanization is providing an opportunity for the economic development of mankind [1], but, on the flip side, increases vulnerability to many illnesses, especially non-communicable diseases (NCDs) and mental health problems [2]. Cities no longer mean neat, clean, well-developed localities with all facilities, high-rise buildings, large shopping complexes, and for the rich or middle class, but there are also urban slums, and pockets of lodgings with overcrowding, stark poverty, and dismal living conditions.

This chapter focuses on CMDs in cities. It also intends to provide examples of any best practices in the prevention and management of CMDs in cities. CMDs, as the name suggests, are the most common psychiatric disorders in the general population. These are also considered to be minor mental disorders, or neurotic and stress-related spectrum disorders. However, in view of urbanization and globalization, it would be interesting to review the details of CMDs in cities, which would help us provide proper service allocation and healthcare budgets. For the sake of this chapter, we have chosen a simple meaning of 'city' as a densely populated urban area with its less-populated surrounding territory, sharing industry, infrastructure, and housing.

CMDs affect individuals in different age groups and, when present in children and adolescents, may be early and less specific manifestations of more serious mental disorders, also impairing the social relationships and school performance of this population. Early identification of CMDs and their main risk factors can contribute to specific interventions and a better prognosis.

CMDs

The CMDs comprise the triad of somatoform, anxiety & depressive disorders, characterized mainly by the presence of symptoms of depression and anxiety, and various non-specific and somatic complaints [3]. CMDs are believed to be a signal of a breakdown in normal functioning and manifest as a mixture of somatic, anxiety, and depressive symptoms, frequently seen in primary care settings. The consequences of CMDs are numerous, often contributing to psychological and somatic distress, discrimination, social isolation, low occupational and academic performance, and increased mortality [4]. A brief description of each of the CMDs is given in the following subsections.

Depressive disorders

Depressive disorders are characterized by feelings of sadness, low mood, lack of interest in surroundings, negative thoughts, low self-esteem, inability to cope with day-to-day stresses, poor sleep, and poor appetite. The stresses are likely to be related to the stresses of living in the city, as mentioned earlier, including difficulties in commuting, transportation, and traffic jams, which a number of cities are famous for. Suicide itself is generally not a feature of such depression in CMDs, but suicidal gestures or attempts may occur frequently [5].

The depressive disorders could be in the form of episodes or continuous, such as a dysthymia. The depression is usually reactive in nature. Given the high prevalence of NCDs in urban areas, depression could also be comorbid with the NCDs and their treatment.

Anxiety disorders

Anxiety spectrum disorders consist of generalized anxiety disorders, panic disorders, and phobias. These are characterized by feelings of tension, fear, and apprehension, anxious foreboding, and nervous tension, stiffness of muscles, worrying thoughts, restlessness, inability to relax, and poor sleep and appetite. Autonomic symptoms of anxiety have also been reported [5].

The first panic attack is often totally spontaneous, characterized by extreme fear and a sense of impending doom. Physical signs include palpitation, tachycardia, dyspnoea, and sweating. The attack is brief, and usually lasts for 10–30 minutes, rarely longer. Comorbidity is common with panic disorder; around 30–90% of patients have other comorbid anxiety disorders, and around 50% have major depression.

Social anxiety and fears of facing crowds in buses, tubes, and metros in the cities are likely to affect city dwellers. Those with claustrophobia may have difficulty in using elevators and lifts. In social phobia, inappropriate anxiety is experienced in situations in which the person is observed and could be criticized. They tend to avoid such situations. The situations include restaurants, canteens, dinner parties, seminars, board meetings, and other public places. Many such situations are likely in cities.

Persons with agoraphobia avoid situations where help is not easily available. Agoraphobia includes fears not only of open spaces, but also situations like crowded stores, closed spaces, busy streets, and wherever there is a difficulty of immediate or easy escape to a safe place. It is one of the most incapacitating of phobic disorders. Severely affected individuals become completely housebound, especially women, making them house-bound housewives.

Somatoform disorders

Somatoform disorders have been described as bodily distress disorders in the 11th Revision of the International Classification of Diseases (ICD-11). These are characterized by physical complaints for which no obvious, serious, or demonstrable organic findings are found. There is some evidence that psychological factors, stresses, or conflicts seem to be initiating, exacerbating, and maintaining the bodily symptoms [5].

The main clinical features are multiple, recurrent, and frequently changing physical symptoms, which have usually been present for several years. Most patients have a long and complicated history of consulting several doctors. Symptoms include gastrointestinal sensations, multiple skin symptoms, sexual complaints, and menstrual irregularities. The presentation of bodily symptoms may constitute an idiom of distress. In many cultures, the presentation of personal or social distress in the form of somatic complaints is the norm. Somatic neurosis is a chronic neurotic syndrome among muslim women in India who report multiple somatic symptoms. This somatic neurosis is different from anxiety neurosis and depressive neurosis. Sociocultural factors contribute to these differences [5].

Clinicians and psychiatrists identify a pattern among women living in the crowded Jama Masjid area in the large city of Delhi, India, as having a locally popular illness, 'Jama Masjid Syndrome', which is characterized by multiple bodily symptoms for which they are permitted by the house elders to move out of the home and visit a medical professional. The women are ordinarily confined to within the household, and seeking medical consultation provides them an opportunity to visit the city [6].

Persons with somatic symptoms are more likely to be recurrent visitors to healthcare systems, go doctor shopping, and are also likely to have a better outcome in terms of survival than those with chronic psychosis or severe mental disorders [7]. It may appear as 'the survival of the sickest', as those with bodily distress are in touch with their physicians and their health anxiety contributes to their survival being better than those with other psychiatric disorders.

Other non-psychotic disorders are obsessive compulsive disorders, dissociative disorders, sleep disorders, and other stress-related non-specific disorders. Of these common dissociative disorders, trance and possession are mainly seen in villages and rural areas, and not in the cities.

Mental health problems associated with social media, mobile technology, the Internet, and the virtual world are likely to result in an entirely new range of mild, CMDs in the days to come, maybe sooner than expected.

Prevalence of CMDs in cities

About 90% of mental disorders are non-psychotic disorders [8]. Because of the high prevalence of these disorders in the general population (20–30%), these are usually called 'common mental disorders' (CMDs) [3]. There is evidence of the high prevalence of CMDs, i.e. 30% in community samples and approximately 50% in primary care samples across a range of settings, especially in low-and-middle-income countries [9–11].

A first meta-analysis published from the data of 20 adult population surveys from developed countries since 1985 found higher rates for CMDs in a pooled total of prevalence rates (38% higher in major depression, 21% higher in anxiety disorder) in urban (mostly cities) than in rural areas [12].

A UK study found the prevalence rate of CMDs in an inner-city population to be nearly double that of a national study estimate. Specific to a depressive episode, a fourfold greater proportion of the inner-city sample had CMDs than the national sample, after adjusting for sociodemographic and socio-economic indicators for all outcomes [13].

A recent large national study [14] compared the prevalence of major depression across four categories of urbanicity—(1) large metropolitan areas, (2) small metropolitan areas, (3) semi-rural areas, and (4) rural areas—with and without adjustment for other demographic risk factors in three consecutive annual samples (2009–11) of adolescents and adults. No association was observed between urbanicity and the prevalence of major depression with or without statistical adjustments in adolescents. However, in adult group, there were no differences in the prevalence of major depression between large metropolitan areas and rural areas, but the prevalence of MDD was slightly higher in the two intermediate urbanicity categories than in large metropolitan areas, suggesting that the move to identify mechanistic explanations for risk associated with the urban environment is premature. The prevalence of mental disorders was not higher in the most urban than in the most rural areas, but there was a slightly higher prevalence in small urban and semi-rural areas—an important finding reported for the first time requires replication studies.

A study from an under-developing country [15] found CMDs in 24% of young adults (aged 15–25 years), using the World Health Organization (WHO) Self Report Questionnaire, in Cali, a major city in Columbia with a population of approximately 2 million. Being a woman, having limited education and experiencing high levels of violence were the main risk factors for CMDs. Social capital did not emerge as a risk factor [15].

The Brazilian Longitudinal Study of Adult Health (ELSA Brasil) [16] from six Brazilian cities reported that 26.8% of the population had CMDs. The most frequent diagnostic category was anxiety disorders (16.2%), followed by depressive episodes (4.2%). More socially vulnerable groups such as women, young, non-white individuals, and those with a lower educational level are at higher risk of CMDs.

Recently published data from the National Mental Health Survey of India from nationally representative samples report that the weighted prevalence of major depressive disorder and neurotic/stress-related disorders in metro samples were 2–3 times higher than in the rural and urban non-metro populations (somatoform disorders specifically not included in this survey) [17].

The prevalence of CMDs in Brazilian adolescents was 30.0%, being higher among girls (38.4%) than boys (21.6%), and older adolescents (33.6%) than in younger adolescent (26.7%). The prevalence of CMDs increased with age for both sexes, always being higher in girls than in boys [18]. In another Brazilian study [19], the overall prevalence of CMDs was 29.6%. It was higher in women and prevalence increased with age, lower income group, lower education, alcohol and smoking habits, and living without a partner (separated/widowed). An interesting finding from this study is the inverse association between physical activities during leisure time with the prevalence of CMDs, after adjusting for confounding variables.

Both psychosocial and physical working conditions, that is, increased and repeated exposure to low job control, high job demands and repetitive movements, and repeated exposure to awkward working postures and rotation of the back, were associated with a higher likelihood of CMDs in midlife and older employees in Helsinki, Finland [20].

In a meta-analysis and systematic review, Das-Munshi et al. [21] reported that migrants to higher-income countries who experienced downward mobility or under-employment were more likely to have CMDs, relative to migrants who were upwardly mobile or experienced no changes to socio-economic position. In general, immigrant populations have an increased risk of psychiatric disease. In support of this, brain-imaging studies of city-dwelling volunteers responded more to social stress, such as disapproval, than those of country-dwellers, clearly showing that people who grow up in cities process negative emotions such as stress differently from those who move to the city as adults [22]. The current issues related to immigration to many of the European countries are not only political, but likely to have mental health implications. Most immigrants end up in the cities of European countries.

In a multicentric study on urban mental health, done in India, the prevalence of CMDs was 37– 50% of all mental health problems [23].

Interactions of biology and environment: focus on CMDs in cities

Despite large amounts of neurobiological evidence for psychiatric disorders, nothing in neurobiology of mental health will become clear unless we can look at the environment through the way in which the brain interacts with it (Jim van Os in [24]). In this way, urban city life is a risk factor for majority of psychiatric disorder, including CMDs.

Even though social causation (environmental breeder hypothesis) is proposed for schizophrenia [25, 26], it is worthwhile discussing this hypothesis with respect to CMDs. Social causation (environmental breeder hypothesis) assumes that various environmental factors are believed to be causative factors for illness. The environmental factors in cities are hypothesized to be risk factors for CMDs. These environmental factors can be physical factors (air pollution, noise pollution, small housing, crowding, population density, etc.) and also social factors (stress, life events, perinatal aspects, social isolation, migration). City-dwellers face more noise, crime, slums, and population density on the road than non-city-dwellers [24]. These urban factors increase the risk of mental disorders such as depression and anxiety disorders [27].

A lot of the stress factors mentioned are more common in urban areas [28, 29]. Urbanization is modestly but consistently associated with the prevalence of psychopathology. The WHO has highlighted stress as one of the major health challenges of the twenty-first century [30]. Stress is the non-specific physiological and psychological reaction to perceived threats to our physical, psychological, or social integrity. Urban living is quickly developing as a major contributor of stress. Our world is shifting towards an urban, small-family or single-person households, and, at the same time, an ageing society. But urban living is not only about getting older; it is also about getting stressed. The following factors are implicated in work-related stress in urban cities:

◆ high work pace, time pressure;

◆ lack of control (work pace, but also related to physical risks);

◆ low participation;

◆ little support from colleagues and supervisor;

◆ poor career developments;

◆ job insecurity;

◆ long working hours;

◆ low income;

◆ sexual and/or psychological harassment;

◆ work–home imbalance.

Persistent stressful working conditions are associated with increasing absenteeism, decreasing performance and productivity, decreasing profit level, decreasing quality of work and products, increasing unsafe working practices and accident rates, increasing complaints from clients/customers, increasing violent events, and increasing occupational diseases [31].

Cities also tend to promote unhealthy lifestyles [1], such as 'convenient' diets that depend on processed foods, sedentary behaviour, smoking, and the harmful use of alcohol and other substances. These lifestyle choices are directly linked to obesity and the rise of conditions like heart disease, stroke, some cancers, and diabetes. And these conditions are increasingly concentrated in the urban poor.

Impact and consequences of CMDs in cities

There is a need to understand the burden of CMDs in cities. The overall implication of 34% of more cases in cities is essential for budget allocation and service distribution, resulting in the allocation of more services to urban areas in view of higher prevalence rates in cities and higher rates of comorbidities in urban areas [32, 33].

Presenteeism is defined in terms of lost productivity that occurs when employees come to work ill and continue to perform their work below standard performance because their illness [34]. This psychological presenteeism is a major issue in workplaces, despite it is not being measured as closely as absenteeism. It is estimated that the costs of presenteeism may be even greater than the costs of absenteeism [35, 36]. This is also true for CMDs like depressive disorders [37].

A city-based study from Silicon Valley on Information Technology and Information Technology Enabled Services (IT/ITES) professionals revealed that psychiatric caseness was noted in 36%: all had features of CMDs and none was receiving any regular medical help [38].

Comorbidity of CMDs in cities

Comorbidity among people with CMDs is higher than expected. In comparison with single illness, patients with multiple disorders are more disabled, more distressed, and use more services in the form of more consultations for mental health problems [39]. CMDs may be comorbid with non-communicable diseases, such as stroke, diabetes, cardiovascular disorders, and respiratory disorders, all of which are more common among urban areas. Patients with CMDs are also noted to have comorbid alcoholism and substance use. These illnesses are linked to non-communicable diseases, HIV, and suicide. Readers who are interested in further reading are referred to the Australian Institute of Health and Welfare [40]. There is a need for interventions to target on primary, as well as comorbid, disorders for better improvement, which eventually reduces the burden on society. Studies have reported higher rates of comorbidities among patients with CMDs in urban areas [32, 33].

Management of CMDs in cities

Most cities have good, even excessive, health facilities. Most psychiatrists and other mental health professionals prefer to work in cities. However, demands are also higher, not only from city dwellers, but also from those in smaller towns and villages seeking help in advanced healthcare facilityies in cities. There is a need to strengthen access to health care based on the expectations of the providers and the clients. These access-to-care characteristics are grouped into five A's: accessibility, affordability, awareness, availability, and acceptability [41]. This concept of access to care best suits the care of patients with CMDs in cities. Availability means the total number of services from which a user can make their choice. Accessibility refers to travel impediments (time or distance or mode of transportation) between a user's residence to service location. Affordability looks at the financial aspects of health care, which involves direct and indirect costs involved in accessing mental health care. Acceptability refers to the cultural and religious beliefs of people who seek mental health services. Accommodation means the extent to which the provider's operation is organized in ways that meet the constraints and preferences of the client [42]. Access to care varies throughout the city [43]. A detailed description of the five A's pertaining to New York is given in ThriveNYC [44].

Treating patients with CMDs at primary care settings is cost-effective. People with CMDs treated in collaborative primary care have good outcomes [45]. Overall, the integration of the care of people with CMDs is better in primary care than that of those with severe mental disorders [46]. Hence, there is need to strengthen the primary care health systems of cities, both in the public and private sectors. In addition, there is need to develop innovative training programmes for primary care physicians [47,48], especially in low-and-middle income countries in view of poor detection by primary care physicians in cities and towns [49].

Recently, the US Preventive Services Task Force has recommended universal screening for depression in all adults, especially in primary care settings [50]. It also recommended for adequate systems to be in place to implement universal screening to ensure accurate diagnosis, effective treatment, and appropriate follow-up. This recommendation also helps in the prevention and early diagnosis of depression in cities especially.

The availability of mental health services in cities in India were reported to be uneven and found to be similar to the pattern generally seen in all health services. The more affluent and well-developed sections of the city got a larger share of the services with larger availability, and the economically poorer sections and the less developed sections get less of the services in their areas [23]. There are likely to be a relatively higher number of mental health professionals in cities, because that is where they would prefer to practice and run their business, in contrast to serving in a rural area with poor facilities.

Standard pharmacological management, along with psychosocial, behavioural, and cognitive behavioural interventions, is effective in the management of CMDs in cities too. Compliance and treatment adherence may be better in cities, owing to accessibility, as compared with those from rural or township areas. Most psychopharmacological agents would be easily available too. There would be more psychologists and counsellors to provide psychosocial interventions.

Promotion and prevention activities for CMDs in cities

In general, the promotional and preventive activities for mental health and CMDs, in particular, can be carried out effectively in given number of mental health professionals and resources. Mental health first aid information can be provided to schools, colleges, industries, workplaces, and housing societies and communities.

Workplace-based interventions can be useful in cities for prevention, as well as for early detection and management, of CMDs. There is a need for an innovation in developing a model organization-based mentally healthy workplace, as well as individual based self-care models for CMDs. A systematic meta-review has evidence for empirically supported workplace interventions that help in the prevention of CMDs and also facilitates the faster recovery of employees suffering from depression and/or anxiety [51].

In view of better mental health with better urban planning, policymakers should focus on better urban planning in the designing and architecture of cities in the future, which is known to reduce CMDs in cities [52]. Successful examples of better urban planning are very few, but include, for example, efforts to improve cities' architecture to minimize the risk of CMDs or to improve safety and reduce the risk of traumatic events that can precipitate CMDs [52].

Conclusions

CMDs in cities are perhaps the most common mode of presentation of mental health problems in cities. Depression, anxiety, and bodily distress disorders present not only in general population, but also in workplaces. Not much research has been carried out on epidemiology, presentation, or outcomes of CMDs in cities. With the growing number of cities, and rapid urbanization and industrialization, demands for mental health care resources would increase rapidly. Newer city-based stresses are likely to create newer presentations of mental health problems related to social media, use of the Internet, and mobile technologies.

References

1. **World Health Organization (WHO).** *Why Urban Health Matters.* Geneva: WHO, 2010.
2. **Whiteford HA, Degenhardt L, Rehm J, Baxter AJ, Ferrari AJ, Erskine HE, et al.** Global burden of disease attributable to mental and substance use disorders: findings from the Global Burden of Disease Study 2010. *The Lancet* 2013; **382**: 1575–1586.
3. **Goldberg DP, Huxley PY.** *Common Mental Disorders: A Bio-social Model.* London: Tavistock/ Routledge, 1992.
4. **Goldberg D, Goodyer I.** *The Origins and Course of Common Mental Disorders.* New York: Routledge, 2005.
5. **Chaturvedi SK, Desai G.** Neurosis. In: **D Bhugra, K Bhui** (eds) *Textbook of Cultural Psychiatry.* New York: Cambridge University Press, 2007, pp 193–206.
6. **Chaturvedi SK, Venugopal D.** Somatisation and somatic neurosis - cross cultural variations. 2010. Available at: http://www.priory.com/psych/somatisation.htm# (accessed 23 October 2016).

7. **Chaturvedi SK, Desai G.** Survival in somatoform disorders in 100 words. *British Journal of Psychiatry* 2016; **208**: 127.

8. **World Health Organization (WHO).** *Towards a Common Language for Functioning Disability and Health – ICF.* Geneva: WHO, 2002.

9. **Shamasundar C, Murthy SK, Prakash OM, Prabhakar N, Krishna DK.** Psychiatric morbidity in a general practice in an Indian city. *British Medical Journal* 1986; **292**: 1713–1715.

10. **Hollifield M, Katon W, Spain D, Pule L.** Anxiety and depression in a village in Lesotho, Africa: a comparison with the United States. *British Journal of Psychiatry* 1990; **156**: 343–350.

11. **Araya R, Rojas G, Fritsch R, Acuña J J, Lewis G.** Common mental disorders in Santiago, Chile: prevalence and socio-demographic correlates. *British Journal of Psychiatry* 2001; **178**: 228–233.

12. **Peen J, Schoevers RA, Beekman AT, Dekker J.** The current status of urban–rural differences in psychiatric disorders. *Acta Psychiatrica Scandinavica* 2010; **121**: 84–93.

13. **Hatch SL, Woodhead C, Frissa S, Fear NT, Verdecchia M, Stewart R,** et al; SELCoH Study Team. Importance of thinking locally for mental health: data from cross-sectional surveys representing South East London and England. *PLoS One* 2012; **7**: e48012.

14. **Breslau J, Marshall GN, Pincus HA, Brown RA.** Are mental disorders more common in urban than rural areas of the United States? *Journal of Psychiatric Research* 2014; **56**: 505.

15. **Harpham T, Snoxell S, Grant E, Rodriguez C.** Common mental disorders in a young urban population in Colombia. *British Journal of Psychiatry* 2005; **187**: 161–167.

16. **Nunes MA, Pinheiro AP, Bessel M, Brunoni AR, Kemp AH, Benseñor IM,** et al. Common mental disorders and sociodemographic characteristics: baseline findings of the Brazilian Longitudinal Study of Adult Health (ELSA-Brasil). *Revista Brasileira de Psiquiatria* 2016; **38**: 91–97.

17. **National Institute of Mental Health and Neurosciences.** National Mental Health Survey 2015-2016: Summary. Bengaluru, India: National Institute of Mental Health and Neurosciences; 2016. Available at: http://www.nimhans.ac.in/sites/default/files/u197/National%20Mental%20Health%20Survey%20-2015-16%20Summary_0.pdf (accessed 6 December 2016).

18. **Lopes CS, Abreu GA, Santos DF, Menezes PR, Carvalho KMB, Cunha CF** et al. ERICA: prevalence of common mental disorders in Brazilian adolescents. *Revista de Saúde Pública* 2016; **50**(suppl. 1): 14s.

19. **Rocha SV, de Araújo TM, de Almeida MM,** Virtuoso Júnior JS. Practice of physical activity during leisure time and common mental disorders among residents of a municipality of Northeast Brazil. *Revista Brasileira Epidemiologia* 2012; **15**: 871–883.

20. **Kouvonen A, Mänty M, Lallukka T, Lahelma E, Rahkonen O.** Changes in psychosocial and physical working conditions and common mental disorders. *European Journal of Public Health* 2016; **26**: 458–463.

21. **Das-Munshi J, Leavey G, Stansfeld SA, Prince MJ.** Migration, social mobility and common mental disorders: critical review of the literature and meta-analysis. *Ethnicity & Health* 2012; **17**: 17–53.

22. **Lederbogen F, Kirsch P, Haddad L, Streit F, Tost H, Schuch P,** et al. City living and urban upbringing affect neural social stress processing in humans. *Nature* 2011; **474**: 498–501.

23. **Desai NG, Tiwari SC, Nambi S, Shah B, Singh RA, Kumar D,** et al. Urban mental health services in India: how complete or incomplete? *Indian Journal of Psychiatry* 2004; **46**: 195–212.

24. **Abbott A.** Stress and the city: urban decay. *Nature* 2012; **490**: 162–164.

25. **Park RE, Burgess EW.** *The City.* Chicago, IL: Chicago University Press, 1925.

26. **Faris R, Dunham H.** *Mental Disorders in Urban Areas.* Chicago, IL: University of Chicago Press, 1939.

27. **American Psychological Association Task Force on Urban Psychology** *Toward an Urban Psychology: Research, Action, and Policy.* Washington, DC: American Psychological Association, 2005.

28. **Freeman H.** *Mental Health and the Environment.* 1st edn. London: Churchill Livingstone, 1984.

29. **Maas J, Verheij RA, Groenewegen PP, Vries Sde, Spreeuwenberg P.** Green space, urbanity, and health: how strong is the relation? *Journal of Epidemiology and Community Health* 2006; **60**: 587–592.

30. **Adli M.** Urban stress and mental health. London: London School of Economics; November 2011. Available at: https://lsecities.net/media/objects/articles/urban-stress-and-mental-health/en-gb/ (accessed 7 October 2016).

31. **Houtman I, Jettinghoff K, Cedillo L.** Raising awareness of stress at work in developing countries: a modern hazard in a traditional working environment: advice to employers and worker representatives. Protecting workers' health, series no 6. World Health Organization, 2007.

32. **Kessler RCP, Chiu WTA, Demler OM, Walters EEM.** Prevalence, severity, and comorbidity of 12-month DSMIV disorders in the National Comorbidity Survey Replication. *Archives of General Psychiatry* 2005; **62**: 617–627.

33. **Peen J, Dekker J, Schoevers RA, Ten Have M, De Graaf R, Beekman AT.** Is the prevalence of psychiatric disorders associated with urbanization? *Social Psychiatry and Psychiatric Epidemiology* 2007; **42**: 984–989.

34. **Biron C, Brun J, Ivers H, Cooper C.** At work but ill: psychosocial work environment and well-being determinants of presenteeism propensity. *Journal of Public Mental Health* 2006; **5**: 26–37.

35. **Goetzel RZ, Long SR, Ozminkowski RJ, Hawkins K, Wang S, Lynch W.** Health, absence, disability and presenteeism cost estimates of certain physical and mental health conditions affecting US employers. *Journal of Occupational and Environmental Medicine* 2004; **46**: 398–412.

36. **The Mentally Healthy Work Place Alliance.** The financial cost of ignoring mental health in the workplace. Jan 23, 2015. Available at: https://www.headsup.org.au/news/2014/05/21/the-financial-cost-of-ignoring-mental-health-in-the-workplace (accessed 7 December 2016).

37. **Cocker F, Martin A, Scott J, Venn A, Otahal P, Sanderson K.** Factors associated with presenteeism among employed Australian adults reporting lifetime major depression with 12-month symptoms. *Journal of Affective Disorders* 2011; **135**: 231–240.

38. **Chaturvedi SK, Kalyanasundaram S, Jagadish A, Prabhu V, Narasimha V.** Detection of stress, anxiety and depression in IT/ ITES professionals in the Silicon Valley of India: a preliminary study. *Primary Care and Community Psychiatry* 2007; **12**: 75–80.

39. **Andrews G, Slade T, Issakidis C.** Deconstructing current comorbidity: data from the Australian National Survey of Mental Health and Well-Being. *British Journal of Psychiatry* 2002; **181**: 306–314.

40. **Australian Institute of Health and Welfare.** *Comorbidity of Mental Disorders and Physical Conditions 2007*. Cat. no. PHE 155. Canberra: Australian Institute of Health and Welfare, 2012.

41. **Penchansky R, Thomas JW.** The concept of access: definition and relationship to consumer satisfaction. *Medical Care* 1981; **19**: 127–140.

42. wyszewianski l. access to care: Remembering Old Lessons. *Health Services Research* 2002; **37**: 1441–1443.

43. **The Office of the Mayor.** Report: Understanding New York City's Mental Health Challenge. Available at: http://www1.nyc.gov/assets/home/downloads/pdf/press-releases/2015/thriveNYC_white_paper.pdf (accessed 7 December 2016).

44. **ThriveNYC.** A Roadmap for Mental Health for All. Available at: https://thrivenyc.cityofnewyork.us/wp-content/uploads/2016/03/ThriveNYC.pdf (accessed 7 December 2016).

45. **Collins C, Hewson DL, Munger R, Wade T.** Evolving Models of Behavioral Health Integration in Primary Care. 2010. Available at: http://www.milbank.org/wp-content/uploads/2016/04/EvolvingCare.pdf (accessed 7 December 2016).

46. **Pike KM, Susser E, Galea S, Pincus H.** Towards a healthier 2020: advancing mental health as a global health priority. *Public Health Reviews* 2013; **35**: 1–25.

47. **Manjunatha N, Singh G, Chaturvedi SK.** Manochaitanya programme for better utilization of primary health centres. *Indian Journal of Medical Research* 2017; **145**: 163–165.

48. **Manjunatha N, Kumar CN, Math SB, Thirthalli J.** Designing and implementing an innovative digitally driven primary care psychiatry program in India. *Indian Journal of Psychiatry* 2018;**60**: 236–244

49. **Manjunatha N, Chaturvedi SK.** POSEIDON study: common mental disorders. *Lancet Global Health* 2016;**4**: e518.

50. **Siu AL; US Preventive Services Task Force (USPSTF), Bibbins-Domingo K, Grossman DC, Baumann LC, Davidson KW,** et al. Screening for depression in adults: US Preventive Services Task Force Recommendation Statement. *JAMA* 2016; **315**: 380–387.

51. **Joyce S, Modini M, Christensen H, Mykletun A, Bryant R, Mitchell PB,** et al. Workplace interventions for common mental disorders: a systematic meta-review. *Psychological Medicine* 2016; **46**: 683–697.

52. **Hartig T, Kahn PH Jr.** Living in cities, naturally. Science 2016; **352**: 938–940.

Chapter 16

Suicide in cities

Kairi Kõlves, Victoria Ross, and Diego de Leo

The City was the acme of efficiency, but it made demands of its inhabitants. It asked them to live in a tight routine and order their lives under a strict and scientific control.

Introduction

Urban populations have increased rapidly in the last 50 years, from 33% of the global population living in cities in 1960, to more than 50% in 2015 [1]. Forecasts indicate a further rise to 70% of the population living in cities by 2050 [2]. Urbanization has traditionally been associated with economic development: the transition from poverty to prosperity. However, such transitions have commonly been associated with high levels of crime, congestion, and contagious diseases [3]. Overcrowding has been linked to stress and illness, and urban living is also related to higher levels of mental health disorders, such as depression, anxiety, and schizophrenia [4]. Furthermore, specific human brain structures have been shown to be associated with city living or upbringing in metropolitan areas, which alters brain responses, resulting in higher sensitivity to social stressors [5]. Given the stressful effects of urbanicity on brain function and mental health, this chapter seeks to investigate the complex relationship between city life and suicide.

Urban versus rural suicides: changing trends

Urban life has been associated with higher levels of suicide, 'By the eighteenth century the city became a metaphor for those habits—intemperance, idleness, melancholy, decline of religious faith, and licentiousness—which sermons since the seventeenth century had connected with suicide' [6, p. 462]. In 1897, Émile Durkheim wrote, 'Suicide is much more urban than rural' [7, p. 320], when comparing suicide to homicide. He also indicated that 'suicide, like insanity, is commoner in cities than in the country' [7, p. 16]. Nevertheless, Durkheim disagreed that there could be a causal link between mental disorders and suicide. Suicide rates by Durkheim's theory are dependent on the levels of social integration and regulation within a group or at societal level rather than on human mental states [7]. Furthermore, in the nineteenth century, Durkheim linked urban life with a reduction in birth rates, weakening of family bonds, changes in gender roles, social alienation, and social disintegration [6–8]. An increase in the number of people leads to a rise of the division of labour in the society. This may heighten isolation as people carrying out specialized tasks may lose a common bond, which is likely to augment the rate of suicide [9, 10]. Durkheim's theory has inspired a wealth of research, major criticisms, and further elaborations. It is also important to consider that throughout the twentieth century, there have been major changes in the social structures of cities and countryside, which may have also impacted on suicide rates. Furthermore, the importance of including psychological factors such as rates of depression and alcohol use in the analysis of cross-cultural differences in suicide rates has been agreed upon [11, 12].

As indicated by Durkheim, suicide rates were historically higher in urban areas [7]. For example, historical data from Poland show that the proportion of suicides and homicides increased from rural areas to urban centres from 1865 to 1913 [13]. Nevertheless, recent figures have shown a different trend. A body of research has observed a general trend of decline in urban suicide rates and an increase in rural trends. In the majority of countries this has led to a growing gap, with suicide rates being lower in urban areas than in rural areas. Such a trend has been noticed in a number of European and Western countries, including Australia [14, 15], Belarus [16], Canada [17], Finland [18], Lithuania [19], New Zealand [20], Scotland [21], and the USA [22, 23]. Overall, this trend seems to be prevailing for males, while in countries like Austria [24] and Hungary [25] it was observed only for males. Despite a convergence in rates between urban and rural females (i.e. a drop in urban and a rise in rural suicide rates), rates were similar for females in urban and rural areas by the end of the 2000s [24, 25]. It has been argued that the female suicide trend is less affected by rurality [24, 26, 27].

Nevertheless, there are some exceptions. In Denmark, suicide rates were shown to increase with urbanicity, with the suicide risk highest in the capital compared with rural areas for both sexes between 1981 and 1997 [28]. This difference was more pronounced for females, although urbanicity was found to be a protective factor for suicide in younger males. In England and Wales, suicide rates were higher in urban areas in the 1980s; this trend was marked in young adults in the 1990s [29].

Recently, a number of studies have employed a detailed spatial patterning. This method builds on previous analyses based on a more aggregated rurality level, but provides further information on a smaller community level as large areas may be heterogeneous and mask variations in suicide mortality [27, 30]. In addition to their earlier results [29], Middleton et al. [30] showed increased suicide rates towards the centres in England and Wales (a 'bullseye' pattern) and also a cluster of increased suicide rates in coastal and/or remote regions. In Australia, suicide rates have been shown to be associated with remoteness; however, a further spatial analysis by postal areas showed a more detailed picture, indicating that rates were significantly higher in rural and remote areas than metropolitan areas for males, but not for females, in 2004–2008 [27]. An exception to this pattern was for New South Wales, which—despite having the lowest rates of all the Australian States and Territories—had higher male suicide rates in metropolitan areas than in rural areas [27].

Urbanization caused significant changes in suicide trends of China during the end of the last century and in the early twenty-first century. Despite evidence of more accepting attitudes towards suicides in urban areas [31], higher suicide rates have been seen in rural areas of China [32]. Given that male suicide rates are generally expected to be higher than those of females (based on Western data), exceptionally, in the 1990s, female rates were higher than those of males in rural China [32]. Throughout the 1990s, suicide rates were shown to decrease for both genders in urban and rural areas, with a strong decline in young females in rural areas [33, 34]. Suicide rates continued to drop in rural areas in the 2000s, and from 2006 on male rates were higher than female rates in rural China. Despite some fluctuations in urban areas, suicide rates remained at similar levels from 2000 to 2010 [6.0 and 6.6 per 100,000, respectively]. Based on estimates by Sha et al. [34], the process of urbanization accounted for 41.8% of the decline in China's suicide rate in the 1990s and 17.7% in the 2000s.

Changes in rural and urban suicide trends have also been observed in South Korea. The association between urbanicity and the geospatial trends of suicide from 1992 to 2012 showed increases in suicide rates over time, varying by age groups across all regions [35]. Increases in suicide rates among young people and working-age adults were greater in both large urban centres and rural areas, and increases in rates for elders were far greater in rural areas. After controlling for age and gender, analyses showed that greater urban density was generally associated with lower suicide rates. This is consistent with other studies, which have observed lower rates in urban rather than rural regions of South Korea [36, 37]. Similarly to China and South Korea, higher rural suicide rates have been observed in Taiwan and Sri Lanka, a pattern shown to be closely associated to suicide methods (i.e. the availability of pesticides in rural and agricultural areas) [38, 39].

Drivers of urban–rural variation in suicide rates

The reasons for lower suicide rates in urban versus rural areas are relatively similar, globally. Somewhat controversially, several researchers have reconsidered Durkheim's views and argued that in recent times rural areas are more *socially isolated* and have lower levels of social integration [34, 40]. Increased isolation in rural areas is associated with migration to cities and other countries; therefore, it is reasonable to expect that this has contributed to changes in the population structure. Additional factors contributing to the population changes and ageing are a decrease in birth rates and longer life expectancies [34, 36, 41]. The majority of studies have also indicated socio-economic differences, rural restructuring, and socio-economic decline as adding to the burden of suicide rates in rural areas versus urban ones [35, 36, 42].

Increased isolation impacts on the availability of mental health services and social support in rural areas [10, 20, 34]. In addition, lower levels of help seeking have been associated with rural attitudes and strong masculine stereotypes in rural areas of Western countries such as Australia, New Zealand, and the USA [20, 26, 43]. These factors are reflected in the results of empirical studies on urban and rural suicide rates. For example, an Australian study found that although male suicide rates were higher in rural than urban areas, these differences became non-significant after adjusting for factors such as migrant status, area socio-economic status, and mental disorder prevalence; the addition of mental health service utilization further reduced suicide risk [40]. Similarly, research from Denmark indicated that people living in more urbanized areas were at higher suicide risk but found this risk was eliminated after adjusting for marital status, income, ethnicity, and psychiatric status [28].

As mentioned earlier, the availability of specific suicide methods in rural areas, such as pesticides in agricultural areas of China, South Korea, Taiwan, and Sri Lanka have also been attributed to differences in suicide rates in rural and urban areas. Restrictions on accessibility of firearms to date have produced mixed outcomes, with Canadian research showing a decrease in firearm suicide rates [44], and research in Australia indicating a reduction in firearm suicides, but an increase in hanging suicides in younger males [45]. Climatic conditions also have an impact on rural suicides, with studies showing an association between risk of suicide and drought in rural Australia [46, 47].

Factors related to city suicides

Although the majority of studies on suicidal behaviour and suicide prevention are conducted in metropolitan areas often linked to large hospitals [29], there is limited analysis of intra-urban factors impacting suicide rates in the city environment. It has to be considered that social processes may differ between urban and rural areas.

Social isolation and fragmentation

Studies on social processes such as social interaction and social fragmentation have provided some insight into the impact of city life on suicides. A recent study by Melo et al. [48] investigated behaviour relative to the scale of city population using three urban indicators: traffic accident fatalities, homicides, and suicides. Available data were analysed from all Brazilian cities from 1992 to 2009 and suicides in US counties from 2003 to 2007. Results showed that doubling the population of cities would result in doubling of traffic accident fatalities and more than double the number of homicides. The opposite was found for suicides, with the rate of suicides decreasing with the population growth. The non-linear trend observed for suicides appears to reflect the complexity of social processes and suggests a beneficial aspect of living in cities [48].

Other recent research has more deeply investigated the complex relationship between suicide rates and social processes in cities. A spatial analysis of suicides in the US found that social fragmentation constructs (including one-person households, one-person household renters, and residential turnover) were highly correlated with suicide in urbanized settings [26].

Deprivation and poverty

Research has shown that the influence of social deprivation and poverty may also impact on urban suicide mortality. An Australian study using individual level information from Queensland found that suicide rates in urban areas showed a positive correlation with a number of deprivation-related measures such as the unemployment rate, median individual income, the tenant households in public housing, and proportion of Indigenous Australians between 2004 and 2008 [49]. Nevertheless, there was an inverse association with the proportion of people below the age of 30 years and households without Internet access [49]. Similarly, analysis of seven South Korean metropolitan cities found that the most deprived districts had a higher risk of suicide after adjusting for individual level socio-economic variables in 2003–08 [42]. Deprivation was measured using the Cairstairs index, which includes low social class, lack of car ownership, overcrowding and male unemployment [42].

Suicide methods in the cities

The important factors in the choice of a suicide method are physical and cognitive availability, acceptability, and lethality. As indicated earlier, moving to urban areas limits access to some suicide methods, such as highly lethal pesticides. Nevertheless, there are some suicide methods that are more strongly associated with suicide in the cities. Concepts such as 'urban' or 'urbanization' do suggest the images of clusters of skyscrapers, big bridges, and subways. One of the methods associated with suicides in metropolitan areas is jumping from a height. Jumping from a height is the most common suicide method in highly urbanized cities such as Singapore and Hong Kong, where nearly 80% of the population live in skyscrapers or tall, multistorey buildings [50]. In Singapore, jumping accounted for more than 70% of suicides in 2000–04 [51], and in Hong Kong for approximately 50% of all suicides in 2002–07 [52]. The majority of people jump from their own apartments; they more frequently have major psychiatric disorders and receive psychiatric treatment than those using other methods [51, 52]. Jumping from a height has also shown to differ by the level of urbanization in Taiwan [50] and has also been found to be the most frequent suicide method in females and the second most frequent method in males in Luxembourg, where the urban population is more than 90% [53].

Subway suicides are also common in metropolitan areas, causing distress to onlookers and train drivers, as well as major delays to subway systems [54]. A systematic literature review of suicidal behaviour in subways found that the majority of those who attempt suicide on the subway were young males living alone, had serious or chronic mental illness, and did receive treatment. In addition, increased numbers of rail suicides have been found in stations in close proximity to major psychiatric hospitals [54]. A recent cluster analysis of Montreal Metro suicides showed that metro suicide cases were not a homogenous group but could be identified in five different clusters: 'isolated persons' (26.3%), characterized by being single persons without a social network and a moderate level of mental health problems; 'family women' (22.8%), who had regular contact with their family and had previous suicide attempts; 'family men with mood disorders' (19.3%), who had some relationships, were in regular contact with their family, and, in addition to mood disorders, also had problems with their work and the police; 'young psychotic men' (16.7%), who had interaction with their family and problems with police; and 'single persons with mood disorder and a social network' (14.9%), who were single persons who lived alone, had a social network, and work problems [55].

Suicide prevention

Suicide prevention in different settings is a challenging task. A recent update about suicide prevention initiatives indicated that there have been major advances in the last few decade [56]. Preventing access to means has been shown to be effective in preventing suicides, especially in cities, where jumping from multistorey buildings and bridges; subway suicides can be prevented through structural changes. Suicide pits, platform screen doors, and blue lights have been found to have potential in preventing rail-related suicides [57]. Physical barriers have also been shown to be effective in preventing suicide from popular jumping sites such as bridges and shopping centres [50, 58]. Appropriate media reporting following the implementation of media guidelines has also shown to reduce the impact of suicide clusters in subways and other 'hotspots', and to avoid the 'popularization' of new methods such as charcoal burning [57, 59]. In addition, current evidence-based programmes include school-based activities, treatment of depression, and chain of care. Further evidence is required for interventions such as gatekeeper and family practitioner's training, Internet-based interventions, helplines, and screening programmes in primary-care settings [60]. In order to get the best results, a combination of the most appropriate strategies should be tailored to the city or suburb context, depending on the socio-economic background, level of deprivation, and demographic composition.

References

1. **World Bank**. Urban population. Available at: http://data.worldbank.org/indicator/SP.URB.TOTL.IN.ZS (accessed 6 February 2017).
2. **Kennedy DP, Adolphs R**. Social neuroscience: stress and the city. *Nature* 2011; **474**: 452–453.
3. **Glaeser E**. Cities, productivity, and quality of life. *Science* 2011; **333**: 592–594.
4. **Krabbendam L, Van Os J**. Schizophrenia and urbanicity: a major environmental influence—conditional on genetic risk. Schizophrenia Bulletin, 2005; **31**: 795–799.
5. **Lederbogen F, Kirsch P, Haddad L, Streit F, Tost H, Schuch P**, et al. City living and urban upbringing affect neural social stress processing in humans. *Nature* 2011; **474**: 498–501.
6. **Kushner HI, Sterk CE**. The limits of social capital: Durkheim, suicide, and social cohesion. *American Journal of Public Health* 2005; **95**: 1139–1143.
7. **Durkheim E**. *Suicide: A Study in Sociology*. London: Routledge, 1897/1951.
8. **Kushner HI**. Suicide, gender, and the fear of modernity in nineteenth-century medical and social thought. *Journal of Social History* 1993; **26**: 461–490.

9. Durkheim E. *The Division of Labor in Society*. New York: Simon and Schuster, 1893/2014.

10. Ritzer G. *Sociological Theory*. New York: Tata McGraw-Hill Education, 1996.

11. Thompson K. *Emile Durkheim*. London: Routledge, 2003.

12. Fernquist RM. How do Durkheimian variables impact variation in national suicide rates when proxies for depression and alcoholism are controlled? *Archives of Suicide Research* 2007; **11**: 361–374.

13. Budnik A, Liczbińska G. Urban and rural differences in mortality and causes of death in historical Poland. *American Journal of Physical Anthropology* 2006; **129**: 294–304.

14. Taylor R, Page A, Morrell S, Harrison J, Carter G. Social and psychiatric influences on urban–rural differentials in Australian suicide. *Suicide and Life-Threatening Behavior* 2005; **35**: 277–290.

15. Page A, Morrell S, Taylor R, Dudley M, Carter G. Further increases in rural suicide in young Australian adults: secular trends, 1979–2003. *Social Science & Medicine* 2007; **65**: 442–453.

16. Razvodovsky Y, Stickley A. Suicide in urban and rural regions of Belarus, 1990–2005. *Public Health* 2009; **123**: 27–31.

17. Ostry AS. The mortality gap between urban and rural Canadians: a gendered analysis. *Rural and Remote Health* 2009; **9**: 1286.

18. Pesonen TM, Hintikka J, Karkola KO, Saarinen PI, Antikainen M, Lehtonen J. Male suicide mortality in eastern Finland-urban-rural changes during a 10-year period between 1988 and 1997. *Scandinavian Journal of Public Health* 2001; **29**: 189–193.

19. Gailiené D, Domanskiené V, Keturakis V. Suicide in Lithuania. *Archives of Suicide Research* 1995; **1**: 149–158.

20. Pearce J, Barnett R, Jones I. Have urban/rural inequalities in suicide in New Zealand grown during the period 1980–2001? *Social Science & Medicine* 2007; **65**: 1807–1819.

21. Levin KA, Leyland AH. Urban/rural inequalities in suicide in Scotland, 1981–1999. *Social Science & Medicine* 2005; **60**: 2877–2890.

22. Singh GK, Siahpush M. Increasing rural–urban gradients in US suicide mortality, 1970–1997. *American Journal of Public Health* 2002; **92**: 1161–1167.

23. Singh GK, Siahpush M. Widening rural–urban disparities in all-cause mortality and mortality from major causes of death in the USA, 1969–2009. *Journal of Urban Health* 2014; **91**: 272–292.

24. Kapusta ND, Zorman A, Etzersdorfer E, Ponocny-Seliger E, Jandl-Jager E, Sonneck G. Rural–urban differences in Austrian suicides. *Social Psychiatry and Psychiatric Epidemiology* 2008; **43**: 311–318.

25. Rihmer Z, Gonda X, Kapitany B, Dome P. Suicide in Hungary—epidemiological and clinical perspectives. *Annals of General Psychiatry* 2013; **12**: 21.

26. Congdon P. The spatial pattern of suicide in the US in relation to deprivation, fragmentation and rurality. *Urban Studies* 2011; **48**: 2101–2122.

27. Cheung YTD, Spittal MJ, Pirkis J, Yip PSF. Spatial analysis of suicide mortality in Australia: investigation of metropolitan-rural-remote differentials of suicide risk across states/territories. *Social Science & Medicine* 2012; **75**: 1460–1468.

28. Qin P. Suicide risk in relation to level of urbanicity—a population-based linkage study. *International Journal of Epidemiology* 2005; **34**: 846–852.

29. **Middleton N, Gunnell D, Frankel S, Whitley E, Dorling D.** Urban–rural differences in suicide trends in young adults: England and Wales, 1981–1998. *Social Science & Medicine* 2003; **57**: 1183–1194.

30. **Middleton N, Sterne JA, Gunnell DJ.** An atlas of suicide mortality: England and Wales, 1988–1994. *Health & Place* 2008; **14**: 492–506.

31. **Li X, Phillips MR.** The acceptability of suicide among rural residents, urban residents, and college students from three locations in China. Crisis. *The Journal of Crisis Intervention and Suicide Prevention* 2010; **31**: 183–193.

32. **Phillips MR, Li X, Zhang Y.** Suicide rates in China, 1995–99. *The Lancet* 2002; **359**: 835–840.

33. **Yip PS, Liu KY, Hu J, Song XM.** Suicide rates in China during a decade of rapid social changes. *Social Psychiatry and Psychiatric Epidemiology* 2005; **40**: 792–798.

34. **Sha F, Yip PS, Law YW.** Decomposing change in China's suicide rate, 1990–2010: ageing and urbanisation. *Injury Prevention* 2016; **23**: 40–45.

35. **Chan CH, Caine ED, You S, Yip PSF.** Changes in South Korean urbanicity and suicide rates, 1992 to 2012. *BMJ Open* 2015; **5**: e009451.

36. **Cheong KS, Choi MH, Cho BM, Yoon TH, Kim CH, Kim YM, Hwang IK.** Suicide rate differences by sex, age, and urbanicity, and related regional factors in Korea. *Journal of Preventive Medicine and Public Health* 2012; **45**: 70–77.

37. **Park BB, Lester D.** Rural and urban suicide in South Korea. *Psychological Reports* 2012; **111**: 495–497.

38. **Chang SS, Lu TH, Sterne JA, Eddleston M, Lin JJ, Gunnell D.** The impact of pesticide suicide on the geographic distribution of suicide in Taiwan: a spatial analysis. *BMC Public Health* 2012; **12**: 1471–2458.

39. **Knipe DW, Padmanathan P, Muthuwatta L, Metcalfe C, Gunnell D.** Regional variation in suicide rates in Sri Lanka between 1955 and 2011: a spatial and temporal analysis. *BMC Public Health* 2017; **17**: 193.

40. **Taylor R, Page A, Morrell S, Harrison J, Carter G.** Social and psychiatric influences on urban–rural differentials in Australian suicide. *Suicide and Life-Threatening Behavior* 2005; **35**: 277–290.

41. **Page A, Liu S, Gunnell D, Astell-Burt T, Feng X, Wang L, Zhou M.** Suicide by pesticide poisoning remains a priority for suicide prevention in China: Analysis of national mortality trends 2006–2013. *Journal of Affective Disorders* 2017; **208**: 418–423.

42. **Lee J, Lee WY, Noh M, Khang YH.** Does a geographical context of deprivation affect differences in injury mortality? A multilevel analysis in South Korean adults residing in metropolitan cities. *Journal of Epidemiology and Community Health* 2014; **68**: 457–465.

43. **Caldwell TM, Jorm AF, Dear KBG.** Suicide and mental health in rural, remote and metropolitan areas in Australia. *Medical Journal of Australia* 2004; **181**: S10–S14.

44. **Lester D, Leenaars A.** Suicide rates in Canada before and after tightening firearm control laws. *Psychological Reports* 1993; **72**: 787–790.

45. **Klieve H, Barnes M, De Leo D.** Controlling firearms use in Australia: has the 1996 gun law reform produced the decrease in rates of suicide with this method? *Social Psychiatry and Psychiatric Epidemiology* 2009; **44**: 285–292.

46. **Hanigan IC, Butler CD, Kokic PN, Hutchinson MF.** Suicide and drought in New South Wales, Australia, 1970–2007. *Proceedings of the National Academy of Sciences U S A* 2012; **109**: 13950–13955.

47. **Page A, Morrell S, Taylor R.** Suicide and political regime in New South Wales and Australia during the 20th century. *Journal of Epidemiology and Community Health* 2002; **56**: 766–772.

48. **Melo HPM, Moreira AA, Makse HA, Andrade JS Jr.** Statistical signs of social influence on suicides. arXiv preprint 2014; **arXiv:1402.2510**.

49. **Law CK, Snider AM, De Leo D.** The influence of deprivation on suicide mortality in urban and rural Queensland: an ecological analysis. *Social Psychiatry and Psychiatric Epidemiology* 2014; **49**: 1919–1928.

50. **Chen YY, Yip P.** Prevention of suicide by jumping. Experience from Taipei City (Taiwan), Hong Kong and Singapore. In: **D Wasserman, D Wasserman** (eds) *Oxford Textbook of Suicidology and Suicide Prevention*. Oxford: Oxford University Press, 2009, pp. 569–571.

51. **Chia BH, Chia A, Ng WY, Tai BC.** Suicide methods in Singapore (2000–2004): types and associations. *Suicide and Life-Threatening Behavior* 2011; **41**: 574–583.

52. **Wong PW, Caine ED, Lee CK, Beautrais A, Yip PS.** Suicides by jumping from a height in Hong Kong: a review of coroner court files. *Social Psychiatry and Psychiatric Epidemiology* 2014; **49**: 211–219.

53. **Värnik A, Kolves K, van der Feltz-Cornelis CM, Marusic A, Oskarsson H, Palmer A,** et al. Suicide methods in Europe: a gender-specific analysis of countries participating in the 'European Alliance Against Depression'. *Journal of Epidemiology and Community Health* 2008; **62**: 545–551.

54. **Ratnayake R, Links PS, Eynan R.** Suicidal behaviour on subway systems: a review of the epidemiology. *Journal of Urban Health* 2007; **84**: 766–781.

55. **Bardon C, Coté LP, Mishara BL.** Cluster analysis of characteristics of persons who died by suicide in the Montreal Metro transit: analysis of variations over time. *Crisis* 2016; **37**: 377–384.

56. **Zalsman G, Hawton K, Wasserman D, van Heeringen K, Arensman E, Sarchiapone M,** et al. Suicide prevention strategies revisited: 10-year systematic review. *The Lancet Psychiatry* 2016; **3**: 646–659.

57. **Barker E, Kolves K, De Leo D.** Rail-suicide prevention: Systematic literature review of evidence-based activities. Asia-Pacific Psychiatry 2017; **9**: e12246.

58. **Pirkis J, San Too L, Spittal MJ, Krysinska K, Robinson J, Cheung YTD.** Interventions to reduce suicides at suicide hotspots: a systematic review and meta-analysis. *The Lancet Psychiatry* 2015; **2**: 994–1001.

59. **Wu KCC, Chen YY, Yip PS.** Suicide methods in Asia: implications in suicide prevention. *International Journal of Environmental Research and Public Health* 2012; **9**: 1135–1158.

60. **Zalsman G, Hawton K, Wasserman D, van Heeringen K, Arensman E, Sarchiapone M.,** et al. Evidence-based national suicide prevention taskforce in Europe: a consensus position paper. *European Neuropsychopharmacology* 2017; **27**: 418–424.

Chapter 17

Sex in the city

Dinesh Bhugra and Antonio Ventriglio

Introduction

Sexual encounters in urban areas are of interest to researchers and clinicians alike. These encounters can be transient, local, and intensely physical. The purpose of sexual encounters is pleasure, intimacy, or procreation. Each purpose can influence the quality, type, and duration of encounters. In urban areas and settings these encounters can occur in highly or lightly organized venues. In this day and age these sexual encounters are also organized through the use of social media, where the sexual encounter is largely transient and purely functional. It is entirely possible that the use of social media in meeting sexual partners and its transient nature reflects the pace of life and immediacy of need rather than prolonged relationships or intimacy. This may well be a by-product in some cases. The urban space in the city may facilitate sexual partnering and sexual transactions, be they financial or emotional. Furthermore, newer approaches may affect and limit the role of traditional approaches such as churches or other social services.

Ellingson et al. [1] remind us that sexual partnerships are fundamental elements of adult social life and inevitably have important social (and personal) outcomes. The purpose of sexual partnering may well vary across cultures and cultural expectations. In sex-negative cultures the main purpose of sex is described as being procreative, whereas in sex-positive cultures the chief function of sexual activity is pleasurable [2]. Therefore, it is theoretically possible that frequency of sexual partnering may also be influenced by social and society's attitudes to sex and sexual activity. Membership of a group and associated activities, along with group norms and expectations, will influence sexual partnering, whether it occurs in the group or outwith the group. It must be remembered that sexual partnering within the group may be only what is the accepted norm; otherwise, individuals may seek sexual release elsewhere, especially if these activities are frowned at within the in-group. How are these activities organized within metropolitan urban spaces? Their understanding can give a clue to the spread of sexually transmitted diseases and associated psychiatric distress.

Another factor that might be worth exploring under these circumstances may be related to migration status, ethnicity, and gender. The vast majority of sexual partnerships originate within tightly circumscribed social settings that produce many partnerships between people with similar social characteristics, and only a few partnerships between people with dissimilar characteristics [3]. These authors go on to point out that sexual behaviour may occur as a result of 'master-status' categories (e.g. race, marital status, etc.) alluded to earlier.

It has been emphasized that sexual partnering is fundamentally a typical local process [1], where two people living in close geographical proximity to each other are more likely to initiate and develop a sexual relationship, although the initiation, in theory, may occur at a distance in terms of establishing contact, but the individual partners may go on to develop the relationship further in close proximity. It is inevitable that for people to form partnerships there needs to be a common place, be it at work, in urban spaces, through friends, or mutual acquaintances. The social factors and forces that may facilitate the formation and maintenance of these relationships and partnerships are likely to be strongly influenced by factors such as group culture, religious affiliation, sex ratios, age, marital status, and group (ethnic or religious) [1]. These sexual partnerships are thus heavily structured by the local organization of social life, the local population mix, and the shared norms guiding the types of relationships that are sanctioned, accepted, or supported. People often meet in social circles and networks where they live or work. In rural areas it may be even closer networks. However, in cultures and societies where individuals' families arrange the match, the relationships are between the families represented by the individuals. These patterns are often seen in traditional societies.

Ellingson et al. [1] illustrate the shared norms guiding the types of relationships that are sanctioned or approved. They note that a young man living in San Francisco may be more likely to consider pursuing a male sex partner than a young man living in Wyoming (p. 7). These transient or temporary sexual encounters are influenced by opportunity and availability of partners, as well as social and sexual expectations. The emphasis in sex markets depends very much upon local, social, and cultural structures, with a limitation put on channelling sexual behaviour.

Hypothetically, in an era of inter-relationship, closely connected through social media and other means, the pool of potential sexual partners is huge, but cultural, social, economic, and religious factors may facilitate or hinder these encounters. Obviously, sexual orientation and sexual behaviour in some areas may be more acceptable than in others. Associated physical illnesses, for example sexually transmitted diseases and consequent mental distress, will need to be taken into account. The attitudes of a particular neighbourhood will be determined by a number of factors, such as socialization processes, closeness of individuals, commercial factors, and so on. These attitudes will be conveyed, and strengthened or weakened, in response to networks and moral beliefs associated with that.

The role of what has been described as master status (e.g. gender, race, age, etc.) [3] is extremely important, but, in the context of urbanicity or city spaces, these characteristics go on to influence sexual partnering and outcomes. Sexual interests, sexual preferences and tastes, and social networks influence sexual relationships. In an urban context, these variables are also influenced by previous experiences and cultural factors. It has been noted that professionals in the city may dress differently and behave differently from non-professionals in the city, as well as among rural inhabitatants [1]. These external stimuli therefore become significant in signalling sexual interest and outcomes.

The sexual market has both men and women in it, but, increasingly, those who are non-binary. It is quite likely that gender variations and non-binary individuals are more common in urban areas, and these communities may further consolidate in urban areas. Dale Mortensen [4] points out that a matching market involves individuals offering themselves as bundles of traits (all or none). Thus, exchange of sexual activities may bring a certain defined value to it. Sex markets by virtue of the gathering of people for purposes of sexual contact take on the role of a business, for example terms such as 'meat market', 'catch', and so on. Are these institutions such as bars, discos, and dance places related to specific sexualities? There is no doubt that traditional market places are giving way to more individualized market places through apps such as Tindr and Grindr in the same way that people are increasingly buying merchandise online. The old marriage algorithms are therefore beginning to change [5–8]. There may be a gap between the actual matching and efficient marriage markets [8, 9]. The challenge to sex markets comes from individual characteristics [8]. It has been argued that searching for sexual partners in educational institutions such as schools, universities, etc (and perhaps in the workplace) can be more cost effective, as search costs are reduced there and information about prospective partners may be better [8]. Such an approach in our understanding of sexual partnering has the advantage of focusing on individuals alone, especially in egocentric and sex-positive cultures, but it also has the negative aspect in that it focuses entirely on individual-level dynamics and characteristics [1]. The balance between the individual and the institution is essential in our understanding of the sexual partnering. The quality and the form of sexual encounter will be determined by both social and individual expectations and cultural norms and values. Cultural, socio-economic status of the individual [10], and educational attainments will also be important factors in not only giving the individuals confidence into sexual partnering, but also in interpreting experiences. Gender [11, 12], age and sex ratio [13], education [14], and propinquity [15–17] need to be remembered.

Using the models of market sociology [18–21], Laumann et al. [22] studied sexual organization in Chicago using a number of investigative strategies. They go on to argue that the sex markets are composed of a varying distribution of role structures for men and women. It is quite likely that different genders will behave in different ways in these places. Gender roles and gender role expectations are very tightly defined by the society and cultures. There is no doubt that some of these encounters will be in public places and, depending upon the type of public place, these encounters may be one-off or may lead to more permanent relationships.

Laumann et al. [22], in their study of sexual organization in the city of Chicago, noted that sex markets are socially bound and each market is distinguished by four organizing features—character of the spatial location, attributes related to other locations, mix of local institutions, local cultural and social ties and ramifying social ties, which produce distinctive neighbourhood-based patterns.

Urban places are meeting places where social interactions take place, which include parks, churches, workplaces, and so on [23–25]. Space and sexual culture are often related, and are influenced by coordinating marketing activities [26]. Specific physical areas in cities have been identified as specified sexual activities [1]. Sexual space is not restricted to market place only. Health clubs, gyms, and churches have become places where sexual encounters, be they transient or leading to something more permanent, may occur.

Sexual cultures have been divided into internal and external. Internal cultures focus on the set of scripts, behaviours, and identities within a particular market. External cultures are paradigmatic assemblies of the social norms impinging on sexual behaviours [27, 28]. Social psychological dynamics play a major role in participants in sexual markets.

One's position in the sex market is likely to change according to age [1]. Men and women may adapt their sexual partnering strategies in response to the ageing process. It is worth noting that in many cultures the age at marriage is increasing. This is further complicated by the fact that these changes vary across the genders. Older individuals may reach their sexual partnering status in different levels and in various changed spaces in urban areas. The possibility of progressing to the marriage market from the sex market is dependent upon a number of factors. Another factor worth bearing in mind in the context of sex in the city is that of criminality. Intimate partner violence and forced sex involve different forms, even though superficially they may be related. Intimate personal violence, as well as forced sex, are related to age, ethnicity, neighbourhood, and so on. Youm and Laumann [29] provide empirical evidence that social networks can reduce the rates of sexually transmitted diseases due to third party embeddedness, which can provide critical information about sex partners [1]. Furthermore, in embedded sexual networks the phenomenon related to 'friends with benefits' may also be seen.

Organizations within the institutional sphere of health care, social service, and law enforcement are seen as controlling sexuality and sex-related health problems [1]. Although on the surface this control appears serious, in reality individuals can override these institutional barriers and expectations [30], but for some individuals this may be very difficult, especially if they have religious connotations. The institutions may attempt to control sexual behaviours, but again these may differ between ego-centric and sociocentric societies. As Ellingson et al. [1] point out, the institution may give a type of moral heterogeneity to guide sex market activity using dis-embeddedness of sexuality, even though it may offer its own definitions of good/safe sex, sexual identities and sexual relationships, cultural norms, and so on. Families, neighbourhoods, friendship networks, and social and physical spaces all provide a kind of structure.

Sex in the city takes place in an environment where search activities are heightened and potential opportunities diverse [31], and with mobile apps it has become even more readily available, and the space for potential contact for potential sexual activity is cyberspace. Such opportunities for both socializing and mixing with sexual partners are not only easily accessible with a certain degree of privacy, but also possibilities of both transient sex and potential long-term sexual partners. Multiple social processes need to be untangled.

Sex markets and sex spaces in urban areas are often well recognized as generally likely to be close to railway termini or bus stations. It is fair to note that with social media these spaces and places are beginning to change fairly rapidly in many parts of the world, although poverty and lack of access to social media still works in favour of these spaces. Grov and Smith [32] remind us that urban centres across the USA are home to concentrations of gay and bisexual men, colloquially known as gay neighbourhoods, gaybourhoods, or gay ghettos (p. 253). These are often seen as attractive places for gay and bisexual men (in particular) to converge to [33, 34], in order (perhaps) to convey a sense of freedom, as well as symbols of gay pride and freedom, as one way of reaffirming one's identity and reclaiming what may have been suppressed. In these neighbourhoods, bars, clubs, gay coffee shops and gay-themed facilities, restaurants, and so on, add to the attractions of living in these neighbourhoods [35]. This large and sometimes extended social environment is gay supportive and gay friendly [32]. These authors note that urban living is more expensive, and in non-gay neighbourhoods individuals may choose to hide their sexuality and sexual identity as they do not feel comfortable in sharing. Gay men may choose to migrate to urban gay neighbourhoods and, although social environments may be changing, younger gay men may wish to escape homophobia in smaller rural communities by moving to larger, anonymous cities. Smith and Grov [36], in their study of male sex workers, found that these individuals had a common goal of material wealth perhaps more easily available in big cities. With the sexualized environment and the commodification of sexuality in gay urban centres, young men may find the idea of sex work less stigmatizing [32].

Sex markets and sex workers

Both male and female sex workers are at risk of violence and sexually transmitted diseases, and physical and mental health consequences thereof.

Laing and Gaffney [37] point out that sex work itself is defined in a number of ways. These definitions depend upon the characteristics related to skills, labour, emotional work, and physical presentations [38]. There is no doubt that sex work exists everywhere, but in rural communities it may be less anonymous. However, it is complex, diverse, and occurs between a variety of people and in multiple settings for a number of complex reasons. The social, cultural, and *geographical* context in which sex work takes place is therefore important in understanding processes of identification in health needs of sex workers.

We do not propose to go into the reasons why people choose to use or become sex workers. The mental ill health of sex workers is often ignored in the broadest possible way by looking at the question of choice. There may be an assumption that those who chose to work as sex workers are healthier. In addition to stigma, dangers of sexually transmitted diseases, violence, and substance abuse can contribute to mental ill health. Stigma related to sex work may lead to 'covering' [39, 40] and can lead to 'concealable stigma' [41]. This puts sex workers at a greater risk of untreated mental ill health [42–46]. These poor outcomes of mental ill health may be related to chronic stress, urban living, and social marginalization and poor social support. It has been argued [41] that cross-sectional samples make it difficult to identify the cause or predictor of mental health outcomes, but male sex workers, even in privileged samples, show higher-than-expected rates of mental ill health [47–49].

Mental health of vulnerable groups (of which sex workers are one) in urban areas requires a public health approach. Bimbi and Koken [50] provide a thorough overview of the history of HIV spread in sex workers (especially male), and propose public health strategies for both sex workers and their clients. Policy changes they recommend include decriminalization of sex work and elimination of stigma through antidiscrimination interventions. Accessible health services are also important, and education of both sex workers and the clients is essential for screening of physical and mental ill health, with early diagnosis and appropriate therapeutic interventions. Of course, the common levels of public health interventions such as universal, targeted (at vulnerable individuals), and individual strategies should be employed.

Conclusion

In this chapter we have provided a brief overview of sex work, sex spaces, and urban spaces in the city. However, with increasing contact through social media, it is essential that our preventive and educational strategies should also change and map onto the needs of the society. For a strategy to be acceptable and successful it has to be culturally appropriate. For subgroups who are in sexual minorities adequate adjustments must be made. Policies at central level have to be translated into action at local levels. In urban areas these may require repetition as transient populations and transient spaces increase.

References

1. **Ellingson S, Laumann EO, Paik A, Mahay J.** The theory of sex markets. In: E O Laumann, S Ellingson, J Mahay, A Paik, Y Youm (eds) *The Sexual Organization of the City*. Chicago, IL: University of Chicago Press, 2004, pp. 3–38.
2. **Bullough V.** *Sexual Variance in Society and Culture*. Chicago, IL: University of Chicago Press, 1976.
3. **Laumann EO, Gagnon J, Michael R, Michaels S.** *The Social Organization of Sexuality: Sexual Practices in the United States*. Chicago, IL: University of Chicago Press, 1994.
4. **Mortensen DT.** Matching: finding a partner for life or otherwise? *American Journal of Sociology* 1988; **94**: 5215–5240.
5. **Gale D, Shapley S.** College admissions and stability of marriage. *American Mathematical Monthly* 1962; **69**: 9–15.
6. **Becker GS.** Theory of marriage. *Journal of Political Economy* 1973; **81**: 813–846.
7. **Becker GS.** *A Treatise on the Family*. Cambridge, MA: Harvard University Press, 1993.
8. **Becker GS, Landes M, Michael R.** An economic analysis of marital instability. *Journal of Political Economy* 1977; **85**: 1141–1187.
9. **Frey B, Eichenberger R.** Marriage paradoxes. *Rationality and Society* 1996; **8**: 187–200.
10. **DiMaggio P, Mohr J.** Cultural capital, educational attainment and marital selection. *American Journal of Sociology* 1985; **90**: 1231–1261.
11. **England R, Farkas G.** *Household, Employment and Gender: A Social Economic and Demographic View*. New York: Aldine de Gruyter, 1986.
12. **England R, Kilbourne B.** Markets, marriages, and other mates: the problem of power. In: R Friedland, PF Robertson (eds) *Beyond the Marketplace Place*. New York: Aldine de Gruyter, 1990, pp. 163–188.
13. **Oppenheimer VK.** A theory of marriage timing. *American Journal of Sociology* 1988; **94**: 563–591.

14. **Mare R.** Five decades of educational assortative mating. *American Sociological Review* 1991; **56**: 15–32.

15. **Kalmijin M.** Status homogamy in the United States. *American Journal of Sociology* 1991; **97**: 496–523.

16. **Lichter D, LeClere F, McLaughlin D.** Local marriage market and the marital behaviour of black and white women. *American Journal of Sociology* 1991; **96**: 843–867.

17. **South S, Lloyd K.** Spousal alternatives and marital dissolution. *American Sociological Review* 1995; **60**: 21–35.

18. **White H.** Where do markets come from? *American Journal of Sociology* 1981; **87**: 517–547.

19. **Faulkner R, Anderson A.** Short term projects and emergent careers: evidence from Hollywood. *American Journal of Sociology* 1987; **92**: 879–909.

20. **Podolony JM.** A status based model of marker competition. *American Journal of Sociology* 1993; **98**: 829–872.

21. **Baker W, Faulkner R, Fisher G.** Hazards of the market: the continuity and dissolution of interorganizational market relationships. *American Sociological Review* 1998; **63**: 147–177.

22. **Laumann EO, Ellingson S, Mahay J, Paik A, Youm Y.** *The Sexual Organization of the City.* Chicago, IL: University of Chicago Press, 2004.

23. **Feld S.** The focused organisation of social ties. *American Journal of Sociology* 1981; **86**: 1015–1035.

24. **McPherson M.** An ecology of affiliation. *American Social Review* 1983; **48**: 519–532.

25. **Wasserman S, Faust K.** *Social Network Analysis.* Cambridge: Cambridge University Press, 1994.

26. **Duyves M.** Framing preferences, framing differences: inventing Amsterdam as gay capital. In: **RG Parker, JH Gagnan** (eds) *Conceiving Sexuality.* New York: Routledge, 1994, pp. 47–66.

27. **Simon W, Gagnon J.** A sexual scripts approach. In **J Greer, WT O'Donohue** (eds) *Theories of Human Sexuality.* New York: Plenum, 1987, pp. 363–383.

28. **Simon W, Gagnon J.** Homosexuality. In: **PM Nardi, BE Schneider** (eds) *Social Perspectives in Lesbian and Gay Studies.* London: Routledge, 1998, pp. 57–97.

29. **Youm Y, Laumann EO.** Social networks and sexually transmitted diseases. In: **EO Laumann, S Ellingson, J Mahay, A Paik, Y Youm**(eds) *The Sexual Organization of the City.* Chicago, IL: University of Chicago Press, 2004, pp. 264–282.

30. **Ellingson S.** Constructing causal stories and moral boundaries: institutional approaches to sexual problems. In **EO Laumann, S Ellingson, J Mahay, A Paik, Y Youm** (eds) *The Sexual Organization of the City.* Chicago, IL: University of Chicago Press, 2004, pp. 283–308.

31. **Van Haitsma M, Paik A, Laumann EO.** The Chicago health and social life survey design. In **EO Laumann, S Ellingson, J Mahay, A Paik, Y Youm** (eds) *The Sexual Organization of the City.* Chicago, IL: University of Chicago Press, 2004, pp. 39–68.

32. **Grov C, Smith M.** Gay subcultures. In: **V Minichiello, J Scott** (eds) *Male Sex Work and Society.* New York: Harrington Park Press, 2014, pp. 242–259

33. **Egan J, Frye V, Kurtz S, Latkin C, Chen M, Tobin K,** et al. Migration neighbourhoods and networks. *AIDS Behaviour* 2011; **15**(Suppl. 1): S35–S50.

34. **Levine MP.** Gay ghetto. *Journal of Homosexuality* 1979; **4**: 363–377.

35. **Lauria M, Knopp L.** Toward and analysis of the role of gay communities in the urban renaissance. *Urban Geography* 1985; **6**: 152–169.

36. **Smith M, Grov C.** *In the Company of Men: Inside the Lives of Male Prostitutes.* Santa Barbara, CA: Praeger, 2011.

37. **Laing M, Gaffney J.** Health and wellness services for male sex workers. In: V Minichiello, J Scott (eds) *Male Sex Workers and Society.* New York: Harrington Park Press, 2014, pp. 261–284.

38. **Sanders T, O'Neill M, Pitcher J.** *Prostitution: Sex Work, Policy and Politics.* London: Sage, 2009.

39. **Koken J, Bimbi D, Parsons J, Halkitis P.** The experience of stigma in the lives of male internet escorts. *Journal of Psychology & Human Sexuality* 2004; **16**: 13–32.

40. **McLean A.** New realm, new problems? Issues and support networks in online male sex work. *Gay & Lesbian Issues and Psychological Review* 2012; **8**: 70–81.

41. **Koken J, Bimbi D.** Mental health aspects of male sex work. In: **V Minichiello, D Scott** (eds) *Male Sex Workers and Society.* New York: Harrington Park Press, 2014, pp. 223–239.

42. **Cole S, Kemeny N, Taylor S, Visscher B.** Elevated physical health risk among gay men who conceal their sexual identity. *Journal of Health Psychology* 1996; **15**: 243–251.

43. **Frable D, Platt L, Hoey S.** Concealable stigma and positive self-perceptions. *Journal of Personality & Social Psychology* 1998; **74**: 909–922.

44. **Huebnes D, Davis M, Nemeroff C, Aiken J.** The impact of internalized homophobia on HIV prevention interventions. *American Journal of Community Psychology* 2002; **30**: 327–348.

45. **Meyer I.** Prejudice, social stress and mental health in lesbian, gay and bisexual populations: conceptual issues and research evidence. *Psychol Bull* 2003; **129**: 674–697.

46. **Shehan D, LaLota M, Johnson D, Celentano D, Koblin B, Torian L,** et al. HIV/STD risk in young men who have sex with men who do not disclose their sexual orientation. *Morbidity and Mortality Weekly Report* 2003; **52**: 82–84.

47. **Smith M, Seal D.** Sexual behaviour, mental health, substance use and HIV risk among agency based male escorts. *International Journal of Sexual Health* 2007; **19**: 27–39.

48. **Mimiaga M, Reisner S, Tinsley J, Mayer K, Safren S.** Street workers and internet escorts. *Journal of Urban Health* 2009; **86**: 54–66.

49. **Mc Cabe I, Acree M, O'Mahony F, McCabe J, Kenny J, Twyford J,** et al. Male street prostitution in Dublin. *Journal of Homosexuality* 2011; **58**: 998–1021.

50. **Bimbi D, Koken J.** Public health policy and practise with male sex workers. In: V Minichiello, D Scott (eds) *Male Sex Workers and Society.* New York: Harrington Park Press, 2014, pp. 199–221.

Chapter 18

Gender and sexual minorities

Richard Bradlow, Neha Singh, Suraj Beloskar, and Gurvinder Kalra

Introduction

The environment in which a person lives can have a profound effect on their mental health outcomes. A person's culture, religion, wealth, education level, country, and urban or rural living settings all make up the milieu that is likely to affect their mental health outcomes. In this chapter, we will focus on the mental health outcomes for lesbian, gay, bisexual, transgender, queer, and intersex (LGBTQI) individuals in an urban setting. An urban setting presents many challenges and advantages to a person's mental health. One could argue that the increased diversity, interconnectivity, opportunities, and the individual city's culture may create an environment conducive to better mental health outcomes. However, it can also be argued that urban environments are more cramped, noisy, congested, and lack the strong sense of community that smaller towns or villages provide, which could contribute to poorer mental health outcomes for those living in cities.

During this chapter, we will use the term 'gender and sexual minorities' (GSM) to refer to the entire gamut of LGBTQI individuals. We also use the word heterosexism, which refers to the assumption that heterosexuality is the normal sexual orientation leading to discrimination against all other sexualities.

A challenge when discussing this topic is the lack of research available, especially in the developing world. As well as a paucity in research around mental health issues affecting GSM, the studies that do exist face many challenges that affect their accuracy. Sexual orientation, for example, is not usually recorded on death certificates, making it hard to monitor suicide among GSM. Fluid definitions in sexuality can also make it difficult to measure mental health outcomes in GSM and different studies define GSM by behaviour, attraction, or identification, with little uniformity. Many people are not comfortable disclosing their orientation in a research setting or, indeed, in any setting and inaccurate self -reporting increases the inaccuracy of studies. As well as those challenges, each country has a different set of cultural values and orientation towards acceptance of diversity of race, sexuality, religion, and so on, which could affect the mental health outcomes of GSM within each country. This can make it difficult to draw conclusions about worldwide mental health issues.

Minority stress and mental health

Poor mental health outcomes have been found to correlate with discrimination or perceived discrimination suffered by all minorities not just GSM [1]. Minorities are more likely to be ostracized and stigmatized by society, which can result in worse mental health outcomes. The minority stress theory is well documented and important in understanding worse mental health outcomes among GSM [2]. It is important to note that there is no evidence to suggest that there is a causative relationship between gender or sexual identity and negative mental health outcomes, rather the evidence available indicates that poor mental health outcomes are a result of the discrimination that GSM are exposed to throughout their lives [3, 4].

This correlative relationship between perceived discrimination and poor mental health outcomes has been found as much in India as in the USA [5, 6]. This is also true in Australia, where GSM report higher rates of verbal and physical abuse than the general population and are up to three times more likely to experience depression compared to the general population [7]. Similarly, in the UK, GSM in England and Wales were found to have higher levels of psychological distress when compared with the general population [8].

In the United States, GSM have been found to have an increased risk of suffering from depression, panic attack disorder, generalized anxiety disorders, and higher levels of psychological distress [9]. GSM in the United States are also at greater risk of expressing suicidality, attempted suicide, and completed suicide than the general population [10]. Young males and transgender young people are the two subgroups with the highest risk of suicidality [11–13]. A 2008 meta-analysis concluded that GSM, when compared with the general population, have higher risks of developing depression, anxiety, and substance abuse disorders, and are at an increased risk of attempting and completing suicide [14].

Thus, the data available suggest that mental health outcomes are not related to how far to the right an individual is on the sexuality spectrum, but how severely individuals are affected by the perceived stress they are subjected to and how accepted they are by their peers [15]. Supporting this is the finding that bisexual young people, a group that is perhaps less understood and accepted by the general population, in the USA and Canada appear to have a slightly elevated risk of suicidal ideation and attempts than their gay and lesbian counterparts [16], and, as previously discussed, transgender young people seem to have a particularly high risk of mental health issues. This could be because there are fewer transgender people than those who identify as gay, lesbian, and bisexual, making them less understood, and that they are more identifiable, making them more of a target [12]. This also makes them a minority within a minority group, thus increasing the overall odds of marginalization and its apparent worse mental health consequences.

Higher rates of recreational drug and alcohol use have been found in urban GSM populations in the US and the UK [17]. In England, 'chemsex'—the combination of sex and illicit drug use—is more prevalent among urban GSM men in London than in GSM in the rest of the UK. Practising chemsex is associated with higher rates of depression and anxiety disorders and practising unsafe sex [18]. Chemsex and the decreased practise of safe sex that comes with it could increase the risk of HIV transmission [19]. Even though it is associated with worse mental and physical health outcomes, men who practise chemsex were found to be unlikely to seek medical help. Fear of judgement by healthcare professionals may be another barrier to seeking help in another example of minority stress [20]. This perceived fear from healthcare professionals is not just 'perceived', as both heterosexism and homophobia have commonly been reported among healthcare professionals, even in the psychiatric community in countries such as India [21] and in South Africa [22], and this has been shown to be a barrier to GSM seeking professional help. Chemsex practices may be different to those of other drug use in the GSM population, as chemsex could be a drug used for sexual enhancement rather than a self-medication for psychosocial stressors, or as a vehicle of escape. This may well explain why it is more common in cities like London, which is seen as a 'gay-friendly' environment. This has been supported by findings that the motivations for drug use in chemsex are founded in enhancing the sexual experience and increasing intimacy rather than separating the participant from reality as would be expected in escapist drug taking [23].

Migration in GSM

The indisputable view of the zeitgeist is that cities are the ideal location for people who are GSM to live. This could be owing to the increased levels of acceptance, tolerance, and diversity in cities. A US survey found that states with the highest percentage of people identifying as GSM are the most liberal and the most urban states [24].

Worldwide, it can be argued that cities are home to the politically left. It would make sense then that GSM communities would migrate to the more 'accommodating' cities from the 'less enlightened' rural areas. This concept of the 'Great Gay Migration' could become a self-fulfilling prophecy. As the idea becomes more pervasive, rural GSM are more likely to feel increased social pressure to move to the city and heteronormative people living in the country may feel that it is more acceptable to openly discriminate against GSM, especially as they see GSM move for perceived greener pastures [25]. GSM migration could lead to cities becoming more sexually diverse in a similar way that ethnic migration has led to racial diversity. In the way that modern multicultural cities challenge past theories of nationalism, future multisexual cities may challenge models of heteronormative sexuality [26].

Those who move to the city owing to their sexual orientation and/or gender identity, to the detriment of other needs, could be greatly disadvantaged. They could be socially isolated, being away from their friends and family support network, and underprepared for most urban jobs, having had previous experience only in rural employment. However, analysis of rural migrants to urban centres in Zhejiang Province, China, found that migrants were not more vulnerable to poor mental health outcomes than the general population [27]. This may not translate to GSM migrants, however, as GSM migrants in cities will no doubt face different challenges than purely economic ones. For some rural GSM in France and the US urban migration is not a permanent move and can be temporary, as although they use the city's anonymity, liberalism, and sexual opportunity to explore their sexuality, they do not identify as urban people [28]. The location of a person's upbringing can have a profound influence on their identity, as much as one's sexuality can have. The identity of a 'rural gay' is distinct from their urban counterpart and a move to the city, while maybe giving them more sexual freedom could be as destructive to their mental health as denying their sexuality [29, 30].

Most people who identify as GSM in Northern Ireland have felt compelled to move to the city and almost half (43%) of those who have done so say that their sexuality has played a role [31]. There is significant anecdotal evidence for the 'Great Gay Migration' occurring in Australia as well. While homophobia/transphobia is not unique to rural areas, smaller communities can increase the attention or perceived attention of harassment. Increased cognisance of an event, such as coming out, may result in a community-wide reaction, which could further increase the stress felt by the person trying to 'come out'.

The increased stigma that GSM may feel in a rural setting is not the only factor affecting their migration to urban settings. As well as factors pushing GSM out of rural settings there may be factors pulling GSM into cities. The urban setting can represent an opportunity for unfettered sexual exploration with more sexual opportunity and anonymity in a highly populated city versus a small rural town [32]. GSM migrants will also be motivated by the same factors that cause urbinization worldwide: better financial and educational opportunities.

In Denmark a correlation has been found between growing up outside of Copenhagen and marrying heterosexually in a first marriage [33]. This could mean that there is some aspect of being raised in an urban environment that makes a person more likely to have a homosexual orientation. Alternatively, it could mean that homosexuality is sufficiently unacceptable outside of Copenhagen, that marrying heterosexually is for reasons of acceptability. This 'development' theory does not imply that homosexuality is a choice, but rather that sexual orientation is influenced by environmental factors that are specific to cities or that individuals are more comfortable in publicly expressing their sexuality in an urban setting [34]. It is possible to postulate from those findings that GSM living in rural areas are less likely to 'come out' and therefore more likely to marry heterosexually, counter to their sexual desires.

The latter explanation may seem more likely based on the available evidence, as marrying a member of the opposite sex can be a poor indicator of sexuality, as Oscar Wilde could attest. A higher level of acceptance is a leading explanation as to why higher education levels are associated with same-sex attraction; the more accepting urban environments could also explain the higher levels of same-sex relationships among people raised there [34].

The *hijra*, a social class/identity group of transgender females in India, have also been found to be concentrated in urban areas—about three-quarters of all *hijras* in India live in urban centres [35]. This is possibly due to migration to urban areas by rurally born *hijras*, which is anecdotally true. There is very little research into the mental health of *hijra* individuals, but up to half of them have been found to have some sort of psychiatric illness and very few have access to psychiatric health services [36]. Research into whether there are differences in access to health care between urban and rural environments for *hijras* would be illuminating.

Challenges for GSM populations in urban settings

Urban environments across the globe have a variety of different advantages and disadvantages. They can be cultural and artistic centres with more opportunity for work and diverse sexual encounters, or they can be overcrowded, noisy, conducive to homelessness, and sex work. The latter environment can present challenges to mental health amongst GSM and non-GSM alike.

The evidence is mixed, in some countries, like Australia and the United States, rural areas have a higher prevalence of suicide. This higher prevalence is attributed to increased isolation, poorer rural communities, better access to means (firearms), closeted GSM who do not feel accepted, and the social expectation of rural men to be strong and self-contained leading them to not reach out for help [37, 38]. Inner-city patients in Ohio were found to come to their general practitioner more often, for longer visits with more complex mental and physical health issues than their rural counterparts. This was believed to be because inner-city patients were more likely to be of a lower socio-economic background [39]. In the United States no psychiatric disorder has been found to have a higher prevalence in a rural setting and some studies have a found lower prevalence of some mental health disorders and substance abuse disorders in rural areas in the United States. This could be due to the higher availability of drugs in cities [40]. Little difference in the prevalence of mental disorders between urban and rural populations has also been found in Iran. In Iran, mental health was more likely to be determined by gender, with women having a much higher prevalence of mental health issues than men. This, too, can be explained by the minority stress model as women are bound to historical social roles in Iran [41]. In contrast, in India, mental health among children was found to be more linked to affluence than location [42]. In the UK, urban settings have been found to be associated with higher levels of mental health morbidity [43].

Mental health statistics among general urban populations include GSM populations; however, GSM face challenges in cities specific to them, although the two are not always separate. In yet another example of the minority stress model, in the United States neighbourhoods with a higher prevalence of hate crimes have higher rates of drug abuse among young GSM [44]. Youth homelessness is an issue focused in cities that disproportionately affects young GSM in the United States [4, 45]. GSM sex workers have higher rates of HIV/AIDS infection in India, Pakistan, and Canada [46].

A 2013 study in the US found no differences in mental health outcomes or life satisfaction of GSM living in urban areas over their rural counterparts [47]. The authors concluded that the general advantages of living rurally, outweighed the increased prejudices they faced for their sexuality.

Another major challenge for this population is violence especially toward transgender people, which is most severe in countries with the strongest and most visible trans political movements and civil organizations [48]. This, again, indicates that easier identification increases the discrimination, perceived or actual, that GSM face. Cities are usually the epicentre of social movements and living in a city may therefore put GSM at greater risk for violent attack due to their more noticeable profile. It is possible that a rural setting, while being less welcoming to GSM individuals, might put them at less risk of violent assaults.

Way forward

Globally, urban GSM face numerous different challenges to their mental health: access to health care, poor social support, victimization and discrimination, and poor education amongst healthcare providers. The most consistent challenge worldwide is the lack of research and academic understanding into mental health issues in GSM. Issues affecting GSM, who may not have as loud a voice in society and may feel marginalized, should be sought out and not avoided. Discrimination often goes unnoticed by those who are not disadvantaged by it and people without lived experiences have little hope of understanding what it means to suffer the slings and arrows that constitute the extreme hurt of the victims of discrimination. There is a paucity of research into the mental health issues amongst GSM, especially in the developing world. More research is required to find out if and where more support services need to be deployed. As heterosexism among healthcare professionals could discourage GSM from seeking help, it is imperative that healthcare professionals are trained in tolerance and acceptance to provide a respectful, accepting and non-judgemental environment for GSM patients.

GSM children of supportive parents have been found to have better mental health outcomes as young people and later in life [49]. Education aimed at the general public making parents more accepting of GSM children could have a profound positive effect on their mental health. The minority stress model would suggest that, as acceptance of GSM in society rises, mental health issues among GSM will diminish. Gay–straight alliance (or gender and sexuality alliance) networks emerging in schools, universities, and companies—primarily in cities—are a product or cause of increasing acceptance of alternate sexualities in the next generation.

Many cities also have 'gay-borhoods', which provide safe spaces to GSM individuals within a city, like the Castro District (San Francisco), Chueca (Madrid), Prahran (Melbourne), or Soho (London). They could provide an access point for health services to provide health care and support to a subpopulation that may be hard to penetrate [26]. These villages within cities have high GSM populations and can have—indeed, some already do have—GSM-specific health services. The larger and more densely packed populations of cities allow for more specialized and targeted services that would not be available in a rural setting. The Fenway Community Health Center and Pride Institute in the United States, the Humsafar Trust and Sakhi Char Chowghi Trust in India, and many smaller family medicine clinics located in 'gay-borhoods' around the world can better serve GSM by offering services tailored to their needs. These institutes are in the best position to reach the knowledge gaps that exist in the scientific literature in regards to GSM. Multinational trials could be possible if organized by well-funded centres using the local clinics that are already there catering to GSM populations. Those specialized clinics are in a unique position to gather information from hard to access communities and should be used so.

GSM drug use, attitudes on HIV, barriers to health care, homelessness, internal migratory patterns, and medical and mental health are areas without enough information for best practice. This lack of research is both a challenge and an opportunity for mental health clinicians today.

References

1. **Williams D, Neighbors H, Jackson J.** Racial/ethnic discrimination and health: findings from community studies. *American Journal of Public Health* 2003; **93**: 200–208.
2. **Meyer I.** Prejudice, social stress, and mental health in lesbian, gay, and bisexual populations: conceptual issues and research evidence. *Psychological Bulletin* 2003; **129**: 674–697.
3. **Rosser B, Bockting W, Ross M, Miner M, Coleman E.** The relationship between homosexuality, internalized homo-negativity, and mental health in men who have sex with men. *Journal of Homosexuality* 2008; **55**: 185–203.
4. **Savin-Williams R.** Verbal and physical abuse as stressors in the lives of lesbian, gay male, and bisexual youths: associations with school problems, running away, substance abuse, prostitution, and suicide. *Journal of Consulting and Clinical Psychology* 1994; **62**: 261–269.
5. **Logie C, Newman P, Chakrapani V, Shunmugam M.** Adapting the minority stress model: Associations between gender non-conformity stigma, HIV-related stigma and depression among men who have sex with men in South India. *Social Science & Medicine* 2012; **74**: 1261–1268.
6. **Mays V, Cochran S.** Mental health correlates of perceived discrimination among lesbian, gay, and bisexual adults in the United States. *American Journal of Public Health* 2001; **91**: 1869–1876.
7. **Hillier L, Jones T, Monagle M, Overton N, Gahan L, Blackman J, Mitchell A.** Writing Themselves in 3. Available at: https://www.acon.org.au/wp-content/uploads/2015/04/Writing-Themselves-In-3-2010.pdf (accessed 26 November 2018).
8. **King M.** Mental health and quality of life of gay men and lesbians in England and Wales: controlled, cross-sectional study. *The British Journal of Psychiatry* 2003; **183**: 552–558.
9. **Cochran S, Sullivan J, Mays V.** Prevalence of mental disorders, psychological distress, and mental health services use among lesbian, gay, and bisexual adults in the United States. *Journal of Consulting and Clinical Psychology* 2003; **71**: 53–61.
10. **Haas A, Eliason M, Mays V, Mathy R, Cochran S, D'Augelli A,** et al. Suicide and suicide risk in lesbian, gay, bisexual, and transgender populations: review and recommendations. *Journal of Homosexuality* 2010; **58**: 10–51.
11. **Paul J, Catania J, Pollack L, Moskowitz J, Canchola J, Mills T,** et al. Suicide attempts among gay and bisexual men: lifetime prevalence and antecedents. *American Journal of Public Health* 2002; **92**: 1338–1345.

12. **Nicholas J, Howard J.** Better dead than gay? Depression, suicide ideation and attempt among a sample of gay and straight-identified males aged 18 to 24. *Youth Studies Australia* 1998; **17**.4: 28–33.

13. **Haas A, Rodgers P, Herman J.** Suicide attempts among transgender and gender non-conforming adults: findings of the National Transgender Discrimination Survey. Available at: https://williamsinstitute.law.ucla.edu/wp-content/uploads/AFSP-Williams-Suicide-Report-Final.pdf (accessed 26 November 2018).

14. **King M, Semlyen J, Tai S, Killaspy H, Osborn D, Popelyuk D,** et al. A systematic review of mental disorder, suicide, and deliberate self harm in lesbian, gay and bisexual people. *BMC Psychiatry* 2008; **8**(1).

15. **Russell S, Fish J.** Mental health in lesbian, gay, bisexual, and transgender (LGBT) youth. *Annual Review of Clinical Psychology* 2016; **12**: 465–487.

16. **Saewyc E, Skay C, Pettingell S.** Suicide ideation and attempts in north American school-based surveys: are bisexual youth at increasing risk? *Journal of Adolescent Health* 2004; **34**: 138.

17. **Stall R, Paul J, Greenwood G, Pollack L, Bein E, Crosby G,** et al. Alcohol use, drug use and alcohol-related problems among men who have sex with men: the Urban Men's Health Study. *Addiction* 2001; **96**: 1589–1601.

18. **Pufall EL, Kall M, Shahmanesh M, Nardone A, Gilson R, Delpech V, Ward H, on behalf of The Positive Voices Study Group.** Sexualized drug use ('chemsex') and high-risk sexual behaviours in HIV-positive men who have sex with men. *HIV Med* 2018; **19**: 261–270.

19. **Bourne A, Reid D, Hickson F, Torres-Rueda S, Weatherburn P.** Illicit drug use in sexual settings ('chemsex') and HIV/STI transmission risk behaviour among gay men in South London: findings from a qualitative study. *Sexually Transmitted Infections* 2015; **91**: 564–568.

20. **Bourne A, Reid D, Hickson F, Torres-Rueda S, Steinberg P, Weatherburn P.** 'Chemsex' and harm reduction need among gay men in South London. *International Journal of Drug Policy* 2015; **26**: 1171–1176.

21. **Kalra G.** Pathologising alternate sexuality: shifting psychiatric practices and a need for ethical norms and reforms. *Indian Journal of Medical Ethics* 2012; **9**: 289–294.

22. **Lane T, Mogale T, Struthers H, McIntyre J, Kegeles S.** 'They see you as a different thing': the experiences of men who have sex with men with healthcare workers in South African township communities. *Sexually Transmitted Infections* 2008; **84**: 430–433.

23. **Weatherburn P, Hickson F, Reid D, Torres-Rueda S, Bourne A.** Motivations and values associated with combining sex and illicit drugs ('chemsex') among gay men in South London: findings from a qualitative study. *Sexually Transmitted Infections* 2016; **93**: 203–206.

24. **Gates G, Newport F.** LGBT Percentage Highest in D.C., Lowest in North Dakota. Available at: https://news.gallup.com/poll/160517/lgbt-percentage-highest-lowest-north-dakota.aspx (accessed 26 November 2018).

25. **Boso L.** Urban bias, rural sexual minorities, and the courts. *UCLA Law* 2013; 60.562.

26. **Kalra G, Bhugra D.** Migration and sexuality. *International Journal of Culture and Mental Health* 2010; **3**: 117–125.

27. **Yang T, Xu X, Li M, Rockett I, Zhu W, Ellison-Barnes A.** Mental health status and related characteristics of Chinese male rural–urban migrant workers. *Community Mental Health Journal* 2011; **48**: 342–351.

28. **Annes A, Redlin M.** Coming out and coming back: Rural gay migration and the city. *Journal of Rural Studies* 2012; **28**: 56–68.

29. **Kazyak E.** Disrupting cultural selves: constructing gay and lesbian identities in rural locales. *Qualitative Sociology* 2011; **34**: 561–581.

30. **Kuhar R, Švab A.** The only gay in the village? Everyday life of gays and lesbians in rural Slovenia. *Journal of Homosexuality* 2014; **61**: 1091–1116.

31. **The Rainbow Project.** OUTstanding In your field exploring the needs of LGB&T people in rural Northern Ireland. Available at: https://www.rainbow-project.org/Handlers/Download.ashx?IDMF=75981d9c-f647-46bf-86e2-a27b566cfe63 (accessed 26 November 2018).

32. **Bianchi F, Reisen C, Cecilia Zea M, Poppen P, Shedlin M, Penha M.** The sexual experiences of Latino men who have sex with men who migrated to a gay epicentre in the USA. *Culture, Health & Sexuality* 2007; **9**: 505–518.

33. **Frisch M, Hviid A.** Childhood family correlates of heterosexual and homosexual marriages: a national cohort study of two million Danes. *Archives of Sexual Behavior* 2006; **35**: 533–547.

34. **Laumann E.** *The Social Organization of Sexuality.* Chicago, IL: University of Chicago, 2002.

35. **Subramanian T, Chakrapani V, Selvaraj V, Noronha E, Narang A, Mehendale S.** Mapping and size estimation of Hijras and other trans-women in 17 states of India: first level findings. *International Journal of Health Sciences and Research* 2015; **5**: 1–10.

36. **Jayadeva V.** Understanding the mental health of the Hijra women of India. *American Journal of Psychiatry Residents' Journal* 2017; **12**: 7–9.

37. **Eberhardt M, Pamuk E.** The importance of place of residence: examining health in rural and nonrural areas. *American Journal of Public Health* 2004; **94**: 1682–1686.

38. **Caldwell TM, Jorm AF, Dear KBG.** Suicide and mental health in rural, remote and metropolitan areas in Australia. *Medical Journal of Australia* 2004; **181**: 10.

39. **Blankfield R.** Addressing the unique challenges of inner-city practice: a direct observation study of inner-city, rural, and suburban family practices. *Journal of Urban Health: Bulletin of the New York Academy of Medicine* 2002; **79**: 173–185.

40. **Vega W, Kolody B, Aguilar-Gaxiola S, Alderete E, Catalano R, Caraveo-Anduaga J.** Lifetime prevalence of DSM-III-R psychiatric disorders among urban and rural Mexican Americans in California. *Archives of General Psychiatry* 1998; **55**: 771.

41. **Noorbala A, Yazdi S, Yasamy M, Mohammad K.** Mental health survey of the adult population in Iran. *The British Journal of Psychiatry* 2003; **184**: 70–73.

42. **Srinath S, Girimaji S, Gururaj G, Shekhar S, Subbakrishna S, Bhola P, Kumar N.** Epidemiological study of child & adolescent psychiatric disorders in urban & rural areas of Bangalore, India. *Indian Journal of Medical Research* 2005; **122**: 67–79.

43. **Paykel E, Abbott R, Jenkins R, Brugha T, Meltzer H.** Urban–rural mental health differences in Great Britain: findings from the National Morbidity Survey. *Psychological Medicine* 2000; **30**: 269–280.

44. **Duncan D, Hatzenbuehler M, Johnson R.** Neighborhood-level LGBT hate crimes and current illicit drug use among sexual minority youth. *Drug and Alcohol Dependence* 2014; **135**: 65–70.

45. **Hunter E.** What's good for the gays is good for the gander: making homeless youth housing safer for lesbian, gay, bisexual, and transgender youth. *Family Court Review* 2008; **46**: 543–557.

46. **Steinbrook R.** HIV in India—a complex epidemic. *New England Journal of Medicine* 2007; **356**: 1089–1093.

47. **Wienke C, Hill G.** Does place of residence matter? Rural–urban differences and the wellbeing of gay men and lesbians. *Journal of Homosexuality* 2013; **60**: 1256–1279.

48. **Trans Respect Versus Transphobia Worldwide**. Comparative research data on190 countries worldwide. Available at: http://transrespect.org (accessed 26 November 2018).

49. **Ryan C, Russell S, Huebner D, Diaz R, Sanchez J.** Family acceptance in adolescence and the health of LGBT young adults. *Journal of Child and Adolescent Psychiatric Nursing* 2010; **23**: 205–213.

Chapter 19

A tale of two cities: urban mental health in Vancouver and New York City

Kerry L. Jang, Michael Krausz
and Michael Jae Song

Introduction

As cities expand worldwide, urban mental health is fast becoming a growing challenge. Rapid migration into urban centres from rural settings in addition to domestic migration and international immigration all contribute to a range of difficulties that can have extremely adverse effects on the mental health of its residents. Pressures not only from finding and keeping adequate housing, employment, love, and transportation are key issues, but also pre-existing issues such as crime, culture, drugs, and the daily 'struggle for survival' all contribute to adverse mental health. Commonly thought of as 'risk factors', these issues are day-to-day realities for those already suffering from mental illness and/or addiction issues. Moreover, with increasing urbanization the limited resources for housing, health care, and social support have to be redistributed and this often leads to social tensions and more unmet needs—especially for poor and vulnerable neighbourhoods.

We want to present and reflect on this perspective of urban mental health. The perspective we speak of is not that of a clinician, mental health service provider, a researcher, or the health authorities. Rather, what is presented is the challenge for local government and public services from the perspective of an elected politician, staff advisor, planner, and a first responder. These perspectives are important not only to understanding key issues in urban mental health, but also the ways and means to address it.

Far too often there is a cry from the general public and the media for politicians to 'do something'—without a clear realization of what they want done or what needs to be done, and often without any appreciation of the constraints local government is under. These constraints are very real, and range from financial resources to service delivery capacity to statutory authority that place significant limits on what local governments can do. With this in mind, both the cities of Vancouver (British Columbia, Canada) and New York City (NY, USA) have created unique approaches to addressing urban mental health based on their fiscal and statutory authorities. Their approaches tend to form the ends of a continuum of civic action. Between these two end points any city, depending on its capacity can adopt aspects of these two approaches that best suit their needs and means. Having some action on urban mental health is far better than no action at all.

Who does what and the orders of government

Most countries have three orders of government: the national or federal; state or provincial assemblies; and city or municipal councils. Each order is relatively independent with its own taxation powers, policy jurisdictions, and responsibilities. Municipal governments typically derive their powers from state or provincial law in the form of a municipal act. This is notable because it places clear statutory limitations on what cities are responsible for, and restrictions on how, and where, the municipality may raise and spend monies. The primary responsibility of municipal governments lies in land use, and within that envelope the actual responsibilities do vary significantly from city to city, but in urban centres local governments are usually responsible for the following:

- *protection of persons and property*, which includes the management of local policing and firefighting services;
- *local transportation*, such as management of public bus and rail services, as well as municipal roadway construction and maintenance;
- *planning and development*, including municipal zoning and industrial/economic development, urban planning, and building form;
- *public utilities*, including the management of local sewage systems, water treatment, and electric utilities;
- *parks, recreation, and culture*, including the development and management of local parks and green spaces, and public recreation facilities, as well as local art and cultural programmes and events;
- *local social-welfare services*, which affect a range of social determinants of health, including management of local health, library and educational facilities, community centres, and other forms of social programmes.

Revenues

Cities and municipalities in North America have very constrained budgets as the primary form of taxation is through property or real estate taxes. These are annual or semi-annual taxes paid by property owners and businesses that are based on the assessed value of privately owned residences, land holdings, or places of business. The tax rate is set to cover the operating expenses of a city and provide for new services as demands present themselves. Cities also charge fees relating to the issuance of permits and licenses (e.g. demolition and building permits, business licenses). Generally, these license fees are revenue neutral covering only the cost of inspection and enforcement of local bylaws.

Development charges are another way cities raise money to provide not only basic infrastructure (e.g. sewers and water), but also community amenities. For example, a rezoning process is triggered when a proposed new building exceeds the local zoning guidelines on height and density. This provides cities with an opportunity to extract community amenity contributions (CACs) from the building's developer based on the increase in property value of the new larger building to fund local area improvements. CACs can be a fixed rate or negotiated. Usually, CACs are used to fund public parks, art installations, or used to help fund housing projects for below-market housing for needy families.

Accessibility of local governments and resident demands

Being local, municipalities are the place where any increased prevalence and incidence of mental health problems, typically manifested by highly visible homeless, mental health incidents, and visible poverty, is first noticed and is the first place residents make demands to address mental health issues. But why do people turn to the cities to address the issues as opposed to higher orders of government who actually have the mandate for the delivery of mental health services?

A primary reason is that municipal governments are the most accessible to residents who often do not understand what order or government is responsible for different services. Local government is often the first place people turn for help and complaints. A telephone call to an emergency number such as 911, 119, or 311 provides residents immediate service (e.g. first responders when they see someone in distress or is a danger to self or others). Moreover, police and fire services are usually the first on scene after a call and are direct employees of a city. A second reason is visibility. As cities grow, especially in areas of rapid urbanization, visible homeless, drug dealing, homeless camps, or mental health incidents become more visible and salient, often resulting in calls to emergency services. The media play a big role, as well highlighting the issues that occurs in a recognizable, often local area bringing the issues 'too close to home'.

Lost in transition: a view of urban mental health from the police

The impact of these calls on municipal service is often the catalyst for action and compels a city to take action outside of its normal jurisdiction. A primary example is the 2008 Vancouver Police Department (VPD) report entitled 'Lost in Transition: How a Lack of Capacity in the Mental Health System is Failing Vancouver's Mentally Ill and Draining Police Resources' [1]. This report provided a quantitative analysis of the prevalence of VPD calls for service that involve mentally ill clients and sought to identify the primary factors that contribute to the frequency of these incidents from a policing perspective. The report is definitely not, and was never meant to be, the type of analysis and report one would expect from public health or academically based researchers. It simply reported the facts as the police saw them.

Over a 16-day period in Vancouver (9–24 September 2007) police incidents in which patrol officers believed that the mental health of an involved person was a factor in their attendance were enumerated. It should be noted that the police officers were not expected to make a specific diagnosis of mental illness but used their judgement in respect to the British Columbia Mental Health Act, which gives officers the power to arrest a person based on their observations. In total, 1154 calls for police service were recorded and, of those, 31% involved at least one mentally ill person. In some areas of Vancouver this figure rose to nearly half of all incidents where police contact was made. The impact of this number of incidents was equivalent to a direct annual cost of $9 million. This estimate was based on the fact that, in 2007, each recorded call for service required an average of 2.6 officer hours. Assuming that calls involving mental health problems require approximately the same police resources as the average police call for service, annually 153,140 officer hours are required to deal with mental health-related calls. This is equivalent to the direct cost of approximately 90 full-time front-line officers but does not include indirect policing costs, or the costs to other agencies such as the ambulance service, hospitals, or the court system.

The impetus for the report was the growing number of mental health calls for service that were clearly overwhelming the existing municipal and police response to mental health. Existing responses are best described as reactive and not ideal in that they may address an immediate issue, but does not address the root problem. For example, city sanitation crews are ordered to clean up homeless camps but that does little but shift the camp to a less conspicuous location, and the only material goods the homeless own are destroyed, increasing poverty and disenfranchisement. In a recent example, city workers in the city of Abbotsford, British Columbia, spread chicken manure in a field to discourage homeless individuals from setting up tents [2]. Police services often create dedicated mental health response units such as specialized patrol cars staffed by an officer and a mental health worker, and enhanced officer training, but these measures are rapidly overwhelmed. An important factor to keep in mind is police culture in which mental health services are not considered police work and fosters resentment among members for becoming *de facto* front line mental health workers. The primary response for the VPD is to apprehend and transport the suspected mentally ill person to hospital emergency, but this simple act significantly impacts on policing because the officer is required to stay with the individual until admitted by an emergency room physician, which has been shown to last several hours to an entire shift.

VPD recommendations

The VPD report made several wide ranging but complimentary recommendations to address the mental health gap. A major recommendation called for a return of institutionalization, and, in particular, a facility that can specifically accommodate moderate-to-long-term stays for individuals who are chronically mentally ill and addicted. The next recommendation was the creation of an 'Urgent Response Center' (URC) by the local health authority. The concept behind the URC is a facility that bypasses traditional emergency wards and is available for police to transport a suspected mentally ill individual and provide direct mental health and addictions treatment, in addition to finding appropriate housing or community supports for individuals before being discharged. Such a facility would speed up the admission process for police by obviating the need for waiting for the emergency physician to examine and admit the patient, allowing police to return to their patrols quickly. A third recommendation called for increased services for people who suffer from concurrent disorders that recognizes the police experience that 50% of people with a mental illness abuse street drugs and alcohol. This recommendation is notable in that it calls upon existing mental health clinics to provide services to people who are also drug addicted, irrespective of which affliction is most severe and breaks down traditionally compartmentalized mental health and addiction care. A final recommendation called for enhanced ability to gather data on all mental health-related calls for service to facilitate research and to establish benchmarks to track change for police in British Columbia, and a system that has readily accessible details of an individual's mental health history (taking into account privacy concerns) that is accessible to police and all mental health service providers.

Politics and politicians

When faced with such requests, how does a politician respond? To understand the politician one has to first understand the word 'optics'. For politicians, it means that one must at the very least appear to be making a difference or at least putting some kind of plan into action. This is why so many municipal approaches to mental health address only the visible symptoms of mental illness and are effective for a very short term. The task ahead of us is to overcome the 'optics' of a situation and to provide the politician with actions that can happen immediately, but at the same time implementing programmes that are based on best practices and research to have a long-term impact. For the politician, the longer-term one will appeal to their sense of vanity because a programme of work can be seen as a legacy project, giving them plenty of things to boast about during the term, and make them appear smarter than they actually are. But every politician needs what is termed 'a quick win', some tangible short-term action that can address immediate suffering, such as food distributions or, in less enlightened jurisdictions, police sweeps to move homeless people from sight.

The challenge facing politicians is best illustrated by example. Politicians are generally adept at understanding the public's perceptions of mental illness and how success is defined in the public eye. Street homelessness is a part of every large city. In the public's eye, they need to see tangible success by having fewer people on the streets. The long-term approach is to build housing and move the people inside—but that relies on a 'trickle-down effect' that is very expensive, and takes time to build and tenant buildings. It will not be seen as a success because for a very protracted period of time visible homelessness remains, and for the politician, issues about costs and raising taxes to pay for it are unpopular, and there is the perception that building housing for homeless people will attract more homeless people to your city. Then there is a politician's political opposition, who will use these issues to fear monger or ridicule attempts in attempt to gain support from the electorate.

Above all, fear is the greatest motivator of public opinion. It is easy to generate, manipulate, and motivate. Because most political terms last 3–4 years, long-term solutions are not politically expedient for the politician. This, of course, does not take into account actual issues as to whether a city has the ability to pay for housing, and if they are willingly accepting a downloading of responsibility from senior orders of government. More locally, NIMBYism or 'Not in My Back Yard' syndrome among vocal opponents to any project to help the homeless, mentally ill, and addicted is a significant factor. NIMBY opposition is usually based entirely on misinformation or lack of information, whose void will be filled by imagination and fear. A vocal NIMBY group is like kryptonite to most politicians. Less skilled politicians will fear the raucus vocal opposition and give into their demands to placate and win their votes in the next election. More skilled politicians will use NIMBYism to punctuate the need and use the opportunity to educate and make the case for the project, but this is a risky proposition for politicians as fear takes many forms. Either way, NIMBYism will garner media attention, which is the milk of political life and can make or break a politician.

The need for a *simultaneous* two-pronged approach is highlighted by the follow-up VPD report to the 2008 'Lost in Transition' (LIT) report, entitled 'Policing Vancouver's Mentally Ill: The Disturbing Truth' [3]:

> The VPD's key finding is that from a 'street cop's' point of view little has changed since the 2008 LIT report. There has been progress and positive outcomes in the areas of supported housing, police record management and analysis, and moderate to long term treatment services for dual diagnosed patients in a quasi-institutional environment … The police, however, are still responding day after day to 'difficult to manage' and 'treat' chronically mentally ill and addicted individuals on the streets of Vancouver. Other issues relating to suicide, suicide attempts and missing persons consume police resources, frustrate police, and in some cases endanger the lives and safety of patients, front-line police officers, other first responders and the public …[1]

It is appropriate here to emphasize that whether long- or short-term initiatives are launched if they were designed to be political in nature, they are doomed to failure. A good example was 'Project Civil City', initiated by the City of Vancouver in December 2006 [4]. The mayor at the time had conducted what he described as an 'informal' poll of residents who noted an upswing in visible homelessness and street disorder attributed (correctly or incorrectly) to the homeless. Sensing a political opportunity, a social engineering project was launched that promised to cut homelessness in half and reduce street-drug use and aggressive panhandling by the year 2010—just in time for the Winter Olympics to be held in that year. Project Civil City made it clear that housing and homelessness were the responsibility of higher orders of government (so any increases in street homelessness could be deflected to them) and that the city would use the powers it had to bring order to the streets. Project Civil City sounded great as a political document and was, in essence, a citizen security

---

[1] Thompson, Scott. (2010). Policing Vancouver's mentally ill: The disturbing truth. Beyond lost in transition. Vancouver Police Department. p. 24.

project that would need the support of the VPD—who did not support this approach.

As such, Project Civil City relied on deterrence measures that could be handled by bylaw enforcement officers targeted at the street homeless. This included increases in bylaw fines for public offences such as jaywalking (increased to $100), failing to wear a bicycle helmet (increased to $50), fighting (increased to $200), not having a dog on a leash (increased to $250), and urinating and defecating in a public place (increased to $100). The project also encouraged and paid for the use of private security guards to keep areas of the city free of homeless individuals. In short, the project devolved into a programme that criminalized homelessness and poverty that a later status report showed that none of the goals was achieved. Instead, the legacy of this project was a decade of litigation led by homeless advocacy groups on how the city actively discriminated against the mentally ill and homeless. Instead of becoming a plan the residents could support, it became an object of ridicule and scepticism shortly after it was launched. Project Civil City is a good example of what not to do because it led with politics rather than solutions based in best practice.

A tale of two cities

Two cities, New York City (NYC) and Vancouver, have created urban mental health plans that approached the problem in unique ways and with different tools, depending on each's capabilities and resources. Their approaches roughly form the ends of the continuum of civic action illustrated in Figure 19.1. As noted earlier, health inequities are often first identified at the local level. At the far left of the continuum the very least thing a city can engage in is targeted advocacy strategies developed to promote health for their residents. Moving further along the continuum, cities and their planning departments that have the capacity and expertise can undertake policy, planning, research, and even provide direct services to meet public health goals.

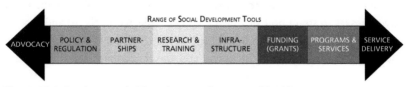

Figure 19.1 Continuum of civic action on urban mental health.

Vancouver's Healthy City Strategy

'The City of Vancouver's Healthy City Strategy' [5] is a policy-based approach that is not focused on urban mental health per se but the *broad* population health needs of its residents. This approach focuses on the social determinants of health and includes all aspects of healthy living, ranging from built environment to access to green space to food to community capacity, to name a few. Unlike other plans, the strategy does not just focus on the needs of the most vulnerable, but on the needs of all residents and accomplishes this by becoming the lens though which all city departments, from engineering and streets, to planning and urban design to first response to social development, must reference as they carry out their work. The strategy sets out an ambitious set of goals, targets, and indicators on topics ranging from early childhood development, food security, the need to create healthy human services, income security, social inclusion, and active living to name a few. Achieving these goals is no easy task, but specific targets and indicators are promoted broadly around city departments and have become a shared framework to direct all City services. The synergy between departments has coordinated some significant advances to reach these goals. For example, between planning and social development departments developed inclusionary zoning practices, official development plans, and local community plans that specify targets for supportive housing and mental health service locations; a programme of offering development grants or waiving of development cost levies to assist in the establishment of mental health centres, and/or services, and supportive or low-income housing. More directly, the City has used its land use roles to promote mental and physical health through urban form and infrastructure design guidelines and bylaws. This ranges from building design, sidewalks, parks, and public spaces, for example, which promotes well-being and healthy activity.

Healthy City Strategy and the Vancouver Police Department

The VPD developed a mental health strategy under the umbrella of the 'Healthy City Strategy' framework to create new police policy and procedure on how to best deal and interact with the mentally ill [6]. The strategy is notable in that it clearly lays out that the primary goal of any police involvement is de-escalation. From there it outlines when the police will engage with, disengage from, or arrest the individual. The strategy also outlines the skills and training a police officer is to have to recognize behaviour that is characteristic of mental illness or a crisis and do the appropriate risk assessments. However, the mental health strategy also makes it clear that the officers are not there to make a diagnosis. Procedures for engagement (e.g. when the police officer will notify supervisors, clear direction on leaving an individual alone, ensuring a suitable support person is in place). Similarly, procedures are outlined for when officers elect to disengage from a situation (e.g. procedures to notify a supervisor, when a supervisor attends the scene and the development of an operational plan, the creation of a police report which includes a follow-up plan and referrals identified to ensure that the individual receives the support they require). The circumstances for arrest are also covered (e.g. when there are reasonable grounds to believe that the individual has committed a serious criminal offence and will ensure subsequent examination by a physician in Vancouver Jail to assess and refer to mental health support). Full details can be found elsewhere [6].

The most important feature of the VPD strategy is their investment in long-term solutions. The VPD has chosen to be a key member of 'assertive community treatment' teams, or ACTs, although not a requirement under the provincial ACT standards. Each team, with a maximum caseload of 80 clients, includes psychiatrists, social workers, nurses, vocational counsellors, occupational therapists, recreational therapists, and peer counsellors, among others.

The goal of ACT is to provide a greater intensity and frequency of support for severe mental health and/or substance use clients where traditional services have been unsuccessful. The primary objective of ACT is to prepare the client who is typically pre-contemplative in their substance use experience severe functional challenges related to community living for a successful transfer to a step-down community service. ACT teams are comprised of 10–12 professionals focused on the well-being of a limited number of clients.

Along with ACT, the police are key players in Assertive Outreach Team (AOT) designed to assist a small cohort of the community that cannot be support by ACT. The AOT programme addresses the needs of clients with moderate-to-severe substance use and/or mental health issues as they transition from the health or criminal justice systems back into the community. The goal of AOT is to reduce the incidences of violence and self-harm, prevent further deterioration in the quality of life of the individual, and reduce re-engagement with the criminal justice system. AOTs function to connect individuals to their primary-care provider over a 1–2-month transitional period, using a collaborative problem-solving approach. AOT is more police-intensive than ACT, allowing the team to assess risk readily, proactively locate individuals in risk-laden environments, and provide input and support for future services. Referrals are received directly through recent police interactions, from health services and the criminal justice system. The VPD have also created an in-house 'early warning system' that identifies individuals with increasing mental illness-related police interactions. An AOT has an average caseload of 40 clients staffed by four full-time officers.

In summary, Vancouver's approach can be best described as a policy-based response that realigns services and functions to better address mental health. Vancouver's approach is a lens through which all city services are examined to ensure urban health goals are met or supported.

NYC Thrive: a roadmap for mental health for all

NYC has recently developed quite a different plan to address mental health. Returning to the continuum of action in Figure 19.1, NYC's plan squarely occupies the opposite end of the continuum that directly encourages and supports the creation of mental health services and their delivery. City governments in United States have much more leverage to affect change in mental health than Canadian municipal governments. In NYC, under the constitution act of New York, the mayor appoints the heads of about 50 departments, including the Department of Health and Mental Health Hygiene (DOHMH). DOHMH is the city public health agency that has collaborated extensively with the mayor and the council to address mental health concerns in the city by creating a plan called 'Thrive NYC'.

Thrive NYC was a response to high mental health demands and inequity of care in NYC. The report notes that New Yorkers often experience economic struggles, violence, discrimination, and racism, which are attributable to concerning rates of depression, anxiety, and other mental illness in the city. In 2013–14, approximately one in five adults in NYC had a mental illness in the past 12 months, and about 524,000 individuals in NYC had depression [7]. However, only 40% of adults with symptoms of depression received mental health treatment in the past 12 months while spending 25.6% of all healthcare expenditures in NYC for patients with mental illness [8]. This mental health crisis led to the $853 million commitment over four years to deliver the roadmap across 20 city agencies on 54 initiatives based on six principles [8].

Starting in January 2015, the City of New York organized 25 focus groups that included treatment specialists, clergy, advocates, educators, researchers, and business leaders representing more than 250 organizations. This coordinated and multi-agency effort was able to gain the support of mental health professionals, which facilitated coordinated actions guided by the roadmap [9]. The six principles represent goals and directions to better allocate resources, and they are not to be understood as an outcome, but as a *process* composed of short-term goals. They collectively address the broad social determinants of mental health, and address various issues, including stigma, education, access to treatment, continuity of care, research, and political will.

The first principle seeks to 'Change the Culture' by reducing stigma with open conversations about mental health. Broad media campaigns will instill the ideas of mental health in public settings such as education, health, and justice. One programme in particular, 'Mental Health First Aid: NYC' is committed to training 250,000 residents in mental health first aid over the next five years. This will equip friends, family members, and co-workers with tools to support those who are suffering from a mental health condition and reduce stigma. The second principle is 'Act Early' and recognizes the value of investing in prevention and early childhood intervention. The initiatives under this principle focus on childhood support. For example, a key initiative is to create a network of mental health consultants serving all schools with NYC hiring 100 School Mental Health Consultants (SMHCs), who are masters-level social workers or counsellors, to advise staff and administrators in schools. These SMHCs will conduct needs assessments, provide support for planning programmes/services, and facilitate emergency response by partnering with other communities. In addition, programmes to increase social-emotional skills for children during critical stage of development by training 9000 teachers, assistants, and school leaders for approximately 100,000 children aged 0–5. Moreover, NYC commits to expanding resources for children with behavioural disorders by providing additional 20,000 clinical visits and consultations for an estimated 3500 children and their parents or caregivers annually.

The third principle is to 'Close Treatment Gaps' that exist because if the huge diversity of ethnic and socio-economic status that exists in NYC. These gaps are to be addressed by increasing treatment and preventative capacity. This will be accomplished by empowering non-specialists to provide support, using technology, and analyzing cost-effectiveness to distribute resources intelligently. The fourth principle is to 'Partner with Communities' to highlight the importance of collaboration with community members and organizations. This principle recognizes that individuals with mental health issues will often seek support from those they are closest to. They will commit to creating a network of community support to not only provide accessible care, but also address the structural violence prevalent in poor neighbourhoods, for example by creating a NYC Mental Health Corps that would consist of approximately 400 physicians and recently graduated Masters and Doctoral-level clinicians working for high-need communities in substance use programmes, mental health clinics, and primary care practices, with the City committing to provide 400,000 additional hours of services.

Principle five is 'Use Data Better' to reflect the commitment to provide more evidence-based decision-making processes, and enhanced surveillance activity using traditional and innovative tools can better identify gaps in care. This would be implemented with the creation of a Mental Health Innovation Lab that is designed to be a research and development arm of the roadmap and will be responsible for collecting information and sharing them to assist and empower stakeholders involved in promoting mental health. The sixth and final principle is 'Strengthen the Government's Ability to Lead', which commits the Mayor's office to a long-term collaborative effort to start systems change by engaging the local community partners and higher orders of state government. This principle recognizes that the City's main role is to collaborate and bring stakeholders together. A key initiative is the creation of a Mental Health Council as the primary vehicle for managing mental health initiatives, policy-making, and problem-solving across City government. It will be comprised of City agencies from every sector of the government, and will work closely with community organizations, other levels of government, clergy, advocates, and individuals with lived experience. Other forms of collaboration with state and federal governments include the creation of new supportive housing for vulnerable populations by committing to bring on 15,000 apartments for supportive housing over the next 15 years.

While Thrive NYC may appear overly ambitious, the roadmap cleverly bridges various short-term goals (initiatives) with long-term goals (principles) to appeal to both the public and politicians. The short-term achievable goals serve as proof of action that satiates the needs of politicians, while long-term goals serve as sustainable action that gains electoral support that will be required to fuel long-term funding and action. At the same time, the roadmap is an evidence-based plan by consulting with various professional stakeholders, addressing the broad issues that are related to mental health. While the future progress of this roadmap will eventually determine its impact, the roadmap itself is an example of establishing consensus between both scientific evidence and political incentives.

Two cities, one goal

The differences in how Vancouver and NYC approach urban mental health show that that urban mental health, which is not an either/or proposition. There are actions to enhance urban mental health, which can be done with existing budgets and powers. It can be a big campaign with new funds and resources. Straightforward policy changes can achieve significant improvements in urban mental health, as shown by Vancouver, as do new programmes, as shown by

NYC. Big or small, any attention to urban mental health takes a commitment from civic politicians to stand up and be the champions. Getting politicians there may be difficult, but by showing how it benefits their cities (and their electoral self-interest!) can help smooth that path. A cynical view perhaps, but whatever the reason it behooves us all to step up to the challenge and actually deliver.

References

1. **Wilson-Bates F.** *Lost in Transition: How a Lack in Capacity in the Mental Health System is Failing Vancouver's Mentally Ill and Draining Police Resources.* Vancouver, BC: Vancouver Police Department, 2008.
2. **Huffington Post.** Manure Dump at Homeless Camp Embarrasses B.C. Mayor. Available at: https://www.huffingtonpost.ca/2013/06/06/abbotsford-manure-dump-homeless_n_3398629.html (accessed 28 November 2018).
3. **Thompson S.** Policing Vancouver's mentally ill: The disturbing truth. Beyond lost in transition. Available at: https://vancouver.ca/police/assets/pdf/reports-policies/vpd-lost-in-transition-part-2-draft.pdf (accessed 26 November 2018).
4. **City of Vancouver.** Project Civil City. Available at: http://www.samsullivan.ca/pdf/project-civil-city.pdf (accessed 26 November 2018).
5. **City of Vancouver.** A Healthy City for All Healthy City Strategy – Four Year Action Plan 2015–2018. Available at: http://vancouver.ca/files/cov/Healthy-City-Strategy-Phase-2-Action-Plan-2015-2018.pdf (accessed 26 November 2018).
6. **Weibe D.** Vancouver Police Mental Health Strategy: A comprehensive approach for a proportional police response to persons living with mental illness. Available at: https://vancouver.ca/police/assets/pdf/reports-policies/mental-health-strategy.pdf (accessed 26 November 2018).
7. **Thorpe LE, Greene C, Freeman A, Snell E, Rodriguez-Lopez JS, Frankel M,** et al. Rationale, design and respondent characteristics of the 2013–2014 New York City Health and Nutrition Examination Survey (NYC HANES 2013–2014). *Preventive Medicine Reports* 2015; **2**: 580–588.
8. **McCray C, Buery R, Bassett MT.** ThriveNYC: A Mental Health Roadmap for All. New York City: The New York City Mayor's Office. Available at: https://thrivenyc.cityofnewyork.us/wp-content/uploads/2016/03/ThriveNYC.pdf (accessed 18 November 2016).
9. **Belkin G, Linos N, Perlman SE, Norman C, Bassett MT.** A roadmap for better mental health in New York City. The Lancet. Available at: http://www.thelancet.com/pb/assets/raw/Lancet/pdfs/S0140673615008302.pdf (accessed 28 November 2018).

Chapter 20

Urban design for mental health in Tokyo

Layla McCay, Emily Suzuki, and Anna Chang

Introduction

The Centre for Urban Design and Mental Health's first city case study considers urban design and planning factors that may impact mental health in Tokyo. An analysis of relevant Tokyo Metropolitan Government (TMG) policies was combined with the interviewing of 11 Tokyo-based urban design and mental health professionals to understand opportunities and challenges around the integration of mental health in urban design policies and plans in Tokyo.

Mental health in Tokyo

The World Mental Health Japan survey found the lifetime prevalence of common mental illnesses to be around one in five people in Japan, and just one-fifth of these seek formal treatment [1]. Mental illness was found to be the second greatest chronic disease cause of severe role impairment, accounting for nearly one-quarter of all-cause disease burden [2]. There was an 8.1% lifetime risk of anxiety disorders, 7.4% substance use disorders (largely alcohol), and 6.5% mood disorders (largely depression). Although gradually improving, Japan has one of the highest suicide rates in the world [3], with a complex mix of drivers, from depression to a tradition of 'honourable suicide' following unemployment, financial problems, or causing a burden for family members.

While Tokyo-specific mental health statistics are less widely available, the city has some particular mental health challenges. A culture of very long working hours restricts time available for socializing, exercising, sleep, and leisure, and is associated with *karoshi* ('death by overwork', usually by heart attacks, stroke, or suicide). The evidence on causality and prevalence of *karoshi* is still incomplete, but high stress is thought to contribute. A further Tokyo-focused issue is *hikkikomori*, acute social withdrawal typified by a young person not leaving their home for more than six months; this affects over a million people each year with a lifetime prevalence of 1.2% [4]. Finally, some of Tokyo's population have been affected by disasters such as the 2011 Tohoku earthquake and tsunami, and everyone lives in recognition that a destructive earthquake could occur at any time.

Urban planning and design for mental health in Tokyo

Tokyo is often considered a city, but it is, in fact, a metropolitan prefecture (region) comprising 23 special wards, each governed as separate cities, plus 26 more cities, five towns, and eight villages, all governed separately (with national and TMG influence), creating a complex picture in terms of urban planning. The city has a population of over 13 million people, and the metropolitan area extends to a population of 36 million, the most populous in the world [5]. The centre has a density of 15,187 people per square kilometer, much less than Manhattan (27,000) and Paris (21,000). Tokyo's urban planning history is characterized by a cycle of city destruction and rebuilding driven by fires, earthquakes, and war. There has been recent decentralization of city planning, and resident consultation and active participation is considered an important element of the planning process.

'Health is always the most important topic in urban planning. When we had the Meiji Restoration, a priority topic was health'—urban planner.

While physical health is addressed, there is less explicit recognition of mental health in urban planning as the concept is not universally recognized. 'Mental health' is often considered to be synonymous with mental illness (for instance, a person with a mental illness is sometimes referred to by the abbreviation 'men-hel'), and is subject to profound stigma. However, concepts of 'stress', 'peace', and 'comfort' are better recognized in Tokyo, and design factors that affect mental health are incorporated into Tokyo projects, such as natural spaces [6, 7], facilitating physical activity [8] and prosocial activity [9], safety (including wayfinding, crime, and traffic), and sleep quality [10, 11]. When asked, interviewees identified design features that they felt might affect mental health in Tokyo: beauty, nature, opportunities for creativity, social connections, opportunities to contribute to the community, access to health care, safety, and confidence that the city is well managed, including efficient, reliable transportation. This is not addressed systematically, and most architects and planners interviewed were not familiar with any specific laws or guidelines that explicitly address mental health, other than those promoting quality of life for older people. However, two of Tokyo's stated goals for urban planning do have relevance for mental health: restoration of green and blue spaces; and creating a city where people can live comfortably, safely, and with peace of mind. Furthermore, at a national level, five goals of Japan's Ministry of Land, Infrastructure, Transport and Tourism have relevance to urban design for mental health: changing social environment to develop people's self awareness on health; promoting elderly people's community participation to help them find the purpose of life; preparing urban functions within walking distance from elderly people's homes so that they can live by themselves; making a city where people can safely walk, for example barrier-free sidewalks; and improving public transportation services.

Access to nature: green and blue places

One of the main ways in which Tokyo's urban design promotes mental health is by increasing citizens' access to green space. In the Edo period, Tokyo was filled with green spaces and waterfront parks. However, with industrialization much of this was lost. Tokyo policies explicitly recognize the health benefits of green space: 'Greenery in urban areas brings pleasant and comfortable features to the lifestyles of residents' and 'greenery brings comfort to the human spirit' (Basic Policies for the 10-year Project for Green Tokyo, TMG 2007).

> 'Plants are a way to improve happiness'—think tank academic.

Tokyo has several public parks, plus several large, landscaped parks that can be visited for a small fee. However, the existing development of the city limits opportunities to integrate further greenery into the cityscape. Nature is recognized as a factor that promotes good mental health and its appreciation is part of Japanese culture; however, Tokyo's green spaces are not always 'useable'. While cherry blossom (hanami) season encourages picnics in the park, a good opportunity to socialize, relax, and meet people beyond one's colleagues and family, at other times of the year, such informal use of green space can be considered inappropriate.

> 'Parks have too many fixed benches, too many plants, and not enough open space. They have early closing times and signs to stay off the grass. And I think guards panic when they see people using a green space that is not designated for that purpose'—urban designer.

The Development Policy for City Planning Park and Green Space (2011) seeks to 'revive beautiful city Tokyo surrounded by water and green corridors' and explicitly recognizes urban greenery 'as a place of relief for Tokyo citizens'. This recognition of the benefits of nature is reiterated in the Metropolitan Area Readjustment Act (1958, frequent revisions), spawning various Green Action Plans, which prioritize the need to 'conserve green spaces that embrace the healthy natural environment'. There is an added in-centive in Tokyo to invest in open green spaces as evacuation locations in the event of natural disasters. A range of laws, including the Urban Park Act, the Landscapes Act, and the Urban Green Space Conservation Act, supports these efforts. The current Tokyo City Planning Vision by the Bureau of Urban Development envisions green roofs, ground-level planting, additional lawns and riverside greenery, and using plants to create more shadow in order to reduce heat.

In the Edo period, Tokyo had many rivers and aqueducts, but many now flow beneath the city. Some of these now form walking and cycling routes, running parallel to roadways, creating green pedestrian pathways and narrow pathways that run alongside houses, and landscaped long, narrow parks with running water. Of the remaining overground rivers and canals, many are now lined by warehouses and other industrial facilities; until recently, the water was polluted, and these areas avoided by residents. Recent improvements in water quality have driven exploration of the opportunities of waterside development [12], spawning new riverside trails for walking and relaxing, yet these are usually only busy for seasonal festivals.

Specific actions to improve access to nature in Tokyo: designating green zones

Tokyo's Comprehensive Policy for Preserving Greenery (2010) has led to the designation of special districts and zones in Tokyo, including those focused on promoting greenery, including special green space conservation districts that conserve and promote urban green spaces; large-scale suburban green space conservation zones that explicitly aim to 'maintain and improve healthy minds and bodies of urban and suburban residents'; and scenic districts that aim to conserve urban scenic beauty and environment.

Incentivizing park development by private companies

In central Tokyo, open space is expensive. While pseudo-public space can have challenges, privately run parks have increased green space across the city. TMG's Guideline for Greenery Development in Privately-Owned Public Spaces encourages the creation of greenery networks and prosocial open spaces as part of large-scale urban development. This includes initiatives like the easing of building regulations for private business projects that include a certain-sized park, which they develop, manage, and make free for public access. TMG also promotes greening through greening requirements in land lease contracts (such as parking lots), and facilitating public-private partnerships such as waterfront projects (Figure 20.1).

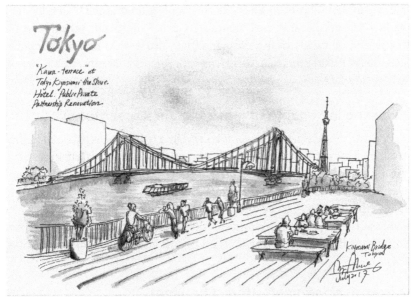

Figure 20.1 Sumida River Terrace Project is a public–private partnership that seeks to deliver a waterside venue for walking, cycling, and socializing in Tokyo.
Courtesy of Ryoji Noritake.

Machizukuri

> 'Machizukuri (街づくり) became popular to stimulate energy of cities by developing good residential environment'—architect.

Machizukuri involves empowering citizens in community design, and a key way in which they do so is in greening the city. Tokyo is remarkable for having relatively few parks, yet a profusion of greenery. Much of this comprises plant pots and tree bases planted and maintained by Tokyo citizens in tiny public spaces near their properties all over the city, ostensibly greening the city at the individual level. TMG has stated that 'the leading players in restoring greenery to Tokyo are its citizens'. They emphasize that to restore greenery of Tokyo 'it is necessary for each citizen of Tokyo to take an interest in greenery. The driving force for creating a verdant Tokyo will be people's wish to nurture green areas in their lives in which greenery is scare and to cherish abundant greenery'. To this end, the TMG has encouraged 'greenery tended carefully by residents', such as the planting of trees (including a practice of 'memorial trees' to celebrate special events like graduation or marriage), and turfing of school playgrounds. TMG recommends approaches to help residents green their neighbourhoods, delivering workshops, and sharing methodology for green rooftops, walls, railroad areas, and parking lots. TMG encourages fundraising to develop new parks, offers tax incentives to encourage residents' efforts, and provides tax incentives on contributions to a 'green fund', and also seeks to 'match' community needs with local business, and citizens with professional urban designers, to achieve green aspirations.

Investing in *Kankyojiku* (environmental green axes)

Kankyojiku are networks of urban spaces around roads, rivers, parks, and infrastructure that are 'lush with greenery' and create a network of 'environmental green axes' throughout the city. The principle of *kankyojiku* spaces is that whenever urban facilities are being developed, deep, wide greenery is integrated to deliver 'pleasant landscapes' and 'scenic beauty' for local communities. TMG published *Kankyojiku* guidelines in 2007 and the *Kankyojiku* Council was established the following year to share lessons and promote development of these areas.

Access to *shinrin yoku* (forest bathing)

Japan has long enjoyed a health tradition of onsen bathing (hot mineral waters). The concept of forest bathing was developed by the Japanese Ministry of Agriculture, Forestry and Fisheries in 1982. This is considered a therapeutic health practice that aims to boost immunity, reduce stress, and promote well-being. *Shinrin yoku* literally means 'taking in the forest atmosphere' mindfully, without any distractions. Japanese research has found this practice to be associated with improvements in physiological and psychological indicators of stress, mood hostility, fatigue, confusion, and vitality [13]. In particular, the research suggests that forests located at high elevations with low atmospheric pressure may help reduce depression. Throughout Japan, there are 48 official forest routes where local research has demonstrated health benefits; five are within Tokyo metropolis and accessible from the city centre by affordable trains. Around a quarter of the Tokyo population are said to participate in *shinrin yoku*, and some companies even include visits as part of their company health plan.

Designing active spaces

Tokyo is a city of commuters but not of car ownership (0.46 cars per household [14]). The metropolis is huge, the housing prices in central areas are expensive, the suburbs are large and sprawling, the public transit system is crowded yet affordable, efficient, and effective, and, as such, many people spend substantial time commuting each day by public transportation (the average one-way commute to work is around 45 minutes).

This means Tokyo's citizens naturally integrate light exercise into their daily routines through active transport (walking, cycling, and accessing public transit).

> 'Increasing walking and pedestrianisation is primarily to ease congestion, improve safety, reduce pollution, and benefit physical health—but of course there is a mental health benefit'—think tank academic.

Walking

TMG's Bureau of Social Welfare and Public Health seeks to increase walking under the tagline 'small efforts, lasting health', stating that 'walking can be a great change of mood and stress-release'. This effort includes publishing walking maps on their website, and encouraging walking in 'urban oases': 'The sound of chirping birds and running water, the sight of beautiful foliage, the fragrance of seasonal flowers, and more—nature has a way of truly refreshing the body and mind'. Japan's Ministry of Land, Infrastructure, Transport and Tourism considers a pedestrian-friendly environment to be a component of healthy ageing, and walkability is explicitly part of living space planning for older people. The guideline emphasizes that people are more willing to walk and exercise if the surrounding environment is planned with social space and facilities, such as resting spots and parks, and recognizes the importance of views and path maintenance.

Walking is the key mechanism by which people access train stations, which are often barrier-free. This naturally integrates physical activity into people's daily routines, although this is not generally considered an exercise opportunity.

> 'You'll see them standing in line for the escalator rather than using the stairs. They don't commute like this for the exercise benefits'—health company employee

The preponderance of walking and cycling, including to access public transport, as the preferred modes of transport in the streets has had the effect of naturally channeling most car traffic onto larger roads; cars use smaller roads at low volume and low speed, primarily for access. This prioritizes pedestrians and cyclists to the extent that in many instances, there is no need for formal pavements, and these roads form largely pedestrian pathways converging into social hubs around stations.

Public transport

Tokyo has the highest usage of public transit in the world. The system's success involves its reach, efficiency, reliability, affordability, and dependability, facilitating access to the full breadth of the city and its suburbs.

'At any station in Tokyo, we have so many passengers on the station platform. However, Japanese people don't feel stress because trains are punctual and come one after another. People know they can get another train soon. In this sense, stress can be reduced by good railway management'—urban planner.

Long working hours, safety, and some of the shortest sleeping times in the world mean that many people commuting to and within Tokyo spend their commuting time having a restorative nap—although this type of sleep can be easily disrupted and of a poorer quality than sleep at home; furthermore, crowded train carriages preclude sleep and other opportunities for relaxation in transit

Overcrowding in train carriages can also cause discomfort and stress, and can facilitate harassment, including unwanted sexual contact from *chikan* (gropers) or voyeuristic 'up-skirt' photography; the latter trend has led to two main design changes in the last two decades: designated women-only carriages, and a loud, compulsory shutter sound for all photographs taken with mobile phones purchased in Japan.

Cycling

Bicycles are another key form of transportation in Tokyo and an important opportunity to integrate physical activity into daily life, but they are used differently than in many other cities. Around 14% of journeys in Tokyo each day are made by bike; however, these are largely short journeys (less than 2 km), and are often undertaken by women undertaking domestic chores such as shopping and picking children up from school. These affordable, light 'mother's bikes', referred to informally as '*mamachari*', have become a cultural icon, affording women independence, physical activity, access to both social and natural settings, and the other benefits of cycling. They emerged in the 1950s and with their space for baskets, luggage racks and multiple child seats have made cycling accessible and convenient for women and their families. They are now ubiquitous. The government sought to impose a limit of one child to be carried per *mamachari*. Mothers complained, and the number of child passengers permissible was increased to a limit of two (although, in reality, three children riders per mamachari are often observed). *Mamacharis* often share pavements with pedestrians, or use smaller roads. It is thought that up to 9% of employees across Japan cycle to work; Tokyo figures are unavailable, but bike commuting is less common than in comparably sized cities overseas, due largely to bureaucratic barriers. Corporate law requires companies to insure their staff for accidents during commuting, and cycling is rarely covered. Companies may also be liable for payment of bicycle repair costs. As a result, many companies impose bans on cycling to work (although some operate a 'don't ask don't tell policy', and occasionally companies do promote cycling for both environmental and health benefits).

> 'In the building next to us, staff members are forbidden from cycling to work, because of the risk of accidents and insurance claims ... Some of the staff do it sneakily anyway'— health company employee.

An important impact of these restrictions has been that formal bicycle infrastructure is limited in Japan. Protected bike lanes are rare, and commuter cyclists commonly cycle on pavements for their safety. This can both restrict the commute's potential efficiency and create hazards for pedestrians. It is unusual for workplaces to provide bike parking, lockers, or showers to facilitate bike commuting. And bikeshare in Tokyo remains sparse, with docking stations far apart and not extending throughout the city, rendering bikeshare practical only for limited routes.

Future plans to facilitate regular physical activity in Tokyo

A series of policies and plans are emerging that contain physical activity promotion and facilitation aspirations. Urban walkability is set to improve. Over the next 13 years, a pedestrian-friendly environment and a new underground network of pedestrian walkways are envisioned in the Toranomon area; 43 km of riverside walking paths by 2024, and the Bureau of Urban Development's road space working group is developing a Rambling Tokyo Strategy, aiming to create a network for walkers in the city, including infrastructure improvements (signs, walkway quality, resting places) and local public transport, alongside encouraging travel by foot by creating and promoting 'charm points', and places of historical, cultural, and entertainment interest on walking routes. Urban bikeability is also set to improve, framed as part of energy-saving policies, including a 264-km bike path (and related facilities) and improved bikeshare facilities. A general citizen fitness programme is also underway to make sports more enjoyable to citizen of Tokyo post-Olympics, using the Olympics facilities, and creating a 'sport-friendly environment'.

Prosocial space

> 'If people feel that they are a part of the society and community through social activities in open public spaces, it is good for their mental health'—architect.

Public spaces are often the epicentre of positive, natural social interaction in a city, and this is widely recognized as an important factor in maintaining good mental health and building resilience. Tokyo tends not to have town squares, which form natural public open spaces in many Western countries; the priority for open-space design is more likely to be evacuation space in case of earthquakes.

Outdoor public places

'There are three types of public places in Tokyo: public parks, train plazas and temples/shrines'—urban planner.

Public parks

'If you go to pachinko (a pinball gambling game) or shopping centre, you will notice the lack of diversity. However, parks are open for anyone. You can see all the generations, including rich, poor, elderly and young people'—architect.

Train station plazas

'Evacuation space for earthquakes takes priority over placemaking. Station plazas are mostly empty other than smoking areas. There is opportunity for development, such as removing smoking areas, and having benches—benches with a more social layout to encourage social interaction'—academic.

Temples and shrines

'Temples and shrines have many community events—matsuri (festivals), markets ...'—urban planner.

Indoor public places

Value is increasingly being recognized in the potential of indoor public spaces to reap the benefits of prosocial interaction. In particular, there is discussion in Tokyo of how to better harness shopping centre design and facilities to improve health and well-being, envisioning the centre of a shopping mall as a new version of a city's town square, how to design bars to facilitate positive social discussions, and how to better design urban workplaces to help counteract the potentially negative health effects of Tokyo's trend for very long working hours.

Shopping places

'Shopping areas next to train stations belong to the train company and generate income—but they are often "placeless spaces", that do not reflect the neighbourhood at all'—academic.

'Shotengai (indoor/covered shopping arcades) feel very connected with their local communities ... shopping malls can be more placeless'—academic.

'Shopping malls have evolved to have more open spaces and high ceilings to reduce stress and let people sit, relax and talk. Sometimes there are classes or markets or other activities'—policy specialist.

'Temples and shrines often have an associated retail corridor. This integrates them with the community'—urban planner.

Bars

'In Akabane, there is a famous drinking place with a ko-shaped counter. The "Ko" shape ['ko' is the pronunciation of the Japanese katakana symbol コ] was invented to increase people's happiness, to share their smiles with other visitors while they drink'—urban designer.

Offices

'Designers are trying to address the stress caused by long working hours—they do that by increasing social interaction, through more open spaces in the office, and by making routes more inconvenient, so that people moving around the office or university have more movement and more social interactions'—policy specialist.

Places for older people

The opportunities of older people to move around their neighbourhoods and socialize is valued, and a new aspect of Tokyo's long-term care policies seeks to bring urban planning into play, with 'designated activity areas', often around a station, that bring together shops and services, home care, health facilities, and social facilities in convenient, barrier-free 'daily activity areas'. There have also been experiments with 'healthy roads' in Tokyo, widening the road to facilitate pedestrian traffic of different speeds, again clustering a range of services in an accessible way.

Post-disaster places

Finally, experiences of disasters in Tokyo and the surrounding regions have led to post-traumatic stress and contributed to the city's focus on opportunities to support people's mental health through architecture and planning, and facilitating prosocial opportunity has emerged as a key factor. One incident that has recently increased interest in the links between urban design and mental health was the March 2011 Great East Japan Earthquake, tsunami, and nuclear accident, from research identifying the emerging benefits of group walking on reducing depression in older people post-disaster to design of temporary housing [15].

'People were traumatised after 3/11 (tsunami and earthquake), so we had to think about city design. People evacuated due to the tsunami were living in temporary housing, which was stressful for most people. We made shared space at the entrance of their temporary housing to increase social interaction and community spaces with gardens. Entrances were designed to face each other rather than side by side to promote sociability'—architect.

Safe space

Tokyo prioritizes the safety of its citizens in terms of maintaining its very low crime rate, and preparing for natural disasters. Design interventions to enhance safety in Tokyo include earthquake-resistant buildings and firebreak belts, along with barrier-free design, to enable the safe movement of older people and those with disabilities around the city.

> 'People feel little stress because Tokyo is safe and clean. If there is an earthquake, we all know what to do, we are all ready, so we do not have to fear; nuclear risks are a big fear'— urban planner.

Although Tokyo is known around the world for being safe, twenty-first-century safety trends have started to drive anxiety leading to reduced prosocial interactions within communities:

> 'I read last week on Twitter that parents of elementary school children suggested a condominium building put up a notice advising residents "Don't say hello to children in this building: they are instructed not to respond strangers to protect themselves from crimes in the building's shared space". Elderly people responded that they feel bad when they say hello to children in the building and nobody responds'—architect.

Measurement of urban mental health

While Tokyo's first policy to link urban living and health was published in 1972, it was not until the 1990s that the city started to measure people's 'life evaluation'. More recently, there has been a trend of promoting the concept of urban 'happiness', particularly in the context of sustainability. In 2011, a prefectural ranking of well-being was published in Japan, leading to a flurry of measurements of well-being across the country. In Shiga prefecture in 2012, residents proposed a 'smile index of wellbeing'; the Tosa Association of Corporate Executives released the Gross Kochi Happiness index; 52 local governments across the country launched a 'Happiness League'; and in 2015, Arakawa City in Tokyo published its first 'Gross Arakawa Happiness Report', inspired by Bhutan's measurement of happiness. These projects tend to use indicators that do not necessarily address urban design factors, and often include few explicit mental health indicators (insert Figure 20.2).

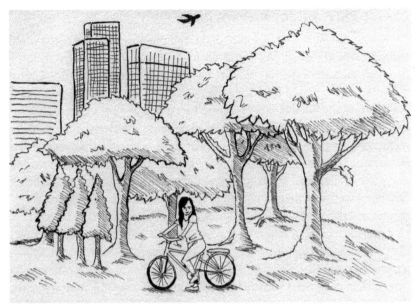

Figure 20.2 Cycling in Tokyo greenery.
Courtesy of Mai Kobuchi.

Case studies

Case study 1: dementia-friendly communities

A dementia-friendly community is one that supports older people with dementia by ensuring they feel included and appreciated in the places they live, helping them remain independent with a good quality of life, reducing stigma, anxiety, and frustration, and reducing the need for higher levels of care. Japan pioneered dementia-friendly communities. These communities combine awareness raising with adaptations to help people with dementia navigate, access, and use local facilities, from shops and banks to pharmacies and public transport. These adaptations can include signage, creating barrier-free access, places to rest and socialize, and toilet availability. The communities also encourage prosocial interaction between all ages. The Dementia-Friendly Japan Initiative helps to deliver these changes: a private sector-led platform of business, local government, academia, non-governmental organizations, and people with dementia and their families. A further policy intervention that supports dementia-friendly communities is Japan's Compact Cities initiative. Developed to cope with depopulation, the initiative clusters government services and other facilities and ensures they are accessible to all by public transport.

Case study 2: suicide prevention

For many years, Japan has had some of the highest rates of suicide in the world, and until recently the subject was taboo. In the last decade, Japan has really focused on suicide prevention, and the rates have decreased. Urban design has played a role in preventing suicide. Part of this has been physical prevention. For example, the installation of platform barriers to prevent access to the train line can deter suicide attempts, or draw attention to suicide attempts, enabling others to press public panic buttons to alert staff before the train approaches. However, other design interventions are being introduced to reduce suicidal intent in certain locations. A Japanese study of installing blue LED lights on platforms seems to suggest an association with a reduction of suicides, although the size of the impact is not clear. It is speculated that this works as blue is associated with calmness or nature; or else it creates associations with the police; or even that it simply causes a disruption in ordinary perceptions and distracts suicidal intention. Blue LED lighting has now been employed by several train companies as a suicide prevention measure [16]. Shin-Koiwa station, a particularly common Tokyo location for suicide by jumping in front of trains, has taken this to another level by covering the roof in blue translucent covering (although covering white light with blue light has also been criticized for degrading lighting quality and reducing safety on the platform). Efforts at Shin-Koiwa station are complemented by measures including the installation of television screens showing nature scenes, and posting information about a free suicide prevention helpline on the walls of station platforms.

Conclusions

While not explicitly designing to promote mental health, Tokyo is interested in reducing population 'stress' and increasing 'comfort'. Furthermore, the city places a high priority on systematically integrating greenery into the urban environment, facilitating safe active transport, and improving older people's quality of life, all key factors in promoting good mental health through the built environment. However, the stigma and lack of awareness and explicit recognition of mental health risks missing opportunities, and the high level of existing development creates placemaking challenges.

Tokyo could help improve urban design for population mental health by:

- *Increasing awareness of the links between urban design and mental health:* awareness-raising and education for policymakers could articulate the opportunity and help create demand for systematic integration of mental health into urban design guidelines, policies, and incentives.

◆ *Realizing the cycling opportunity:* To reap fully the productivity and physical and mental health benefits of cycling (including counteracting the effects of long working hours), companies' insurance policies could evolve to facilitate commuting by bike, and investments could be make in cycling infrastructure in the city (such as more protected bike lanes, cycle routes that go through natural settings, and bike parking) and in the workplace (such as showers, lockers, and bike parking).

◆ *Harnessing waterways for better mental health and well-being:* Tokyo's waterways remain largely untapped natural spaces that could provide more green and blue spaces for walking, watersports, relaxing, and socializing.

◆ *Designing public spaces for social interaction:* innovative design can help increase opportunities for positive, natural social interactions. This may include street seating, street games, outdoor gyms, nature installation, and public gathering spaces for festivals, markets, and other local events.

◆ *Optimizing the workplace for better mental health:* Tokyo's practice of having long working hours compared with other cities, along with often long commutes, means that Tokyo citizens are missing out on quality time for leisure, nature access, exercise, and socializing on work days. Urban designers can help integrate these protective factors into the 'work pathway' to help promote good mental health. This includes the commute to/from work (opportunities for physical activity, nature exposure, relaxing setting, and efficiency, including management of overcrowding on public transport), and in the work setting (access to nature—including views of nature, pictures of nature, office gardens and office greenery, circadian lighting, opportunities for social interaction, privacy, choices about workspaces and settings, physical activity within the office, and support of physical activity in office commute).

Lessons from Tokyo can be applied in other cities:

◆ *Empower and incentivize city users to install nature everywhere:* to green a city where large park spaces may not be available, it is possible to empower the general public to take personal responsibility in contributing to street greenery. A combination of education and incentive programmes can also help to encourage businesses to invest in innovative greening of available spaces, including roofs, walls, and public parks.

◆ *Nudge vehicles into main streets to achieve natural pedestrian-friendly superblocks:* encouraging motor vehicles to use large, efficient roads and avoid smaller roads other than for access prioritizes pedestrian and cyclist safety, public street events and activities, and development of green space.

- *Make active transport the most convenient way to get around:* an affordable, efficient, reliable, and extensive public transport system can nudge a natural reduction in cars and prioritize pedestrians and bicycles around station residential, shopping, social, and service hubs. Combined with a culture of biking as a family transport method, this:
    - promotes walking and biking, delivering regular physical activity;
    - drives demand for pedestrian infrastructure (such as overpasses and underpasses to access stations and services);
    - drives demand for fine-grained, human-scale streetfronts with welcoming, interesting engaging aspects for pedestrians, which help reduce negative thoughts, improve walkability and prosocial engagement with neighbours, and increase feelings of safety;
    - reduces light and sound from traffic on residential streets, promoting better sleep.
- *Make social exercise easy:* public transit access to exercise locations (from sports facilities to hiking) plus publicly accessible drinking water, lockers, and shower facilities for jogging, and convenient public transport accessibility for sports facilities, can help facilitate social exercise.
- *Integrate spiritual centres with the wider community:* temples, shrines, and other types of spiritual centres often contain potentially welcoming public spaces in cities otherwise lacking in available public spaces; communities can be drawn in with local festivals and retail corridors that connect their open spaces to the rest of the community.
- *Harness indoor public spaces for better mental health:* where wide-open urban public spaces are not available outdoors, innovative investment in interior placemaking for indoor, densely frequented places such as shopping malls can deliver green, active, prosocial spaces.
- *Use innovative design to help prevent suicide:* suicide reduction is not simply about physical barriers; psychological deterrents may be explored, such as blue lights and images of nature at high-risk train stations.

References

1. Ishikawa H, Kawakami N, Kessler RC, World Mental Health Japan Survey Collaborators. Lifetime and 12-month prevalence, severity and unmet need for treatment of common mental disorders in Japan: results from the final dataset of World Mental Health Japan Survey. *Epidemiology and Psychiatric Sciences* 2016; **25**: 217–229.
2. Health Japan. Available at: http://www.mhlw.go.jp/seisakunitsuite/bunya/kenkou_iryou/kenkou/kenkounippon21/en/kenkounippon21/data03.html (accessed 27 November 2018).

3. **Organisation for Economic Co-operation and Development.** Suicide rates. Available at: https://data.oecd.org/healthstat/suicide-rates.htm (accessed 27 November 2018).

4. **Koyama A, Miyake Y, Kawakami N, Tsuchiya M, Tachimori H, Takeshima T.** Lifetime prevalence, psychiatric comorbidity and demographic correlates of 'hikikomori' in a community population in Japan. *Psychiatry Research* 2010; **176**: 69–74.

5. **Koyama A, Miyake Y, Kawakami N, Tsuchiya M, Tachimori H, Takeshima T; World Mental Health Japan Survey Group, 2002–2006.** Lifetime prevalence, psychiatry comorbidity and demographic correlates of "hikikomori" in a community population in Japan. *Psychiatry Research* 2010; **176**: 69–74.

6. **Roe J.** Cities, green space and mental wellbeing. *Environmental Science* 2016; DOI: 10.1093/acrefore/9780199389414.013.93.

7. **Gascon M, Triguero-Mas M, Martínez D, Dadvand P, Forns J, Plasència A, Nieuwenhuijsen MJ.** Mental health benefits of long-term exposure to residential green and blue spaces: a systematic review. *International Journal of Environmental Research and Public Health* 2015; **12**: 4354–4379.

8. **Morgan AJ, Parker AG, Alvarez M, Jimenez AF, Jorm AF.** Exercise and mental health: an Exercise and Sports Science Australia commissioned review. *JEP Online* 2013; **16**: 64–73.

9. **Francis J, Wood LJ, Knuiman M, Giles-Corti B.** Quality or quantity? Exploring the relationship between Public Open Space attributes and mental health in Perth, Western Australia. *Social Science & Medicine* 2012; **74**: 1570–1577.

10. **Clark C, Myron R, Stansfeld S, Candy B.** A systematic review on the effect of the built and physical environment on mental health. *Journal of Public Mental Health* 2006; **6**: 14–27.

11. **Litman T.** Urban Sanity: Understanding Urban Mental Health Impacts and How to Create Saner, Happier Cities. Available at: http://www.vtpi.org/urban-sanity.pdf (accessed 27 November 2018).

12. **Tokyo Construction Bureau.** On the Progress of River Restoration and the Future View in Japan and Asia. Available at: http://rwes.dpri.kyoto-u.ac.jp/~tanaka/APHW/ APHW2004/proceedings/FWR/56-FWR-A782/Resubmit%2056-FWR-A782.pdf (accessed 27 November 2018).

13. **Park BJ, Tsunetsugu Y, Kasetani T, Kagawa T, Miyazaki Y.** The physiological effects of Shinrin-yoku (taking in the forest atmosphere or forest bathing): evidence from field experiments in 24 forests across Japan. *Environmental Health and Preventive Medicine* 2010; **15**: 18–26.

14. **Hongo J.** Number of cars per household stagnates in Japan. *Wall Street Journal.* Available at: https://blogs.wsj.com/japanrealtime/2014/08/18/number-of-cars-per-household-stagnates-in-japan/ (accessed 27 November 2018).

15. **Tsuji T, Sasaki Y, Matsuyama Y, Sata Y, Aida J, Kondo K, Kawachi I.** Reducing depressive symptoms after the Great East Japan Earthquake in older survivors through group exercise participation and regular walking: a prospective observational study. *BMJ Open* 2017; **7**: e013706.

16. **Matsubayashi T, Sawada Y, Ueda M.** Does the installation of blue lights on train platforms prevent suicide? A before-and-after observational study from Japan. *Journal of Affective Disorders* 2013; **147**: 385–388.

Challenges in urban settings

Chapter 21

Urban mental health strategies

Todd Litman

Introduction

Urban living can impose special mental health risks such as crowding and reduced privacy, fear of crime, reduced physical activity, economic stress, unpleasant transport conditions, and inadequate interaction with nature. New research helps experts understand and respond to these risks. Urban healthcare professionals can use this information to protect and enhance their own mental health, to better address their patients' mental health problems, and to guide policymakers and urban planners to enhance mental health in their communities.

By understanding these effects, health professionals can help inoculate their cities against mental health risks the same way they support strategies that reduce physical health risks such as infectious diseases and unhealthy lifestyles. This chapter examines mental health risks associated with urban living, the degree that they are associated with or caused by urban conditions, and possible ways for individuals and communities to reduce these risks and enhance urban mental health. These issues are important in both developed and developing countries.

Concentrated mental illness risk factors

Many cities areas have concentrations of people with elevated mental illness risk factors, including poverty, homelessness, physical and mental disabilities, drug and alcohol abuse, and social alienation [1]. This partly occurs because urban areas offer better services and opportunities, so disadvantaged people rationally choose to live in cities. This can create a self-reinforcing cycle, called *social drift*, when certain areas have more poverty and mental illness services, and become more tolerant of deviant lifestyles, which attracts high-risk residents and repels more affluent households [2].

Association or causation?

The concentration of higher risk groups in urban areas is mainly an *association* rather than a *cause* of mental illness. This concentration may exacerbate some mental health problems, for example, vulnerable people may abuse drugs and alcohol more if surrounded by people with that propensity, but they may also find more economic opportunities and specialized treatment services that reduce their risks. Although such neighborhoods may have high mental illness rates, mentally ill residents may be better off than if they located in more isolated areas.

Potential individual responses

Vulnerable people may want to avoid urban neighbourhoods with concentrated poverty and social problems.

Potential community responses

Cities should recognize that they tend to attract people with mental health risk factors, and so should provide appropriate support services, including suitable housing, community-based mental health and addiction services, job training and placement that targets higher-risk groups, and targeted law enforcement. In some situations it may be appropriate to discourage excessive concentration of social services and poor households in urban neighbourhoods.

Substance (alcohol and drug) abuse

Substance abuse is both a cause and symptom of mental illness. Alcohol and drug abuse patterns differ by geography: cocaine and heroin addiction is more common in cities, whereas prescription drug, methamphetamine, and alcohol abuse rates tend to be more common in rural areas. As alcohol and marijuana abuse is more common than heroin and cocaine addiction, total substance abuse rates tend to be higher in rural areas.

Association or causation?

The relationships between geography and substance abuse are complex, including cultural traditions (some communities are more accepting of drug and alcohol use), ease of obtaining drugs and alcohol, and access to treatment. The concentration of substance abuse can create a self-reinforcing cycle as that area becomes more tolerant, and attracts more users and related services. To the degree that such areas attract people who would abuse drugs or alcohol regardless of where they live, this is association; to the degree that it enables addiction it may cause substance abuse; and to the degree that such areas attract treatment services it may reduce total abuse. Similarly, as rural areas tend to have high prescription drug, methamphetamine, and alcohol abuse rates, rural living may cause such abuse.

Potential individual responses

Individuals susceptible to substance abuse may avoid geographical areas with high availability and abuse rates, and may use various personal prevention strategies. For example, somebody prone to cocaine and heroin addiction may avoid living in urban neighbourhoods where such drugs are easily available, and somebody prone to methamphetamine or alcohol abuse may avoid living in suburban and rural areas where their abuse is more common.

Potential community responses

Communities can provide targeted substance abuse prevention and treatment programmes. For example, urban areas may focus on cocaine and heroin addiction risks, whereas rural areas may focus on methamphetamine, prescription drug, and alcohol abuse prevention and treatment.

Social isolation and loneliness

Urban residents, particularly newcomers, sometimes experience social isolation, often described as 'lonely in a crowd', which may contribute to mental illness and unhappiness (Griffin 2016). Several factors may contribute to this.

Urban residents are more likely to be interregional migrants (new to a community). Only a third of urban residents spend their entire lives in one area, compared with half of rural residents, resulting in fewer local friends and family members [3]. Urban residents are often described as less welcoming than smaller communities [4].

Compact, walkable urban neighbourhoods provide excellent opportunities for daily, informal social interactions, which can create ongoing relationships. These are particularly important for people with disabilities and low incomes. For example, describing why he plans to retire to a busy city, one expert explains, 'Chance encounters brighten the day. They're like little love affairs without consequences. They keep you alert. This is what any senior citizen needs' [5].

Association or causation?

Some of the factors that contribute to urban loneliness are associations. Cities tend to have high rates of interregional migrants, and people living alone, who tend to be vulnerable to these effects, regardless of community size. Those people would experience similar isolation and loneliness if they moved to a rural area.

Lower marriage rates and higher divorce rates probably reflect a combination of association and causation, but these differences are disappearing. Cities offer more social opportunities, including specialized subcultures, which can reduce isolation and loneliness.

Visible minorities probably experience less stress in cities than they would in smaller communities where other residents are less accustomed to diversity; for those groups, city living probably increases mental health and happiness [6].

Potential individual responses

People who move to a new community should recognize the risks of isolation and loneliness, and take advantage of appropriate social opportunities to create friendships. People who have severe difficulties making new friends may be better off staying in their original communities in order to maintain their familial and social networks, but most people who move to cities can create new social networks. Conversely, people who feel alienated in a small community may be less lonely in a city where they can find more people with similar interests.

Potential community responses

Urban communities can encourage community cohesion (positive interactions among neighbours) by creating a welcoming public realm such as sidewalks and public parks, encouraging neighbourhood social activities, and by providing inclusive community and sports events [7]. Specific strategies include neighbourhood parks, improved walkability, and community festivals. It may be appropriate to sponsor special programmes to welcome and engage new residents, and monitor newcomers for possible isolation and loneliness.

Noise and light pollution

Urban areas tend to have more ambient noise and light pollution, which can induce stress and interrupt sleep. However, these problems are not unique to cities; suburban areas also have landscaping and vehicle noise, and rural areas experience farming activities and highway traffic noise. Rural residents experience about 10% more light exposure but have less 'social jet lag' (sleep and wake at times that are out of sync from their internal, biological clock) than urban residents [8].

Association or causation?

Noise and light pollution exposure tends to increase with density, and so can be considered as inherent to cities, but can often be managed and reduced with improved design.

Table 21.1 Community noise and light reduction strategies

Noise	Light
◆ Regulate on noise generation ◆ Restrict noisy vehicles (gasoline motorcycles and diesel trucks and buses) and reduce traffic speeds ◆ Restrict on sirens and alarms ◆ Restrict noisy industrial, construction, and landscaping activities ◆ Establish building noise insulation standards ◆ Develop street trees, walls, and other noise barriers	◆ Orient street lights downward ◆ Sign and building lighting restrictions ◆ High-quality window covers ◆ Sun glasses and eye shades ◆ Light design education

Various strategies can reduce urban noise and light pollution.

Potential individual responses

Urban residents can choose home locations away from roads with high speeds and traffic volumes (particularly heavy diesel vehicle routes), and homes with noise insulation and good window covers. People who are very noise or light sensitive may wear ear plugs or dark glasses. People who are very noise sensitive may need to avoid wood-frame multifamily housing.

Potential community responses

Table 21.1 lists various community strategies for reducing ambient noise and light pollution. Many of these strategies provide co-benefits; for example, shifts from diesel to electric buses reduce air and noise pollution, and double-pane windows reduce energy consumption.

Toxic pollution

Exposure to some toxins may increase mental illness. High childhood lead exposure, a common problem in some urban neighbourhoods increased adolescent aggression and behaviour problems, and adult criminal behaviour [9]. Fine particulate exposure is associated with increased anxiety, impaired cognition, and depressive behaviors [10, 11]. Prenatal polycyclic aromatic hydrocarbons (an air pollutant) exposure increases children's attention deficit disorder rates [12]. These impacts can increase mental illness directly, and indirectly by increasing crime rates. Because many of these toxins originate from industrial activities and vehicles, they tend to increase with density, highway proximity and highway travel. Suburban and rural residents also experience toxic pollutants, including motor vehicle travel, agricultural chemicals, and, in some areas, wood smoke. Control programmes are reducing some of these risks. For example, childhood lead exposure peaked in 1970 and subsequently declined after lead was phased out of gasoline and paint.

Association or causation?

To the degree that toxic pollution exposure increases with development density and mix, it can be considered to be caused by urban living. Exposure to lead paint tends to be common in older, poorly maintained housing in both urban and rural areas. Suburban residents that frequently travel on major highways may also suffer from toxin exposure and resulting illnesses.

Potential community responses

Communities can reduce toxic emissions by reducing total vehicle travel and shifting to less polluting vehicles; locating houses, worksites, schools, and playgrounds away from busy highways; and reducing the time people spend travelling on congested highways.

Excessive stimulation and stress

Some people speculate that urban living causes 'relentless' stimulation (also called *cognitive overload*) imposes mental stress [13–15]. This is understandable as urban environments tend to be busy and noisy, cities contain competitive industries and jobs, urban areas offer more economic and social opportunities than rural areas, and many people work in cities but live and recreate in suburban and rural areas, and so associate cities with responsibility and stress. However, these effects are largely associations rather than being unique to cities: a rural job can impose as much stress as an urban job, and, except for ambient noise, there is no reason that urban residents cannot engage in relaxing activities, such as knitting and reading, as they could in rural areas.

Cities may also increase psychological stress by causing frequent interactions with unfamiliar, diverse, and sometimes unfriendly people [4]. In a typical day, urban residents interact with hundreds of unfamiliar people, which exceeds *Dunbar's Number*, the number of close relationships that most people can maintain, which is generally estimated at 150–250 people. Urban populations tend to be diverse, so many of these interactions involve very different, and therefore frightening, people. The frequency and anonymity of these interactions may cause city residents to be less friendly than in smaller communities. Although most urban social interactions are benign or positive, their large numbers and diversity of may cause discomfort and stress, particularly for urban newcomers unaccustomed to these conditions [16]. A survey of urban neighbourhood residents found that many, particularly older, people consider 'a diverse mix of people in the precinct' to be undesirable [17]. Respondents indicated that they were afraid of increased density because it would increase unpredictable social interactions and possibly crime rates.

Association or causation?

Much of the stimulation and stress in cities is association rather than causation, reflecting the types of people and activities that locate in cities rather than a unique condition of urban living. Except for additional noise, few relaxing activities are significantly more difficult in cities than smaller communities. Increased interactions with unfamiliar and diverse people may cause mental stress to some people, particularly urban newcomers, but this is likely to decline as residents become more accustomed to urban social conditions. Many minorities and non-conformists probably experience less stress in cities than in small communities.

Potential individual responses

People who find diversity stressful can make an effort to become more familiar and comfortable with different groups in their community. Urban residents can organize their lives and homes to encourage calming and stress-reducing activities.

Potential community responses

If cultural diversity increases stress, communities can support community cohesion programmes that encourage people to become more familiar and comfortable with different groups. Planning can increase quiet and calm urban environments through noise reduction and greenspace development, and support calming and reassuring community activities such as local art and recreation programmes.

Crime

Crime is both a cause and effect of mental illness. Real or perceived fear of crime tends to increase stress and distrust, which reduces mental health and happiness. Because crime receives considerable media attention, many people have exaggerated perceptions of actual crime risks.

Reported crime rates are often higher in cities than rural areas. Several factors may contribute to this. Cities contain activities that have unique crime risks, such as fighting and assaults in entertainment districts, and robberies at banks and stores. Social isolation and anonymity in cities increase criminal behaviour by reducing social interdependencies that create community solidarity, that is, the chances that a crime will affect somebody the offender cares about. In addition, crime reporting may be more common in cities.

Cities also have features that can reduce crime rates. All else being equal, crime rates decline in more compact, mixed, walkable neighbourhoods, apparently due to more passive surveillance (also called *eyes on the street*) by non-criminal by-passers [18–20], increased economic opportunities for disadvantaged residents, and more specialized policing.

Association or causation?

High urban crime rates probably reflect a combination of special risks such as entertainment and commercial districts, causal factors such as social isolation and anonymity, associations due to concentrated poverty and drug addiction, plus higher reporting rates.

Potential individual responses

Individuals can reduce their personal crime risk through rational crime reduction strategies, and reduce excessive fear by learning about actual urban crime rates.

Potential community responses

Urban communities can reduce crime risks through better intervention programmes for at-risk residents, and urban design features that create more compact, walkable neighbourhoods with passive surveillance. Because many people have exaggerated sense of their actual crime threat, it may be helpful for better communicate actual crime risks and reduce excessive fear of crime.

Crowding and reduced privacy

Some researchers argue that mental illness and unhappiness increase with population density [21], sometimes citing a *Scientific American* article, 'Population density and social pathology' [22], which described how rats in extremely crowded colonies demonstrated pathological behaviour, but critics point out that *crowding* (excessive people in confined spaces) is very different from *density* (people per hectare), that the degree of crowding in that study was many times greater than what is commonly associated with urban living, and humans respond to problems differently than rats.

Studies find that crowding is associated with mental illness [23], particularly for young people [24], but, as space per resident tends to increase with income it is difficult to isolate this effect from confounding factors such as poverty [25]. There is no evidence that typical urban densities (20–60 residents per hectare) cause social problems [26]. Because mid-rise (3–6 storey) apartments generally have the cheapest cost per square foot (including land, construction, and operating expenses), such housing can reduce crowding compared with more expensive, lower-density single-family housing.

Increased densities and multifamily housing can reduce the privacy of activities such as arguments and outdoor parties, but small-town residents may also lack privacy because 'everybody knows your business' [27].

Association or causation?

High urban land prices tend to increase building costs per square meter, which can lead to crowding, but many other factors that affect mental health also increase with density, and households can often afford larger houses in cities than in smaller communities due to higher wages. As a result, positive relationships between density and mental illness probably reflect confounding factors rather than density itself.

Potential individual responses

Households can choose housing that enhances mental health, including adequate space to minimize crowing, and design features that provide adequate privacy, natural light, and attractive views.

Potential community responses

Policy reforms that reduce housing development costs can allow households to afford larger, less crowded homes [28]. Since mid-rise (3–6 storey) multifamily housing tends to have the lowest costs per square meter, allowing more of this type of housing tends to reduce crowding, particularly if some units accommodate larger families.

Economic stress

Economic stresses may contribute to mental illness and unhappiness [29, 30]. Rural and urban areas have different economic stresses. Rural areas tend to have higher poverty rates, and fewer education and employment opportunities (particularly for non-drivers), higher transportation costs, and less access to affordable goods and services, such as bulk retailers. Many cities have high living costs and economic disparity rates (differences between high- and low-income households), plus concentrated poverty, and urban residents tend to have limited opportunities to build their houses and grow food. Although urban areas tend to have less *absolute poverty* (residents cannot afford essential goods), they may have more *relative poverty* (expectations concerning what income level is sufficient) because residents are exposed to wealthier neighbours and expensive commercial activities that make them feel poor.

Association or causation?

Some urban economic stresses, such as less ability to build houses and grow food, are inherent to urban areas, but because urban areas are more productive and provide more economic opportunities, particularly for physically and economically disadvantaged groups, urban living probably reduces economic stresses overall [31]. Relative poverty may currently be greater in urban areas, but this difference is likely to decline as rural residents become more exposed to consumer marketing.

Potential individual responses

Individuals should make informed and rational decisions when deciding where to live: cities offer better education and employment opportunities, and therefore greater long-run incomes, but have higher living costs. Urban households can minimize economic stresses by choosing affordable housing and transport options, and developing financial support systems for periods of low income. Fixed-income households may be better off living in lower living cost areas.

Potential community responses

Communities can increase disadvantaged groups' economic opportunities, and improve affordable housing and transport options, and develop support services for economically distressed residents, particularly those with other mental health risks.

Inadequate physical activity

Several studies suggest that physical exercise and fitness can increase mental health, and prevent mental illness such as dementia [32]. Increased neighbourhood walkability is associated with reduced symptoms of depression [33], and reduced frequency of dementia [34]. A study of 299 older adults found significantly higher rates of grey matter volume and cognitive ability in those who previously walked more than 72 blocks a week [35].

Although there are many ways to exercise, many, such as organized sports and gym workouts, require special time, money, and effort, which discourages use, particularly by people who are low income and sedentary. For groups that are most at risk of physical inactivity, neighbourhood walking and cycling are among the most practical ways to increase daily, lifelong exercise. Urban living tends to increase physical activity compared with sprawled, automobile-dependent areas [36]. As most public transit trips include walking links, physical fitness tends to increase with transit travel [37]. A study of residents in 14 international cities found that controlling for other factors, net residential density, intersection density, public transport density, and number of parks was significantly positively related to physical activity [38]. Residents of the most activity-friendly neighbourhoods reported about 75 more weekly minutes of physical activity, half the target recommended by experts to maintain basic fitness and health. This suggests that, to improve public fitness and health, cities should be designed for walkability.

Association or causation?

Many people walk and bicycle for transportation because they cannot afford motorized transport. As incomes increase, so does motor vehicle ownership and the risks of sedentary living. This tends to occur first in cities and eventually in rural areas. To the degree that cities offer better walking and cycling conditions, they tend to increase physical activity by affluent residents, providing physical and mental health benefits.

Potential individual responses

Residents can choose homes in walkable and bikeable neighbourhoods, with appropriate parks and recreation facilities nearby, and choose physically active transport and recreation options, for example, walking and cycling rather than driving for errands, commuting, and social activities when possible.

Potential community responses

Cities can be designed to maximize physical fitness with compact and mixed development, good walking and cycling conditions, pro-transit policies, and appropriate parks and recreation facilities located close to most homes.

Transport conditions

Local transport conditions affect mental health and happiness [39]. Improved walking conditions and increased walking activity can increase community cohesion (positive interactions among neighbours), community security (more passive surveillance), public fitness, and health [40]. Reduced vehicle travel also reduces per capita traffic casualty and crime risks, which can cause mental stress to victims and their families.

Commute stress tends to be lowest for walkers and cyclists, higher for comfortable public transit travel, and highest for driving in congestion and uncomfortable public transit travel [41, 42]. Data from 18 waves of the British Household Panel Survey indicate that after accounting for various potential confounding factors relating to work, residence, and health, psychological well-being was significantly higher for active-mode commuters compared with car travel or public transport [43]. Switching from car travel or public transport to active travel was associated with an improvement in well-being. A UK Office of National Statistics study also found that commute duration is negatively related to personal well-being [44]. The data indicate that automobile commutes exceeding 15 minutes are associated with reduced happiness and increased anxiety, while public transport commuting does not reduce personal well-being until journey times exceed 30 minutes. Improving local mobility and accessibility options tends to reduce rates of depression, and walking provides mental health and happiness benefits [45].

A Gallup Healthways Index study found that large, compact, multimodal cities such as Boston, San Francisco, Chicago, New York, and Washington DC have significantly higher rates of exercise, and lower rates of depression, obesity, diabetes, and smoking than sprawled, automobile-dependent cities such as Fort Wayne, Indianapolis, Oklahoma City, Tulsa, and Durham-Chapel Hill, and controlling for age, education, and income levels, longer commutes reduce subjective well-being [46].

Association or causation?

City living generally increases walking and cycling, and reduces total time spent driving, causing positive impacts, but commute duration tends to increase with city size, and public transit is sometimes crowded and dirty, causing negative impacts. Net impacts depend on the trade-offs between these factors.

Potential individual responses

Individuals can choose to live in accessible and multimodal areas with good walking, cycling and public transit services, and shorter travel distances. They can also support policies that improve active transportation.

Potential community responses

Cities can increase mental health and happiness by improving walking, bicycling, and public transit conditions, particularly reducing the most uncomfortable conditions such as excessive crowding, harassment and extreme temperatures. They can also improve housing options in multimodal neighbourhoods, which reduces total travel time.

Inadequate interaction with nature

Some experts argue that urban living deprives people of frequent interactions with nature, leading to *nature deficit syndrome,* and exposure to nature improves mental health [1, 47]. Using Wellbeing Index data and controlling for other geographical and demographic factors, US residents' well-being increases significantly with the portion of urban land devoted to parks (ranging from 2.0% to 23%), park quality (per capita parks spending), and accessibility (percentage of residents within half a mile of parks) [48].

A major study of 1287 Southern California adolescent twins found that, after controlling for socio-economic factors such as age, gender, and race, and geographical factors such as neighbourhood quality, traffic density, and ambient temperatures, more greenspace (parks, golf courses and fields) within 1000 meters of a subject's home is associated with significant reductions of aggressive behaviours, equivalent to 2–2.5 years of behavioural maturation [49]. The researchers suggest that this results from increased physical activity, reduced pollution exposure, and possibly more exposure to positive microbial biodiversity, which improves brain health. Another study found that Los Angeles residents' physical and mental health ratings increased with proximity to public parks [50].

Association or causation?

Various factors may contribute to the positive associations between greenspace and mental health, including reduced noise and air pollution exposure, and positive associations many people have with natural environments. Although many cities have significant greenspace, including street trees, public parks, private gardens, and indoor plants, they generally offer less access to nature than suburban and rural areas.

Potential individual responses

People who value nature can choose urban homes close to public parks, with gardens and indoor plants, and they can regularly visit natural areas.

Potential community responses

Cities can increase resident's access to nature by devoting sufficient land (generally more than 15% of total area) to public greenspace, ensuring that most houses are located within a five-minute walk of public parks and recreational facilities, incorporating trees and planters into street and building designs, providing community gardens, and sponsoring nature visiting programmes.

Impacts summary

Table 21.2 summarizes various mechanisms through which urban living can affect mental health and happiness, whether these are associations or inherently caused by urban conditions, and strategies for reducing negative impacts in order to create saner, happier cities.

This analysis suggests that these risk factors are mostly *associated with* rather than *caused by* urban conditions, and they can be reduced through the following strategies:

- *Targeted social service.* Recognize that cities tend to attract people with elevated mental illness risk factors (poverty, mental and physical disabilities, minority and immigrant status, alienation, etc.), and provide appropriate social services.

- *Affordability.* Improve affordable urban housing and transportation options to reduce residents' financial stress. Ensure that houses are large enough to avoid crowding.

- *Prosocial places.* Create public spaces (streets, parks, public buildings, etc.) that promote community and encourage positive interactions among residents, particularly vulnerable groups, including people who are poor, have disabilities, or are visible minorities, migrants, young or are seniors.

- *Create cohesion communities and calming environments.* Support programmes that encourage residents to become more familiar and comfortable with different groups. Create quiet and calm urban environments through noise reduction and greenspace development, and support calming and reassuring community activities such as local art and recreation programmes.

- *Design for physical activity.* Integrate physical activity by providing good walking and cycling conditions, high-quality public transit (as transit travel complements walking and cycling), compact and mixed neighbourhoods (so common destinations, such as schools and shops, are located within walking and cycling distance of most homes and worksites), local parks, and recreational facilities, plus appropriate community sports and recreation programmes.

- *Greenspace.* Design cities with appropriate greenspaces, including local and regional parks (15–25% of urban land should be devoted to public parks, and most homes should be within a five-minute walk of neighbourhood parks or appropriate recreational facilities), green infrastructure (e.g.

Table 21.2 Summary of urban mental health impact mechanisms

Risk factor	Causation or association	Mental health and happiness strategies
Concentrated mental illness risk factors	Primarily association, although this concentration may exacerbate mental illness in some residents	Recognize that cities tend to attract people with mental health risk factors and provide appropriate support services
Substance (alcohol and drug) abuse	Mainly association. Cities have more cocaine and heroin addiction, rural areas more prescription drug, methamphetamine, and alcohol abuse	Provide targeted substance abuse prevention and treatment programmes
Social isolation and loneliness	Mixed. Urban residents tend to be more mobile and less welcoming, but cities offer more opportunities for social interactions	Design cities to encourage positive interactions among neighbours, and develop special programmes to welcome newcomers
Noise and light pollution	Increases with density but can be minimized with policy and design changes	Regulations and designs that reduce noise and light pollution
Toxic pollution	Increases with density but can be reduced	Toxic pollution reduction strategies
Excessive stimulation and stress	Mixed. Urban areas have more activities and social interactions	Plan for quiet and calm urban environments, and reassuring community activities
Crime	Mixed. Some urban areas have high crime rates, but this is declining	Support crime reductions and more accurate crime risk information
Crowding and reduced privacy	High housing costs can increase crowding, particularly for low-income households	Increase affordable housing supply in cities, including larger units for families
Economic stress	Mixed. Urban areas tend to have high housing costs but better economic opportunities	Support affordability and economic opportunities
Inadequate physical activity	Mainly causation	Support active transport and local parks
Transport conditions	Mixed. Urban residents usually experience more walking and cycling, and less driving but sometimes experience unpleasant transit services	Improve walking, cycling, and public transit, and support Smart Growth policies
Inadequate access to nature	Mainly causation but can be reduced	Increase greenspace and opportunities to visit natural areas

Urban living can affect mental health and happiness in several ways. Some are inherent to urban conditions, but many are associations related to confounding factors.

Reproduced from Todd Litman (2017), Urban Sanity: Understanding Urban Mental Health Impacts and How to Create Saner, Happier Cities, Victoria Transport Policy Institute (www.vtpi.org); at www.vtpi.org/urban-sanity.pdf. Todd Alexander Litman © 2016–2018.

street landscaping and rooftop gardens), and out-of-city wilderness access programmes.

Conclusions

The human experience is increasingly urban so it is important to understand how city living affects our sanity and happiness. This analysis indicates that city living has mixed mental health impacts: urban residency tends to increase some mental health risks but reduces others. Higher mental illness rates in cities result largely from the concentration of risk factors such as poverty and disability in cities, because urban areas offer better services and opportunities. This can create a self-reinforcing cycle of urban poverty and mental illness, and associated social problems, called *social drift*. Higher urban mental illness rates may also partly reflect better reporting. As a result, the *association* between cities and mental illness does not really mean that cities *cause* these problems. In fact, many people are saner and happier living in cities than they would be in smaller communities that offer less opportunity and support.

References

1. **Hartig T, Kahn PH.** Living in cities, naturally. *Science* 2016; **352**: 938–940.
2. **Lederbogen F, Haddad L, Meyer-Lindenberg A.** Urban social stress – risk factor for mental disorders. the case of sschizophrenia. *Environmental Pollution* 2013; **183**: 2–6.
3. **Taylor P.** American Mobility Who Moves? Who Stays Put? Where's Home? Available at: http://www.pewresearch.org/wp-content/uploads/sites/3/2010/10/Movers-and-Stayers.pdf (accessed 27 November 2018).
4. **Milgram S.** The experience of living in cities: adaptations to urban overload create characteristic qualities of city life that can be measured. *Science* 1970; **167**: 1461–1468.
5. **Spiegelman W.** For a Long Life, Retire to Manhattan. *New York Times*. Available at: www.nytimes.com/2016/09/04/opinion/sunday/for-a-long-life-retire-to-manhattan.html (accessed 27 November 2018).
6. **Ray B.** The Role of Cities in Immigrant Integration. Available at: www.migrationpolicy.org/article/role-cities-immigrant-integration (accessed 27 November 2018).
7. **Community and Faiths Unit.** Community Cohesion: Seven Steps; A Practitioner's Toolkit. Available at: http://bit.ly/1XVARGX (accessed 27 November 2018).
8. **Carvalho FG, Hidalgo MP, Levandovski R.** Differences in circadian patterns between rural and urban populations: an epidemiological study in countryside. *Chronobiology International* 2014; **31**: 442–449.
9. **Wolpaw Reyes J.** Lead Exposure and Behavior: Effects On Antisocial And Risky Behavior Among Children and Adolescents, Working Paper 20366, National Bureau Of Economic Research. Available at: www.nber.org/papers/w20366 (accessed 27 November 2018).

10. **Power MC, Kioumourtzoglou M-A, Hart JE, Okereke OI, Laden F, Weisskopf MG.** The relation between past exposure to fine particulate air pollution and prevalent anxiety: observational cohort study. *BMJ* 2015; 350.

11. **Fonken LK, et al.** Air pollution impairs cognition, provokes depressive-like behaviors and alters hippocampal cytokine expression and morphology. *Molecular Psychiatry* 2011; **16**: 987–995.

12. **Perera FP, et al.** Early-life exposure to polycyclic aromatic hydrocarbons and ADHD behavior problems. *PLoS ONE* 2014; 9.

13. **Palti I, Bar M.** A manifesto for conscious cities: should streets be sensitive to our mental needs? *The Guardian.* Available at: http://bit.ly/1hkyYjJ (accessed 27 November 2018).

14. **Abbott A.** Stress and the city: urban decay. *Nature* 2012; **490**: 162–164.

15. **Patil MP.** Overload and the City. Available at: www.urbandesignmentalhealth.com/blog/overload-and-the-city (accessed 27 November 2018).

16. **Freeman D, Emsley R, Dunn G, Fowler D, Bebbington P, Kuipers E, et al.** the stress of the street for patients with persecutory delusions: a test of the symptomatic and psychological effects of going outside into a busy urban area. *Schizophrenia Bulletin* 2015; **41**: 971–979.

17. **Nematollahi S, Tiwari R, Hedgecock D.** Desirable Dense Neighbourhoods: An Environmental Psychological Approach for Understanding Community Resistance to Densification. *Urban Policy and Research* 2015; **34**: 132–151.

18. **Christens B, Speer PW.** Predicting violent crime using urban and suburban densities. *Behavior and Social Issues* 2005; **14**: 113–127.

19. **Gilderbloom JI, Riggs WW, Meares WL.** Does walkability matter? An examination of walkability's impact on housing values, foreclosures and crime. *Cities* 2015; **42**: 13–24.

20. **Humphrey C, Jensen ST, Small D, Thurston R.** Analysis of Urban Vibrancy and Safety in Philadelphia. Available at: https://arxiv.org/pdf/1702.07909.pdf (accessed 27 November 2018).

21. **Okulicz-Kozaryn A, Maya Mazelis J.** Urbanism and happiness: a test of wirth's theory of urban life. *Urban Studies* 2016; **55**: 349–364.

22. **Calhoun JB.** Population density and social pathology. *Scientific American* 1962; **306**: 139–148.

23. **Urist J.** The Health Risks of Small Apartments: Living in Tiny Spaces Can Cause Psychological Problems. *The Atlantic.* Available at: www.theatlantic.com/health/archive/2013/12/the-health-risks-of-small-apartments/282150 (accessed 27 November 2018).

24. **Solari CD, Mare RD.** Housing crowding effects on children's wellbeing. *Social Science Research* 2012; **41**: 464–476.

25. **Fitts AS.** The Psychology of Living in Small Spaces. Available at http://undark.org/2016/05/31/psychology-living-small-spaces (accessed 27 November 2018).

26. **Ramsden E.** The urban animal: population density and social pathology in rodents and humans. *Bulletin of the World Health Organization* 2009; **87**: 82–82.

27. **Preston DB, D'Augelli AR.** *The Challenges of Being a Rural Gay Man: Coping with Stigma.* London: Routledge, 2013.

28. **Burda C, Collins-Williams M.** Make Way For Mid-Rise: How To Build More Homes In Walkable, Transit-Connected Neighbourhoods. Available at: www.pembina.org/reports/make-way-for-mid-rise.pdf (accessed 27 November 2018).

29. **Tobin B.** Rural Poverty and Urban Poverty. Available at: http://borgenproject.org/rural-poverty-urban-poverty (accessed 27 November 2018).

30. **Winters J, Li Y.** The bigger and denser the city you live in, the more unhappy you're likely to be. Available at: http://blogs.lse.ac.uk/usappblog/2016/05/12/the-bigger-and-denser-the-city-you-live-in-the-more-unhappy-youre-likely-to-be.

31. **Glaeser EL.** *Triumph of the City: How Our Greatest Invention Makes Us Richer, Smarter, Greener, Healthier, and Happier.* London: Penguin Press.

32. **Robertson R, Robertson A, Jepson R, Maxwell M.** Walking for depression or depressive symptoms: a systematic review and meta-analysis. *Mental Health and Physical Activity* 2012; **5**: 66–75.

33. **Berke EM, Gottlieb LM, Vernez Moudon A, Larson EB.** Protective association between neighborhood walkability and depression in older men. *Journal of the American Geriatrics Society* 2007; **55**: 526–533.

34. **Larson EB, Wang L, Bowen JD, McCormick WC, Teri L, Crane P, Kukull W.** Exercise is associated with reduced risk for incident dementia among persons 65 years of age and older. *Annals of Internal Medicine* 2006; **144**: 73–81.

35. **Erickson KI, Raji CA, Lopez OL, Becker JT, Rosano C, Newman AB,** et al. Physical activity predicts gray matter volume in late adulthood: The Cardiovascular Health Study. *Neurology* 2010; **75**: 1415–1422.

36. **Ewing R, Hamidi S.** Measuring Urban Sprawl and Validating Sprawl. Available at: https://www.smartgrowthamerica.org/app/legacy/documents/measuring-sprawl-2014.pdf (accessed 27 November 2018).

37. **Lachapelle U,** et al. Commuting by public transit and physical activity: where you live, where you work, and how you get there. *Journal of Physical Activity and Health* 2011; **8**: S72–S82.

38. **Sallis JF, Cerin E, Conway TL, Adams MA, Frank LD, Pratt M,** et al. Physical activity in relation to urban environments in 14 cities worldwide: a cross-sectional study. *The Lancet* 2016; **387**: 2207–2217.

39. **Montgomery C.** *Happy City: Transforming Our Lives Through Urban Design.* New York: Farrar, Straus & Giroux, 2013.

40. **Appleyard D, Appleyard B.** *Livable Streets.* Berkeley, CA: University of California Press, 2012.

41. **Hilbrecht M, Smale B, Mock SE.** Highway to health? Commute time and well-being among Canadian adults. *World Leisure Journal* 2014; **56**: 151–163.

42. **Wei M.** Commuting: 'The Stress that Doesn't Pay'. Available at http://bit.ly/2ciqEmt (accessed 27 November 2018).

43. **Martin A, Goryakin Y, Suhrcke M.** Does active commuting improve psychological wellbeing? Longitudinal evidence from eighteen waves of the British Household Panel Survey. *Preventive Medicine* 2014; **69**: 296–303.

44. **Office of National Statistics.** Commuting and Personal Well-being, 2014. Available at: http://bit.ly/24PlONm (accessed 27 November 2018).

45. **Melis G, Gelormino E, Marra G, Ferracin E, Costa G.** The effects of the urban built environment on mental health: a cohort study in a large northern Italian city. *International Journal Of Environmental Research And Public Health* 2015; **12**: 14898–14915.

46. **Gallup**. Active Living Environment in U.S. Communities; State of American Well-being. Available at: http://info.healthways.com/hubfs/Gallup-Healthways_State_of_American_Well-Being_2015_Community_Impact_vFINAL.pdf?t=1476384420877 (accessed 27 November 2018).

47. **Berto R**. The role of nature in coping with psycho-physiological stress: a literature review on restorativeness. *Behavior Science* 2014; **4**: 394–409.

48. **Larson LR, Jennings V, Cloutier SA.** Public parks and wellbeing in urban areas of the United States. *PLoS ONE* 2016; **11**.

49. **Younan D, Tuvblad C, Li L, Wu J, Lurmann F, Franklin M**, et al. Environmental determinants of aggression in adolescents: role of urban neighborhood greenspace. *Journal of the American Academy of Child and Adolescent Psychiatry* 2016; **55**: 591–601.

50. **Sturm R, Cohen D.** Proximity to urban parks and mental health. *Journal of Mental Health and Policy and Economics* 2014; **17**: 19–24.

Chapter 22

Re-conceptualizing urban spaces: towards recovery and reintegration of women living with mental disorders

Shubhada Maitra

Introduction

Shanti, currently 28 years of age, hails from rural Bihar. She lost her parents at a young age and never went to a formal school. She began working in a brick kiln, packing bricks. She married at a young age and had a son whom she doted on. However, she was unhappy in her marriage; her husband drank heavily and beat her regularly. Her in-laws were unsupportive when conflicts took place between the couple. 'The tension was too much', she says. One day her husband threw her out of the house and took away her son. Shanti remembers the sense of loneliness and emptiness that engulfed her. She began roaming around the village, surviving on dole that people gave her. She slept in the open, taking shelter occasionally in places of worship. She dreamt of her dead mother often, gradually seeing her and hearing her voice even during the day. She has no memory of what happened to her after that.

Mental hospital records where she was admitted show that she was brought by the police in 2010 and was diagnosed to be suffering from schizophrenia. She did not know what the label meant or what the consequences of being admitted to the mental hospital meant in the long run. When asked her name, she would introduce herself as 'I am Shanti, not known'.

There are many women like Shanti who wander off from their place of residence, mostly a far-flung Indian village, fed up with life, sometimes in a fit of rage after fights in the home or as a result of 'hearing voices, seeing people', not knowing where they are going. Landing up in an unknown city, disheveled, emaciated, and hardly coherent, they end up in a mental hospital. Patients whose whereabouts and family details are not known at the time of admission are given a name by the hospital staff, adding 'not known' as their family name. This becomes their identity, coupled with a tag of 'madness'.

How does the city, an urban space, respond to women with mental disorders? How do they add up to the statistics as urban residents, migrants, homeless persons?

Urbanization, urban spaces, and mental health

According to the United Nations 2014–15 report, globally more people live in urban areas than in rural areas, with 54% of the world's population residing in urban areas in 2014. It projects that by 2050, 66% of the world's population will be urban [1]. Africa and Asia are urbanizing faster than other regions and are projected to become 56 and 64% urban, respectively, by 2050. Asia, despite its lower level of urbanization, is home to 53% of the world's urban population. The urban population of the world has grown rapidly since 1950, from 746 million to 3.9 billion in 2014. Urbanization at this rapid pace is unequal and thus unplanned, thereby drawing on the regions' resources, threatening sustainable development when the necessary infrastructure is not developed or when policies are not implemented to ensure that the benefits of city life are equitably shared. Urban living is often associated with higher levels of literacy and education, better health, greater access to social services, and enhanced opportunities for cultural and political participation, and people move towards cities with this vision in mind.

In addition to natural population growth, urbanization is driven mainly by rural–urban migration and migration between cities. Urban migrants form a hugely diverse group that comprises internal migrants originating from rural areas in search of better employment and education opportunities in cities, cross-border migrants, internally displaced persons and urban refugees, as well as victims of trafficking and forced labour [2]. Migration can therefore create specific psycho-social vulnerabilities that, if combined with other risk factors, can affect the mental health of migrants. Being separated from family and friends and possibly exposed to exploitation, discrimination, xenophobia, or sexual and gender-based violence in countries of transit and destination can heighten the vulnerability of migrants to psychological illnesses [3].

Migration to cities has increased dramatically over the past few decades. Most migrants come from rural areas, bringing values, beliefs, and expectations about mental health that are often very different from the ones they encounter in their new location. In many instances, people coming from rural areas have endured years of isolation, lack of technological connection, poor health, poverty, unemployment, and inadequate housing [4].

The links between urbanization and mental disorders have been extensively documented [5–8]. Mental disorders have been linked with poverty, alienation, and powerlessness. These conditions are more frequently experienced by women. The influence of patriarchy and gender discrimination resulting in women's lower status, lack of physical, mental and emotional nurture, poor access to resources, and basic needs such as education, employment, income, housing, role overload, domestic and sexual violence, malnutrition, and a poor living standard has been researched widely. Women's vulnerability to mental distress and common mental disorders has been explored through community-based surveys and other clinical studies [9–14].

While there is substantial research around urbanization and mental health, writings on urban spaces and mental health are scant. The few that are available are focused on urban space as a green space, the need to enhance the presence of nature in urban spaces, including structural design and the contribution of a green environment, not only to feelings of well-being, but also in alleviating symptoms associated with several mental health conditions such as childhood attention deficit disorder, improving the quality of life of patients living with Alzheimer disease and dementia, and reducing stress and depression [15]. However, research and documentation on mainstream urban spaces as responsive to those with mental disorders along a continuum of marginalization to acceptance and integration is hard to locate.

People with mental disorders are often found wandering on the streets. Many leave their homes and families during an active episode and stray far from their place of residence. Some are brought by the police to mental hospitals where they are admitted as 'not known' patients, while others end up on the streets. This constitutes a group of migrants to the city that goes undocumented, unaccounted for. The city responds in a variety of ways to such individuals: most ignore them, thus rendering them invisible; a few pelt stones at them or make fun of them; some good Samaritans offer food, clothes, and first-aid/medication for open wounds or other visible conditions; a minority may go through the process of getting them admitted to a mental health facility or another institutional set-up for destitutes.

There is universal agreement that mental health programme and policy needs are gender-sensitive, taking into consideration not only the biomedical aspects, but also sociocultural factors and issues around social development. This chapter describes one such intervention: a community-based recovery and reintegration project with women living with mental disorders. The project links self and psycho-social issues, shelter, and livelihoods to facilitate recovery and reintegration. The project illustrates how space and people can interact with each other. The chapter highlights the project's experience of negotiating urban spaces to reduce the stigma and discrimination associated with mental disorders. Partnering with community-based structures, the project aims at bringing about a change in these very structures to make them more responsive to mental health needs of women diagnosed with a mental disorder.

About *Tarasha*

Initiated in 2011, *Tarasha* (meaning chiseled or sculpted in Hindi) is a field action project of the Tata Institute of Social Sciences, Mumbai, India, and partners with the Directorate of Health Services, Maharashtra. *Tarasha* works collaboratively with working women's hostels, vocational training centres, and daycare centres to facilitate recovery and reintegration. *Tarasha* was conceptualized in response to a study, 'Status of Women in Mental Hospitals in Maharashtra', undertaken for the Maharashtra State Commission for Women [16]. The study utilized a mixed-methodology design; all case records (approximately 2000) of women admitted at the time of data collection to the four mental hospitals in Maharashtra were studied to understand their sociodemographic and medical profiles. In addition, four focus group discussions and 10 in-depth interviews with women who were asymptomatic were conducted across the four hospitals. The objective was to hear the women's voices, understand their illness experiences, and trajectories of recovery and relapse, as well as aspirations for the future. Key informant interviews were conducted with psychiatrists, social workers, nursing staff, and ward attendants to explore treatment, care, and rehabilitation issues. Some of the key findings were that:

- Nearly 70% women were admitted by their families, yet less than half were currently in touch with their families. Although women were asymptomatic, families either did not want to take them back or had 'disappeared', their addresses untraceable.
- Women were admitted in their early 30s, and a majority had spent nearly 10 years in the hospital.
- Each of the 10 women interviewed in depth revealed a history of violence and abuse.
- Women's aspirations centred around standing on their own feet and making a life for themselves such that they were economically independent.

Abandoned by the family, with little education and no skills to make a living in the outside world, women grew old in the institution. However, their dreams centred around leading a productive life outside, making a living, getting a roof over their head, and going beyond the identity of a 'mad' woman, labelled with a psychiatric diagnosis and incarcerated in the institution for years.

The authors' engagement with the mental hospitals continued beyond the study. Following dissemination of the findings, some changes were brought about within the hospital in terms of treatment and care issues. However women's life issues and aspirations beyond the illness and institution remained unmet and unanswered. It was at this time that the challenge to operationalize the findings of the study was deliberated upon. *Tarasha* was thus intended to be a pilot project to help us establish 'proof of concept', linking shelter, livelihoods, and psycho-social issues of women living with mental disorders.

Theoretical perspectives

Tarasha uses the feminist and ecological frameworks in principle and practice to understand and operationalize recovery. Recovery from mental disorders encompasses both internal processes such as aspirations, personality traits, and symptom management, as well as external factors, such as interaction with the environment and social support. Independence, or rather, interdependence, employment, and fulfilment of community roles are all part of that recovery process. An ecological framework helps us to organize and interpret the phenomenon of mental health recovery that is emerging. Ecological perspective incorporates both the individual and the environment and focuses on the relationship between the two, with emphasis on interactions and transactions [17]. Thus, recovery can be viewed as facilitated or impeded through the dynamic interplay of forces that are complex, synergistic, and linked [18]. Individual characteristics such as aspirations, hope, and empowerment; environmental characteristics, such as safe shelters, employment, and opportunities for social interaction; and the characteristics of exchange between the two, such as freedom and choice, can facilitate or hamper recovery.

Social connectedness, social inclusion, and economic participation are key determinants of mental health and recovery. Social connectedness is meant to include a valued social identity that goes beyond the diagnostic label, ability to form and sustain social support networks, and personally meaningful relationships; social inclusion addresses issues of discrimination based on gender and (dis)ability, the freedom to exercise one's choice and a sense of control over one's life, opportunities and access to key societal/ community resources; and economic participation encompasses the ability to be engaged in fulfilling and productive work, the ability to afford safe and secure housing, health care, and vocational training/ education based on one's aspirations and choice.

The philosophy of *Tarasha* focuses on the fact that women recovering from mental disorders are entitled to an independent and a dignified life outside of an institution. *Tarasha* supports women recovering from mental disorders in building and sustaining social networks and livelihoods, and locating safe, non-stigmatized, non-segregated shelters in the community.

Feminist critique of the family as an institution that offers love, safety, and security for its members resonates well with the experiences of women living with mental disorders. Socialization into stereotypical gender roles and behaviour, limited access to education and economic resources, and discrimination and violence in both the natal and marital family disadvantages women and limits them from attaining their full potential. Aspirations are lauded if they are in the context of one's family and children but rarely for the woman's strategic needs. As long as the woman behaves in accordance with her gender role, she is appreciated and accepted. But if she develops a mental disorders or experiences distress due to the very circumstances of her living, the family is quick to dump her in an institution. This was amplified by the research on Status of Women in Mental Hospitals mentioned earlier. A key informant from one of the mental hospitals narrated an incident where the father had come to admit his 21-year-old daughter to the hospital. She was single, and diagnosed to be suffering from paranoid schizophrenia; she was pregnant at the time of hospital admission. Being single, pregnant, and mentally ill, the young girl (and more importantly her family) had no place to hide their shame and stigma. Once the admission process was over, the father turned to the key informant and stated, 'Maylee tar aamchi, jagli tar tumchi'('If she dies, she is ours, if she lives, she is yours'), making it abundantly clear that he did not wish to be in his daughter's contact in her lifetime. This is just one of the many narratives of discrimination and abandonment by the family on grounds of mental disorders. With no family support, little education and absence of employable skills, women were destined to become 'long-stay patients' in the mental hospital. *Tarasha* adopts the feminist perspective to move women towards self-determination, economic/financial autonomy, building and valuing social networks beyond the 'family', understanding life experiences that contribute to emotional distress, nurturing the self and believing in one's abilities and attributes despite a diagnostic label. Thus, *Tarasha* works towards helping women recovering from mental disorders in making a transition from institutions back into the community. This is done by addressing social exclusion, stigma, and discrimination thereby facilitating the process of breaking the cycle of unemployment, poverty, marginalization, and disability.

The Beginning

Tarasha's first partnership was with the Directorate of Health Services (DHS), Maharashtra. Setting up the project meant seeking permission to work with women within the mental hospital, orienting the hospital team to our work modalities, and building the hospital's association with *Tarasha*. Women who had received a diagnosis of mental disorders and abandoned by their families continued to reside as 'mental patients' within the hospital. The State typically did not discharge such women as it had assumed guardianship in the absence of their own families. The logic for this was the fact that the hospital provided a roof and meals to the women who were not in a position to fend for themselves. The danger of being violated and abused on the streets of a large metropolitan city prevailed. Operating from a feminist strengths-based perspective, *Tarasha* believed in self-determination and freedom of choice. Besides, the United Nations Convention on Rights of Persons with Psychosocial Disabilities (UNCRPD) had laid the context for operationalizing 'legal capacity' on the ground. We believed that adult women who were currently asymptomatic and on the path to recovery can seek their discharge from the hospital. (Typically, when women have no family and the State has assumed guardianship, women are not discharged. They can only obtain leave of absence for short durations to return to the hospital at the end of this period.) The State urged us to take guardianship of the women and seek leave of absence to facilitate re-admission in case of a relapse. However, we rejected this, given our critique of the family and belief in the 'legal capacity' of the women. We were able to convince the DHS to discharge asymptomatic women who wished to join *Tarasha* and work towards living a life outside an institutional set-up. Owing to processes of the women being examined by the Visitors' Committee (a body that comprises legal, social, and medical experts which decides on issues related to discharge/ leave of absence following an interview with the woman) prior to discharge were to be followed by us. It was not until the first five women discharged from the hospital had been employed in mainstream occupations that the hospital staff was convinced about *Tarasha's* work. The DHS and the mental hospital were the first urban spaces we worked with towards making them responsive to the needs of women living with mental disorders.

Tarasha's cornerstones

Self

Tarasha views recovery as a non-linear process that is characterized by linking selfhood issues, shelter, and livelihoods (see Figure 22.1). Given women's experiences of trauma and mental disorders, getting in touch with oneself and ones' psycho-social issues assumes importance.

Work on selfhood issues incorporates group and individual sessions within the hospital prior to and after discharge. The sessions encourage women to move

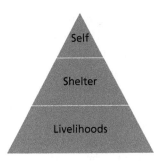

Figure 22.1 Tarasha.

towards an identity beyond illness and achieve a greater degree of autonomy in making choices and decisions that concern their lives. It addresses issues related to their illness experience, symptoms of distress, recovery maintenance, emotions, communication, and social skills. Their goals, aspirations, and dreams are addressed, and women are helped in charting out ways to achieve these. An important aspect of selfhood issues that we address is disclosure about history of mental disorders. Believing that 'The Personal is Political', the power to generate a discourse around women's distress and mental disorders through personal disclosures is discussed in group sessions. However, women are free to choose whom, when, and what to tell.

Aspects of daily living such as familiarizing with and negotiating the city, use of public transport, handling and managing money, and managing the self with respect and dignity are learnt through experiential methods and role plays. It is in the process of negotiating the city that women's contact with urban spaces increases. For many of the women who are discharged from the hospital after several years, the openness, vastness, and unfamiliarity of the city is overwhelming. One way to overcome this is to know the city, own the city, and believe it is your home. Following discharge from the hospital, the first couple of weeks are devoted to 'knowing your city'. Women, accompanied by *Tarasha* team member(s) take public transport, walk, go to beaches, malls, eateries, places of worship, and other places of interest (prominent among these are visits to residential areas of Bollywood stars). This is followed by attending the day care centre located approximately 5 miles away from their place of residence. In less than a couple of months, women feel at home in the city, increasing their sense of safety and confidence.

Shelter

Recovery and reintegration is difficult to facilitate in the absence of safe, secure, warm shelters. Segregated spaces such as shelters for women in distress or half-way homes continue to attract the stigma and discrimination experienced by marginalized populations. Social inclusion and access to community spaces that are not stigmatized enhance the processes of recovery. *Tarasha* therefore partners with non-segregated, mainstream spaces like working women's hostels in the city. The choice of such a space was deliberate: it allowed *Tarasha* women to interact with other women who were single, living on their own, and working for a living. Interacting over meals and television time was an opportunity to forge social connections, sometimes friendships. It emphasized the value of living a life with dignity where nurturing and looking after one's self and other room mates were goals in themselves. Working women's hostels also have an optimal mix of sensitivity to women's needs and issues, and can also offer a certain degree of clinical supervision if the need arises. It also provided an opportunity for *Tarasha* and the women to talk about mental health issues and distress thereby breaking the stereotypes and silence around 'madness'.

Contrary to our initial misgivings about using working women's hostels as 'shelter' for women discharged from the mental hospital, our access to the hostels was fairly smooth. Our proposal for partnership was accepted by two women's hostels in the city. Our institutional affiliation, a social work degree, and our professional work were key facilitators. However, beyond this, it was the novelty of the project and the desire to push the boundaries that excited the office-bearers of the hostels. While we were open and transparent about our project, we had decided that we would not disclose women's illness history to anyone without their permission and knowledge. Thus, we were quite surprised to hear that several women would share with their hostel mates, matter of factly, that they had come to the hostel from the mental hospital. The women had clearly begun to 'occupy' the hostel space.

Livelihoods

Tarasha believes that attaining economic autonomy through a steady, mainstream job facilitates a positive sense of self and confidence. It also increases one's social skills and widens perspectives through interaction with colleagues in a formal set-up. Employment is known to promote mental health by facilitating social inclusion, clarifying an individual's identity, providing economic remuneration, enhancing social status and giving a sense of contribution to the individual in addition to a basic structure of their day.

The concept of 'rehabilitation' in the field of mental health is contested. Evidence-based practice favours supported employment to sheltered workshops and other traditional vocational rehabilitation programmes. Research and practice shows that most clients will plateau in segregated settings.

Tarasha partners with vocational training institutes which provide skill-training over a period of 3 months based on women's interest and aptitude. At the end of the training period, the institute facilitates job placement. Given that women discharged from the hospital are older than the cohort of trainees and do not possess any documents such as educational certificate, the challenge is to find appropriate job placement opportunities. Despite this, *Tarasha* women have been employed in mainstream occupations, earning a monthly salary between Rs. 7000 to Rs. 10,000 (USD$100–150). Unlike the hostel space, women often choose not to share their background with their colleagues and employers. Once they build a closer relationship, they share their experience of institutionalization and are able to draw support from the 'friend' at the workplace.

The following section elaborates on the phases through which recovery and reintegration is facilitated.

Phase I: towards de-institutionalization

Phase I is a stage of screening, selection, capacity building, and a move towards de-institutionalization. This stage includes intensive group and individual sessions with women at the hospital. Women who are interested in attending the sessions are invited to a common space where group sessions are held. Social workers, psychiatrists, and occupational therapists often recommend women to the *Tarasha* team. The group is an open one, with women having the freedom to participate in the therapeutic sessions. The content of the sessions is non-linear and is often decided on a 'needs basis' depending on where the group is in terms of their interest, information, and readiness to absorb the discussions. All sessions are designed with an emphasis on an experiential, participatory approach. The sessions can be broadly categorized as introductory, informative, exploratory, and reflective. The sessions facilitate group interactions, sharing, assessing, and enhancing strengths and capacities, as well as cognitive and body functioning, building awareness about the self; exploring boundaries, emotions, responses, and the body; building trust; addressing societal norms, notions, constructs, gender, and mental disorders; understanding mental disorders, distress and symptoms, medication, managing conflict, and relationships; exploring what recovery means to women; and so on. The women are encouraged to form and share their own opinions, and listen to those put forth by other group members.

Group sessions are conducted 2–3 times a week for 6 months, with approximately 15- 20 women. In addition, women who wish to share their experiences or talk to the team are met once a week in individual session. A subset of these women, depending on the degree of family support available (*Tarasha* works primarily with women who are abandoned in the hospital and have minimal or no family support), level of functioning, current symptoms, and willingness to join *Tarasha* are helped towards de-institutionalization.

Phase II: psycho-social recovery and support

This phase of the project is marked by two events: (1) moving into a working women's hostel and (2) beginning psycho-social recovery through attending a day-care centre (DCC) for persons recovering from mental disorders.

The hostel provides a safe, secure environment that fosters women's recovery. This is one of the first spaces wherein they begin to meet and interact with other women from different backgrounds, learn to follow a routine, look after themselves and their space, and move towards living in a community. This is when the women begin to shape an identity for themselves outside the bracket of a diagnosis, and apart from their disorders. The idea of the 'future' starts to become more concrete. A major challenge is readjusting to a life outside the hospital, with a regular schedule to follow, negotiating time and space, and living an 'urban' life in a large metropolitan city.

For the first three months after discharge, women attend a DCC for persons living with mental disorders. Women participate in group and individual sessions, art and recreation, yoga, and pet therapy, where the focus is on the self: understanding oneself, the illness, developing social and emotional competence, and so on. The DCC, unlike the hostel, is a mixed-gender space. It is for the first time, after years of institutionalization that women begin to interact with men on a daily basis. Friendships, attraction, and fondness are emotions women experience and discuss, awkward as it might be to begin with. However, given women's short duration at the DCC and restricted mobility on the part of the men attending the DCC, long-term relationships do not develop in this space. Work on psycho-social issues and the learning at the DCC prepares the women for the next phase.

Phase III: vocational training

Our vocational training partners offer training in retail and sales, housekeeping, hospitality, printing technology, and home-based care. Negotiating training for women who have no educational certificates (some of them learn reading and writing after their association with *Tarasha*), and are usually older than other students undergoing training, was a challenge. Once again, the project design and philosophy, besides institutional affiliation, paved the way for a smooth partnership. The vocational training institutes worked around their policies to help women access training. Instructors spent time and efforts to ensure that women kept pace with other students. Women's own motivation and desire to stand on their own feet propelled them to get the best out of the training. The training typically lasts about 3 months. Following successful completion of training, women appear for interviews and are selected for job placement.

Besides vocational training, this phase also sees women interact with other 'students' in a learning environment, appear for job interviews, and get selected on a competitive basis. Just as opportunities open up in this phase, it also brings several challenges. Women have to go beyond their identity of a person with a diagnosis of mental disorders to someone who is a student-learner, a potential employee, a colleague, and so on. (At the DCC, women mix with others who also have a history of mental illness). It is at such times that self-doubt and fear surface often. This is the time when *Tarasha* counsellors begin to see the deeply internalized stigma of their condition and institutionalization. Women re-learn and re-adapt their understanding of boundaries and relationships. Distinguishing between friends and colleagues, identifying strengths that set them apart from the rest of the student group, learning new behaviours benefi-cial to the workspace and absorbing what is taught during the training become important indicators for the women.

Phase IV: job development and job support

Once women are employed, the project team works with them to help them maintain their jobs and work efficiently as per their job role. Support is offered in terms of regularity and punctuality at the workplace, developing professional work relationships, managing money and travel to the work place. Women dis-charged since 2012 are successfully managing their job and workplace issues. The team is in regular touch with the women and with their employers on a need/demand basis. In an effort to build ownership over their recovery, and maintain autonomy, support and counselling sessions are also scheduled upon a client's request. Positive reviews about women's performance and work ethics from our partners and workplace supervisors foster self-confidence and motivation.

One of the women managed to create her own networks and acquired a new job with a different company, and now works as a sales and marketing execu-tive. This is reflective of her independence and resourcefulness, no longer re-quiring the support of the project to create her own success story. We view this as an example of true reintegration.

Phase V: exit

The entire process from discharge to reintegration requires approximately 18 months. Once the women are independent and able to fend for themselves,

Tarasha urges them to 'exit' the project. The exit is symbolic, a tangible way for women to acknowledge contracting with themselves, and taking responsibility for their recovery, seeking help when needed. The exit procedure includes a formal meeting with the woman in the presence of a third party, usually the hostel warden, wherein the woman is provided with a printed document, much like the one they sign indicating their consent when entering the project. The document highlights the woman's work and accomplishment in the time she has been a part of *Tarasha*, acknowledging her participation, efforts, and commitment to recovery. In addition, we include a maintenance plan based on our work with the woman, usually including insights that she has provided through the counselling sessions.

The team keeps in touch with women who exit the project, monitoring their progress. In case of any signs of a relapse, the project team works with the woman towards accessing medical help and providing psycho-social assistance as required.

Challenges

One of the biggest hurdles in the process of reintegration is the issue of 'undocumented persons'. The women *Tarasha* works with have a long history of institutionalization—anywhere between three to eight years, and a prior history of wandering from one place to the other, sometimes through other mental hospitals in the country. As such, they have no papers to prove their identity, place of residence, educational qualifications, and citizenship. In the first year of our work we realized the importance of this aspect of their lives. Since then, citizenship rights and identity are at the core of *Tarasha's* work. Perhaps for the first time in India, in 2013, *Tarasha* was able to open bank accounts, procure *Aadhar* cards (Unique Identity Document), and PAN cards (permanent account number, which is a code that acts as identification for Indian nationals, especially those who pay income tax) for women discharged from the mental hospital.

The other challenge is the fact that non-institutional spaces for treatment and care of persons with mental disorders in the city of Mumbai are almost non-existent. General Hospital Psychiatric Units treat severe mental disorders through their inpatient units. However, the patient needs to be accompanied by an attendant at all times during admission to the hospital. This is beyond the current resources of the project. Thus, in case of a relapse, women are required to be re-admitted to the mental hospital. While we at *Tarasha* see this as a short-term arrangement until the woman recovers from the episode, women themselves respond negatively to re-admission. It is through a process of discussion and negotiation that women may agree to treatment within the hospital. In all such instances, it is the woman's wish that is upheld.

Conclusions

One of *Tarasha's* broader objectives is the expansion of safe and legitimate spaces across communities for women living with mental disorders. To this end, the project has worked extensively to locate mainstream community-based spaces for women—to be, to live, to connect to work, and enjoy. While most spaces have been responsive and openly inclusive, much effort needs to go into making work spaces accepting of people living with mental disorders. While the discourse around mental health issues and rights has gained momentum, stigma and discrimination in the workplace needs to be understood in depth. It is perhaps for this reason that women associated with *Tarasha* hesitate to disclose their history of institutionalization. Perceived stigma and self-stigma operate together to create a culture of silence among women with lived experiences of mental disorders. For *Tarasha* it poses a barrier to discuss mental health issues at the workplace and enter into formal spaces to create a dialogue and an enhanced understanding of upset, distress, and disorder. We are exploring ways of starting these discussions without 'outing' the women. Living spaces, for example working women's hostels, are also not permanent solutions for women surviving mental disorders. Low-cost housing and subsidized housing such as Housing First [19], along with supportive services and other community spaces need to be available to women for sustainable existence, to cement their autonomy and fully embrace independent living.

Acknowledgements

I would like to thank *Tarasha* team members Ashwini Survase, Anindita Bhattacharya, Rohina Naikody, Rosanna Rodrigues, and Sargam Jadhav for their work on the ground. *Tarasha* is what it is today as a result of their efforts.

References

1. **United Nations, Department of Economic and Social Affairs, Population Division.** World Urbanization Prospects: The 2014 Revision. Available at: https://esa.un.org/unpd/wup/Publications/Files/WUP2014-Report.pdf (accessed 28 November 2018).
2. **Schultz C.** Migration report 2015: Migration, Health and Cities. Migration, health and urbanization: Interrelated challenges. Available at: https://www.iom.int/sites/default/files/our_work/ICP/MPR/WMR-2015-Background-Paper-CSchultz.pdf (accessed 28 November 2018).

3. **Bhugra D, Jones P.** Migration and mental disorders. *Advances in Psychiatric Treatment* 2001; 7: 216–223.

4. **Trivedi JK, Sareen H, Dhyani M.** Rapid urbanization—its impact on mental health: a South Asian perspective. *Indian Journal of Psychiatry* 2008; **50**: 161–165.

5. **Srivastava K.** Urbanization and mental health. *Industrial Psychiatry Journal* 2009; **18**: 75–76.

6. **Dekker J, Peen J, Koelen J, Smit F, Schoevers R.** Psychiatric disorders and urbanisation in Germany. *BMC Public Health* 2008; **8**: 17.

7. **Sundquist K, Frank G, Sundquist J.** Urbanisation and incidence of psychosis and depression. *The British Journal of Psychiatry* 2004; **184**: 293–298.

8. **Bhugra D, Mastrogianni A.** Globalisation and mental disorders: overview with relation to depression. *The British Journal of Psychiatry* 2004; **184**: 10–20.

9. **Davar BV.** *Mental Health of Indian Women: A Feminist Agenda.* New Delhi: Sage Publications, 1999.

10. **Davar BV** (ed.) *Mental Health from a Gender Perspective.* New Delhi: Sage Publications, 2001.

11. **Addalakha R.** *Deconstructing Mental Disorders: An Ethnography of Psychiatry, Women and the Family.* New Delhi: Zubaan Books, 2008.

12. **Kessler RC, Sonnega A, Bromet E, Hughes M, Nelson CB.** Posttraumatic stress disorder in the National Comorbidity Survey. *Archives of General Psychiatry* 1995; **52**: 1048–1060.

13. **Reddy MV, Chandrasekhar CR.** Prevalence of mental and behavioural disorders in India: a metanalysis. *Indian J Psychiatry* 1998; **40**: 149–157.

14. **Wright C, Nepal MK, Bruce Jones WD.** Mental health patients in PHC services in Nepal. *Journal of Institute Medicine* 1990; **12**: 65–74.

15. **Wolf KL, Flora K.** *Mental Health and Function—A Literature Review. Green Cities: Good Health* 2010. Seattle, WA: College of the Environment, University of Washington.

16. **Maitra S.** Status of Women in Mental Hospitals in Maharashtra. Unpublished Report. Mumbai: Tata Institute of Social Sciences, 2002. DOI: 10.13140/RG.2.2.11348.09604 (unpublished report).

17. **Onken SJ, Craig CM, Ridgway P, Ralph RO, Cook JA.** An analysis of the definitions and elements of recovery: a review of literature. *Psychiatric Rehabilitation Journal* 2007; **31**: 9–22.

18. **Onken SJ, Dumont JM, Ridgway P, Dornan DH, Ralph RO.** *Mental health REcovery: What Helps and What Hinders?* Alexandria, VA: National Technical Assistance Centre for State Mental Health Planning, 2002.

19. **Padgett DK, Henwood BF, Tsemberis SJ.** *Housing First: Ending Homelessness, Transforming Systems and Changing Lives.* Oxford, NY: Oxford University Press, 2016.

Chapter 23

Work, worklessness, and mental health

Jed Boardman and Tom K. J. Craig

Introduction

The relationships between work and health, both of which are important to individuals, communities, and economies, have long been a source of interest to medicine for many reasons: the value of work for health, as well as its hazards; the detrimental effects of lack of work; the use of work as a rehabilitative tool; and the connections of work and health to economic and social changes and to economic inequalities. In this chapter, we will look at the current evidence for the mental ill-effects of unemployment and the effects of economic cycles on employment and mental health. We also consider barriers to employment for people with mental health disorders and the evidence for schemes to improve employment opportunities for these people.

Work and employment

We usually contrast *work* with *leisure*. Work is traditionally seen as something that you do for others, and leisure activities as those where you can 'please yourself'. Work is an activity that involves the exercise of skills and judgement, taking place within set limits prescribed by others [1]. Many work activities may not provide financial rewards, for example childcare, housework, or looking after elderly or sick relatives, but *employment* is work you get paid for [2]. When considering worklessness, a distinction is often made between the 'unemployed' as referring to those out of work but looking for re-employment and the 'inactive' who are no longer in the job market. But, people who have been out of work for a long time when jobs are scarce, as during a widespread recession or from trades that are no longer wanted by society, may give up job searching but nevertheless suffer as much as others who meet the narrow definition.

Work, and particularly paid employment, is central to personal identity. In most social encounters, questions about occupation follow closely on who we are and how we reply to questions about our employment coveys a great deal about our social standing in the world, our wealth, and even whether we are likely to share common values with the enquirer. Employment provides financial rewards, structure, and purpose to the day, opportunities for socialization, and friendship. The social networks established in the workplace often extend beyond it and are a core component of social capital. It is therefore not that surprising that the loss of employment can be traumatic and precipitate mental illness, especially when unemployment is prolonged and where opportunities for returning to the labour market are curtailed. However, gaining employment can be beneficial to those suffering from mental health problems as it can offer a role valued by society with the potential benefits outlined earlier. It is hardly surprising, therefore, that people with mental health problems frequently put work at the top of their goals for life [3, 4].

Of course, there is a dark side to employment too. Much is now known about aspects of work environments that are bad for health [5]. Overcrowded, poorly ventilated 'sweatshops' that pay a pittance to their workers while demanding long hours of work, regardless of laws mandating minimum wages, still exist even in affluent societies [6]. Bullying in the workplace is another pernicious problem but one that is not always easy to identify where it emerges within an organizational culture that rewards managers based on the performance of the team they manage, leading to unfair pressure or 'punishment' of a low-performing team member [7]. For people who develop ill health while in work this may result in a period of sick leave ('absenteeism') or they may underperform at work ('presenteeism') and struggle on despite ill health, making matters worse both for themselves and the employer, who uncaring or unaware of the underlying health problem responds punitively to the perceived incompetence.

Job loss and unemployment as a cause of mental ill health

Cross-sectional studies typically find higher rates of common mental disorders (CMDs) such as depression and anxiety among the unemployed than among those in work, even after adjusting for age and sex [8]. Suicide rates are up to three times higher in the unemployed than in those in work, especially among the long-term unemployed, and the risk of suicide or attempted suicide is also greater in the long-term unemployed than those unemployed for a shorter time [9, 10]. Job loss can lead to problematic alcohol consumption for around one in five men and two in five women [11], and rises in alcohol consumption and alcohol-related deaths are reported during periods of economic strain [12–15].

However, causality is difficult to establish because the association is often bi-directional and difficult to disentangle. Mental disorder may be the response to job loss, but it can also be the underlying reason for unemployment. There are, however, several persuasive longitudinal studies. A systematic review identified 16 longitudinal studies carried out between 1986 and 1996, of which 12 reported sufficient data for meta-analysis. Of these, seven studies involving 1500 individuals looked at the effect of returning to work from a period of unemployment and found significant reductions in measures of CMD, with an overall effect size of 0.56. Five studies, with some 600 individuals, showed that the effect of moving from employment to unemployment was associated with worsening mental health albeit with a somewhat lower effect size of 0.36 [16]. More recently, data from five countries (UK, Australia, Canada, Switzerland, and South Korea) showed that becoming unemployed had a significant negative impact on mental health, particularly for men, whereas returning to work was associated with improved mental health [17].

Unemployment may have different impacts, depending on gender and the age at which it occurs. In an analysis of data collected as part of a Canadian national health survey with a two-year follow-up, becoming unemployed was associated with clinically significant depression among those aged 31–55 years but was not found in the under-30s of either sex [18]. Similarly, data from the Swedish Longitudinal Occupational Survey of Health compared the mental health of 196 workers who lost their jobs through redundancy when an employing organization 'downsized' to 1462 who held on to their jobs and 1845 employees in non-affected organizations. Job loss consistently predicted depression in both men and women. While there was also evidence for selection effects, it was striking that among those with pre-existing depression it was women not men who lost their jobs [19].

It seems reasonable to conclude that there is a causal association between losing employment and subsequent mental distress and ill health. Reasons for this include income loss, stigma, reduction of social networks, shame, loss of status, and subjective satisfaction gained through with employment [20]. Conversely, many studies show benefits of returning to work, although this may depend on the psychosocial quality of the job gained. Moving to a job with low psychosocial quality was no better, and may have even more adverse effects on mental health than remaining unemployed [21].

Effects of economic recessions

Mental ill health and suicide

One of the earliest scholarly studies of the consequences of job loss was reported by Marie Jahoda and colleagues [22], who described the impact of the closure of the 'Marienthal' factory on the population of the Austrian village of Gramatneusiedl in 1929. An effect of the Great Depression, the final closure of the factory left the village with 1300 of its approximately 1400 inhabitants without work. At the time of the survey these ex-industrial workers were getting by as allotment gardeners, collecting firewood, and rearing rabbits for the cooking pot. The majority were in a state of intense apathy, no longer utilizing the few opportunities that came along. Paul Lazerfeld, the project lead, subsequently migrated to the USA and continued his studies of mass unemployment, compiling more than 100 reports and concluding that such mass unemployment led, with near inevitability, to emotional instability, depression, hopelessness, and apathy, which, in turn, contributed to other social and interpersonal problems, including domestic discord [23].

These observations have been confirmed by many later studies. In the UK, around two in every five of those who lost their jobs in the 1991 and late 2008 recessions experienced mental health problems such as depression and anxiety [24]. The global financial crisis of 2008–9 was the deepest recession in the UK since World War II precipitating an upsurge in unemployment, debt, and housing repossessions that particularly affected young people and those at the bottom of the employment market, many of whom were already struggling with high levels of personal debt. As in previous recessions, the downturn was associated with increased rates of suicide and mental health problems. In England, there was a reversal in previously falling suicide rates, as well as increases in suicide attempts and depression, particularly in men [25]. A review of 287 suicides in that period showed about 14% could be attributed to unemployment and financial difficulties [26]. In some countries the impact was even worse, as, for example, in Greece, where suicides shot up by 60% [27].

The effects of a recession can show a lagging effect on unemployment [28]. For example, following the recession of the 1980s, it took 19 years before unemployment returned to the rate at the onset of the recession. After the recession of the 1990s, it took five years and nine months before unemployment returned to the rate at the onset. While most people move back into work swiftly, certain groups are more at risk of negative social outcomes as a consequence of the recession, including young men with low skills, younger couples on a low income who have high debts, and older men who lack transferable skills [28].

Wider impacts of a recession that influence health

In recessions, there are many social consequences that affect individuals, families, close social networks, and even entire communities [22–24, 28–31]. People who lost their job in 1991 and late 2008 were between 4–6 times more likely to find it difficult to get by financially than those who remained employed, with 24% reporting financial hardship for 3–6 years [24]. Unemployment increases the risk of marital dissolution by 70% [30]; Men and women who lose their jobs are 33% and 83%, respectively, more likely to experience relationship breakdown than those who stay in their jobs [31]. Family strain may increase the likelihood of domestic violence and child abuse [29]. Households that experience job loss are around three times more likely to be evicted from their accommodation than households that remained in employment [28]. People with mental health conditions are particularly vulnerable to accruing debts and debt can directly cause mental health problems [32]. Figures from the second British National Survey of Psychiatric Morbidity found that a quarter of people with common mental health problems, a third of those with a diagnosis of psychosis, a quarter of those with alcohol dependency, and over a third with drug dependency had debts compared with 8% of the general population [33].

These consequences have disproportionate effects on certain sections of society. Those who are poor or near the poverty line are likely to be hit the hardest. Other vulnerable groups include children and younger people, single-parent families, black and ethnic minorities, migrants, older people, and the mentally ill. A recession is likely to increase the social exclusion of these groups. There may be an impact on future generations: extreme poverty may affect the cognitive, emotional, and physical development of children with longer-term consequences on their health and well-being [34].

One psychological experience that links unemployment, receiving social security benefits, poverty, lack of basic necessities, and income inequality with poor mental health and stigma is that of shame [35–38]. It is shame 'that erodes the self-esteem, self-worth, agency and confidence that are essential to flourishing wellbeing' [38].

The impact of mental ill health on employment

In general, people with all forms of disability are more than twice as likely as non-disabled people to be without work [39]. This group contains many people with mental health conditions and those with intellectual disabilities. People with psychoses have particularly low levels of employment, lower than those with physical disabilities. While people with common mental health conditions, largely mild-to-moderate severity depression and anxiety, have higher levels of employment, these are still significantly lower than those of the general population [8, 40–41].

People with mental health conditions have more than double the risk of losing their jobs than people without mental health problems [42]. They represent the highest number of those claiming sickness and disability benefits [8].

Many people experience their first episode of a mental health problem in their late teens or early 20s, which can have serious consequences for their education and employment prospects [43]. In an economic downturn they have a lower re-entry rate into the labour market [44, 45].

Surveys in the UK have shown that adults with CMD were 4–5 times more likely than those without such a disorder to be permanently unable to work. Overall, 61% of men with one CMD and 46% with two disorders were working, compared with 77% of those with no disorder; the equivalent figures in women were 58%, 33%, and 65%, respectively [40].

Rates of employment are much lower in people with a diagnosis of a psychosis, even where this is broadly defined to include full- or part-time open employment (working and supporting oneself with earnings only), as well as sheltered employment. A European study of people with schizophrenia who were in contact with psychiatric services in England, Germany, and France found that broad rates of all employment varied from 6.7% in London to 60% in Heilbronn, Germany, possibly reflecting the greater availability of vocational rehabilitation services in the latter. The rates for open employment were much lower, from 2.7% in London to 18.3% in Hemer, Germany. Rates also differed within countries, for example Leicester, in the East Midlands of England, had a broad employment rate of 19% and an open employment rate of 15.1% [46].

These variations in the employment rates for people with schizophrenia are dramatically demonstrated in a large population-based study in China [47]. This compared the employment rates of 370 people with schizophrenia in urban and rural areas. They found an overall open employment rate of 77.6%, with the rural rates of employment being three times that of the urban areas (93.9% vs 26.7%). In the rural areas, 90% of the jobs obtained by people with schizophrenia were as farmers or fishermen, (only one person in an urban area was thus employed). These striking differences could not be explained by differences in the severity of disorders between the urban and rural groups. Cultural and contextual factors may explain these contrasts. The rate of open employment in people with schizophrenia in the urban areas approximates to that found in Europe, suggesting that they may face similar barriers to employment. Rural China may provide a more supportive context for people with schizophrenia, for example, a plentiful availability of agricultural work, greater flexibility allowing fluctuations in disability to be accommodated, and the involvement of extended family networks. This contrasts with Europe, North America, and urban China, where employment is more formal, structured, and regulated.

The costs of mental ill health in the workplace

While unemployment is costly to individuals, families, communities, and the broader economy, mental ill health has a cost to employers. At any one time, nearly one in six of the workforce is affected by a CMD, and one in five if alcohol and drug dependence are also included. Approximately 137.3 million working days are lost as a result of sickness or injury in the UK in 2016 [48]. Common mental health problems contributed 15.8 million of these days, representing 11.5% of the total. Only 'minor illnesses', such as coughs and colds, (34.0 million days lost—24.8% of the total) and musculoskeletal problems (30.8 million days—22.4% of the total) exceeded this.

The costs of these disorders to businesses have been estimated to be in the order of £26 billion each year [49]. The bulk of these costs are made up by the loss in productivity that occurs when employees come to work but function at less than full capacity because of ill health ('presenteeism'): £15.1 billion a year. Sickness absence contributes £8.4 billion a year and £2.4 billion a year is spent in replacing staff who leave their jobs because of mental ill health.

Getting people with mental health problems into employment

Supported employment for people with severe mental disorders

Historically, work has played an important part of rehabilitation for people with severe mental health conditions. In the asylum era this typically involved unpaid work on the hospital farm or industrial unit. As the hospitals closed, these resources transformed into sheltered workshops and factories intended to provide training and work experience that would equip patients with the skills needed for open employment (jobs based in ordinary settings alongside others without disabilities and that are not reserved for people with disabilities). But, in practice, very few of those in this 'train then place' model ever achieved this goal. In contrast, two approaches have proven more effective. Firstly, are small businesses operating commercially in the open market that are set up to facilitate employment of people with mental health problems. Referred to variously as social enterprises, social firms, or affirmative businesses, all employees, whether or not disabled, are paid the going rate for the job they do. The disabled members can also hold managerial positions. While all are expected to operate as commercial enterprises, most also receive some state funding. Most provide jobs in service industry, catering, and manufacture. Although this model does provide properly paid work in the open market, they are small organizations addressing only part of the wider need [50]. The second model, 'supported employment', starts with the primary aim of helping people get into a job that pays at least the minimum wage and is available on the open market (i.e. not specifically set aside for people suffering from mental ill health).

The most widely researched supported employment approach is Individual Placement and Support (IPS) [51].

Based on eight principles (Box 23.1), a great deal of the effort of an IPS service is in finding job opportunities for clients, including working with potential employers to create suitable vacancies and providing ongoing support to the employee. There are now 17 international randomized trials providing positive evidence for the success of IPS in helping people achieve open employment [52]. IPS is cost-effective, has low dropout rates, and generates positive outcomes across several domains (into work quicker, work more hours per week, longer job tenure), and gives good personal outcomes, fewer hospital admissions, and quicker recovery [51]. Working in line with these eight principles ('fidelity to the model') results in better employment outcomes [51], while lack of fidelity hampers the success of IPS programmes and their dissemination [53]. Schemes have been designed to supply technical support to services and staff to aid the effective implementation of IPS [54, 55].

Such a high level of evidence for the value of IPS when used for people with severe mental illness is unusual in vocational rehabilitation studies, but, despite this, IPS schemes have proved difficult to implement internationally partly due

---

Box 23.1 The principles of Individual Placement and Support (IPS)-supported employment

1. Competitive employment is the primary goal.
2. Eligibility is based on patient choice.
3. Integration of vocational and clinical services.
4. Job search guided by individual preferences.
5. Personalized benefits counselling.
6. Rapid job search.
7. Systematic job development.
8. Time-unlimited support.

Adapted from Robert E. Drake, Gary R. Bond, and Deborah R. Becker, *Individual placement and support: an evidence-based approach to supported employment*, pp. 33–38. Copyright (2012) by permission of Oxford University Press, USA.

to low expectations, but also structural factors [56]. These include labour market fluctuations [57]. For example, as high local unemployment rates reduce the effectiveness of these programmes [58, 59], although even in these conditions the IPS schemes perform better than control conditions. Other structural factors, such as the levels of tax on labour or regulations on job security, reduce the likelihood of employers taking on workers with mental health problems [57, 58]. The 'benefits trap', where people lose payments when moving into paid work, is another barrier. In general, social security systems need to be sufficiently flexible to encourage people with fluctuating conditions to enter employment while protecting them in periods of crisis and avoiding unnecessary coercion (e.g. benefit payment sanctions) and problems such as in-work poverty.

Moving people with common mental health conditions off benefits

Since the early 2000s consecutive UK governments have made changes to the social security systems to reduce the number of people receiving invalidity benefits and to encourage more people with health conditions into work. Many of these policy initiatives have been met with criticism. Changes to the assessment and eligibility criteria have been opposed by all disability groups as unjust, with sanctions said to have been disproportionately used for people with mental health conditions and the failure of these welfare-to-work programmes to get people with mental health conditions off benefits and into work [60–63]. A recent study across 149 local authorities in England showed an association between the number of welfare reassessments and rises in rates of suicide, mental health problems, and antidepressant prescribing, such that the adverse consequences seem to outweigh any benefit from moving people off disability allowances [64]. In contrast, countries with better social support through welfare policy show less evidence for the link between unemployment and suicide than countries with less comprehensive support [65], and there is good evidence for the benefit of active labour market programmes such as job clubs and targeted support for people who experience sudden job loss, as well as wider measures including more control over access to alcohol [66].

There have been no trials of IPS for people with common mental health conditions, but there is no reason to believe that this approach would not be helpful and has been suggested as a possible way forward in a recent report from RAND Europe [67].

Keeping people in work

The longer a person is off work due to sickness, the lower the likelihood of returning. Keeping people in work when they take time off for sickness reasons involves cooperation between the employer, employee, and clinician (and occupational health department, if this exists). In the UK, the general practitioner is the key clinician who signs the 'sick note' to excuse people from work because of their health condition. Employers use this as evidence of the validity of claims for sick pay and the State uses it as evidence for benefit claims. This system of sick certification has been criticized in recent years, because of the costs of sickness absence, its ineffectiveness in getting people back to work, and its failure to inform employers about the necessary adjustments that can be made to help people return to work [68]. A new 'Fit Note' certification was introduced in 2012 to try and remedy some of these problems, but it did little for people with mental health conditions [69–72]. It was implemented without prior piloting and now requires a stronger evidence base to justify its continuation. Possible improvements include the addition of partial sickness absence, which has been successfully tested in Finland and Norway, and appears to be an effective way to improve a return to work [73, 74]. Unlike the fit note, partial sickness absence involves legislation that encourages the employee and the employer sign a fixed-term work contract for part-time work.

Part of the rationale for the changes to sickness certification was to improve discussions between doctors and patients about fitness to work and how best to return to work, for example by advising on 'reasonable adjustments' to the workplace. For many people with mental health problems these adjustments are concerned with helping them negotiate the social and interactional aspects of work and may involve changes in working hours or patterns, support with their workload, and support from others [75, 76]. Awareness of these, prompt treatment of the health condition, discussion of means of returning to work, and the provision of advice are all part of the clinician's role in helping keep people in work.

The changing nature of employment

Many of our assumptions about healthy work begin with the notion of employment stability: people leave school and find a job and are expected to remain with that employer in the long term, with some prospect of advancement and improved income with seniority. Large mining and manufacturing employers ran businesses targeted on primary domestic markets—automobiles in Detroit or coal mining in Britain. But globalization has brought unprecedented levels of international competition. Companies have moved operations to where labour costs were lower or were driven out of business. The development of robotics and information technologies also made many manual trades more or less redundant. The consequence of the climate of insecurity that results from these systemic changes is that the old 'permanent' positions are being replaced by greater numbers of temporary, part-time, and flexible employment, including so-called 'zero-hour' contracts in which people are placed on a contract under which the employer has no obligation to offer regular work and in which rights to paid holiday, maternity leave, or protection against unfair dismissal are not provided [77]. These jobs are low in psychosocial quality and many workers will have little or no sense of obligation to their employer. The result is potentially a far more mobile workforce with most people expecting to have several jobs in the course of their life and increasingly have to make their own arrangement for pensions. One consequence of these changes is said to be an increase in employment-related mental health problems [78, 79].

Traditionally, employment has been seen as providing a protection against poverty, but it may no longer provide such a guarantee. In the UK, there has been an increase in precarious employment and a rise in the number of households experiencing 'in-work poverty' [80]. Between 2004–5 and 2014–15, the risk of being in poverty has risen by 26.5% from 12.4% to 15.7% in working-age adults living in working households [81]. By 2015, 60% of people of all ages living in poverty were living in working households—over 3.8 million workers.

Conclusions

That there is a relationship between employment and health does not seem in doubt, but the nature of this is multifaceted. Unemployment, especially when prolonged, is bad for physical and mental health, reducing social networks and social functioning and sapping motivation and interest. In general, employment (or at least engaging in some valued or meaningful activity) has a positive effect on health and well-being. It provides more than just monetary reward, it also has non-financial, latent, gains. However, certain jobs, especially those with poor psychosocial quality, can be as bad for a person's mental health as unemployment.

People with mental health conditions, particularly those with long-term and severe conditions, are less likely to be in open employment than the general working-age population. Individuals with these conditions are especially sensitive to the negative effects of unemployment, highlighting the importance of structure and valued activity in their daily life. Stigma and discrimination play a significant role in producing the low employment rates seen in people with mental health problems and the workplace can provide a useful environment for tackling stigma and public education on mental health [82].

For people with mental health conditions, and for many people who are unemployed, vocational rehabilitation forms an important part of their recovery journey and contributes to their opportunities to participate in their communities [83, 84]. For mental health services, helping people to gain or retain good and appropriate work is a valid recovery goal. Supporting people into employment or other valued activities can improve their sense of hope and agency, as well as offering them important opportunities, all of which are key components in personal recovery [83].

References

1. **Bennett D.** The value of work in psychiatric rehabilitation. *Social Psychiatry* 1970; **5**: 224–230.

2. **Hartley JF.** The impact of unemployment upon the self-esteem of managers. *Journal of Occupational Psychology* 1980; **53**: 145–147

3. **Secker J, Grove B, Seebohm P.** Challenging barriers to employment, training and education for mental health clients: the client's perspective. *Journal of Mental Health* 2001; **10**: 395–404.

4. **Dunn EC, Wewiorski NJ, Rogers ES.** The meaning and importance of employment to people in recovery from serious mental illness: results of a qualitative study. *Psychiatric Rehabilitation Journal* 2008; **32**: 59–62.

5. **Dalton AJP.** *Safety, Health and Environmental Hazards in the Workplace.* London: Cassell, 1998.

6. **U.S. Government Accountability Office.** Garment Industry: Efforts to Address the Prevalence and Conditions of Sweatshops. Available at: http://www.gao.gov/products/HEHS-95-29 (accessed 16 June 2017).

7. **Sewell G, Wilkinson B.** Empowerment or emasculation? Shopfloor surveillance in a Total Quality Organization. In: **P Blyton, P Turnbull** (eds) *Reassessing Human Resource Management.* London: Sage, 1992, pp. 97–115.

8. **McManus S, Bebbington P, Jenkins R, Brugha T.** (eds) Adult Psychiatric Morbidity Survey 2014: Survey of Mental Health and Wellbeing, England, 2014. Available at: https://digital.nhs.uk/data-and-information/publications/statistical/adult-psychiatric-morbidity-survey/adult-psychiatric-morbidity-survey-survey-of-mental-health-and-wellbeing-england-2014 (accessed 28 November 2018).

9. **Platt S, Hawton K.** Suicidal behaviour and the labour market. In: **K Hawton, K van Heeringen** (eds) *The International Handbook of Suicide and Attempted Suicide.* Chichester: Wiley, 2000, pp. 309–384.

10. **Maki N, Martikainen P.** A register-based study on excess suicide mortality among unemployed men and women during different levels of unemployment in Finland. *Journal of Epidemiology and Community Health* 2012; **66**: 302–307.

11. **Eliason M, Storrie D.** Job loss is bad for your health—Swedish evidence on cause-specific hospitalisation following involuntary job loss. *Social Science & Medicine* 2009; **68**: 1396–1406.

12. **Norström T, Ramstedt M.** Mortality and population drinking: a review of the literature. *Drug and Alcohol Review* 2005; **24**: 537–547.

13. **Zaridze D, Brennan P, Boreham J, Boroda A, Karpov R, Lazarev A,** et al. Alcohol and cause-specific mortality in Russia: a retrospective case-control study of 48,557 adult deaths. *The Lancet* 2009; **373**: 2201–2214.

14. **Dee TS.** Alcohol abuse and economic conditions: evidence from repeated cross-sections of individual-level data. *Health Econoics* 2001; **10**: 257–270.
15. **Johansson E, Böckerman P, Prättälä R, Uutela A.** Alcohol-related mortality, drinking behavior, and business cycles: are slumps really dry seasons? *The European Journal of Health Economics* 2006; **7**: 215–220.
16. **Van Der Noordt M, Ijzelenberg H, Droomers M, Proper KI.** Health effects of employment: a systematic review of prospective studies. *Journal of Occupational and Environmental Medicine* 2014; **71**: 730–736.
17. **Organisation for Economic Co-operation and Development.** Are all jobs good for your health? The impact of work status and working conditions on mental health. Available at: https://www.oecd-ilibrary.org/employment/oecd-employment-outlook-2008/are-all-jobs-good-for-your-health-the-impact-of-work-status-and-working-conditions-on-mental-health_empl_outlook-2008-6-en (accessed 28 November 2018).
18. **Breslin FC, Mustard C.** Factors influencing the impact of unemployment on mental health among young and older adults in a longitudinal, population-based survey. *Scandinavian Journal of Work, Environment and Health* 2003; **29**: 5–14.
19. **Andreeva E, Magnusson Hanson LL, Westerlund H, Theorell T, Brenner MH.** Depressive symptoms as a cause and effect of job loss in men and women: evidence in the context of organisational downsizing from the Swedish Longitudinal Occupational Survey of Health. *BMC Public Health* 2015; **15**: 1045.
20. **Helliwell JF, Putnam RD.** The social context of well-being. *Philosophical Transactions of the Royal Society of London. Series B, Biological Sciences* 2004; **359**: 1435–1446.
21. **Butterworth P, Leach LS, Strazdins L, Olesen SC, Rodgers B, Broom DH.** The psychosocial quality of work determines whether employment has benefits for mental health: results from a longitudinal national household panel survey. *Occupational and Environmental Medicine* 2011; **68**: 806–812.
22. **Jahoda M, Lazarfeld PF, Zeisel H.** *Marienthal: The Sociography of an Unemployed Community* (J Reginall, T Elsasser, English translation). London: Tavistock, 1974.
23. **Eisenberg P, Lazarfeld PF.** The psychological effects of unemployment *Psychological Bulletin* 1938; **35**: 358–390.
24. **Barnes M, Mansour A, Tomaszewski W, Oroyemi P.** Social impacts of recession: the impact of job loss and job insecurity on social disadvantage. *National Centre for Social Research* 2009; **39**: 1–25.
25. **Gunnell D, Donovan J, Barnes M, Davies R, Hawton K, Kapur N,** et al. The 2008 Global Financial Crisis: effects on mental health and suicide. Policy Report 3/2015. Available at: http://www.awp.nhs.uk/media/757861/policyreport-3-suicide-recession.pdf (accessed 28 November 2018).
26. **Coope C, Donovan J, Wilson C, Barnes M, Metcalfe C, Hollingworth W,** et al. Characteristics of people dying by suicide after job loss, financial difficulties and other economic stressors during a period of recession (2010–2011): a review of coroners' records. *Journal of Affective Disorders* 2015; **183**: 98–105.
27. **Kentikelenis A, Karanikolos N, Papanicolas, Basu S, McKee M, Stuckler D.** Health effects of financial crisis: omens of a Greek tragedy. *The Lancet* 2011; **378**: 1457–1458.
28. **Social Exclusion Task Force.** *Learning from the Past: Tackling Worklessness and the Social Impacts of Recession.* London: Cabinet Office, 2009.

29. **Wahlbeck K, McDaid D.** Actions to alleviate the mental health impact of the economic crisis. *World Psychiatry* 2012; **11**: 139–145.

30. **Lampard R.** An examination of the relationship between marital dissolution and unemployment. In: G Gallie, C March, C Vogler (eds) *Social Change and the Experience of Unemployment*: Oxford: Oxford University Press, 1994, pp. 264–298.

31. **Blekesaune M.** Unemployment and Partnership Dissolution. Working Paper Series. Colchester: Institute for Social and Economic Research, 2008.

32. **Fitch C, Chaplin R, Trend C, Collard S.** Debt and mental health: the role of psychiatrists *Advances in Psychiatric Treatment* 2007; **13**: 194–202.

33. **Jenkins R, Bhugra D, Bebbington P, Brugha T, Farrell M, Coid J,** et al. Debt, income and mental disorder in the general population. *Psychological Medicine* 2008; **38**: 1485–1493.

34. **Marmot MG, Bell R.** How will the financial crisis affect health? *BMJ* 2009; **338**: b1314. doi:10.1136/bmj.b1314.

35. **Jones C, Burstrom B, Marttila A, Canvin K, Whitehead M.** Studying social policy and resilience in families facing adversity in different welfare state: Britain and Sweden. *International Journal of Health Services* 2006; **36**: 425–442.

36. **Wilkinson RG, Pickett KE.** The enemy between us: the psychological and social costs of inequality. *European Journal of Social Psychology* 2017; **47**: 11–24.

37. **Walker R, Kyomuhendo GB, Chase E,** et al. Poverty in global perspective: is shame a common denominator? *Journal of Social Policy* 2013; **42**: 215–233.

38. **Friedli L.** *Mental Health, Resilience and Inequalities*. Copenhagen: WHO Regional Office for Europe, 2009.

39. **All Party Parliamentary Group on Disability.** *Ahead of the Arc – A Contribution to Halving the Disability Employment Gap*. London: All Party Parliamentary Group on Disability, 2016.

40. **Marwaha S, Johnson S.** Schizophrenia and employment. *Social Psychiatry and Psychiatric Epidemiology* 2004; **39**: 337–349.

41. **Meltzer H, Gill B, Petticrew M.** *OPCS Surveys of Psychiatric Morbidity in Great Britain. Report No. 3. Economic Activity and Social Functioning of Adults with Psychiatric Disorders*. London: HMSO, 1995.

42. **Boardman J.** Work, employment and psychiatric disability. *Advances in Psychiatric Treatment* 2003; **9**: 327–334.

43. **Kim-Cohen J, Caspi A, Moffitt TE, Harrington H, Milne BJ, Poulton R.** Prior juvenile diagnoses in adults with mental disorder: developmental follow-back of a prospective longitudinal cohort. *Archives of General Psychiatry* 2003; **60**: 709–717.

44. **Gardiner L, Gaffney D.** *Retention deficit. A new approach to boosting employment for people with health problems and disabilities*. London: Resolution Foundation, 2016.

45. **Farre L, Fasani F, Mueller H.** *Feeling Useless. The Effects of Unemployment on Mental Health in the Great Recession. Working Paper 774*. London: Queen Mary University of London, 2015.

46. **Marwaha S, Johnson S, Bebbington P, Stafford M, Angermeyer MC, Brugha T,** et al. Rates and correlates of employment in people with schizophrenia in the UK, France and Germany. *British Journal of Psychiatry* 2007; **191**: 30–37.

47. **Yang LH, Phillips MR, Li X, Yu G, Zhang J, Shi Q**, et al. Employment outcome for people with schizophrenia in rural v. urban China: population-based study. *British Journal of Psychiatry* 2013; **203**: 272–279.

48. **Office for National Statistics (ONS).** *Sickness Absence in the Labour Market: 2016. Analysis Describing Sickness Absence Rates of Workers in the UK Labour Market.* London: ONS, 2017.

49. **Sainsbury Centre for Mental Health.** *Mental Health at Work: Developing the Business Case. Policy Paper 8.* London: Sainsbury Centre for Mental Health, 2007.

50. **Gilbert E, Marwaha S, Milton A, Johnson S, Morant N, Parsons N**, et al. Social firms as a means of vocational recovery for people with mental illness: a UK survey. *BMC Health Services Research* 2013; **13**: 270.

51. **Drake R, Bond G, Becker DR.** *Individual Placement and Support: An Evidence-based Approach to Supported Employment.* Oxford: Oxford University Press, 2012.

52. **Modini M, Tan L, Brinchmann B, Wang M-J, Killackey E, Glozier N**, et al. Supported employment for people with severe mental illness: systematic review and meta-analysis of the international evidence. *British Journal of Psychiatry* 2016; **209**: 14–22.

53. **Bond GR, Drake RE, Becker DR.** Generalizability of the Individual Placement and Support (IPS) model of supported employment outside the US. *World Psychiatry* 2012; **11**: 32–39.

54. **Becker DR, Drake RE, Bond GR, Nawaz S, Haslett WR, Martinez RA.** Best practices: a national mental health learning collaborative on supported employment. *Psychiatric Services* 2011; **62**: 704–706.

55. **Centre for Mental Health.** *Implementing What Works: The Impact of the Individual Placement and Support Regional Trainer.* London: Centre for Mental Health, 2012.

56. **Boardman J, Rinaldi M.** Difficulties in implementing supported employment for people with severe mental health problems. *British Journal of Psychiatry* 2013; **203**: 247–249.

57. **Warner R.** *Recovery from Schizophrenia: Psychiatry and Political Economy.* 3rd ed. Abingdon: Brunner-Routledge, 2004.

58. **Cook JA, Blyler CR, Leff HS, McFarlane WR, Goldberg RW, Gold PB**, et al. The employment intervention demonstration program: major findings and policy implications. *Psychiatric Rehabilitation Journal* 2008; **31**: 291–295.

59. **Burns T, Catty J, Becker T, Drake RE, Fioritti A, Knapp M**, et al. The effectiveness of supported employment for people with severe mental illness: a randomised controlled trial in six European countries. *The Lancet* 2007; **370**: 1146–1152.

60. **Hale C.** *Fulfilling Potential? ESA and the Fate of the Work-Related Activity Group.* London: Mind, 2014.

61. **National Audit Office.** *Benefit Sanctions.* London: National Audit Office, 2016.

62. **Dorsett R.** *Pathways to Work for New and Repeat Incapacity Benefits Claimants: Evaluation Synthesis Report. Research Report No 525.* London: Department for Work and Pensions, 2008.

63. **McCartney M.** The disturbing truth about disability assessments. *BMJ* 2012; **345**: e5347.

64. **Bar B, Taylor-Robinson D, Stuckler D, Loopstra R, Reeves A, Whitehead M.** 'First do no harm': are disability assessments associated with adverse trends in mental health?

A longitudinal ecological study. *Journal of Epidemiology and Community Health* 2016; **70**: 39–345.

65. Stuckler D, King L, McKee M. Mass privatisation and the post-community mortality crisis: a cross-national analysis. *The Lancet* 2009; **373**: 399–407.

66. Haw C, Hawton K, Gunnell D, Platt S. Economic recession and suicidal behaviour: possible mechanism and ameliorating factors. *International Journal of Social Psychiatry* 2015; **61**: 73–81.

67. van Stolk C, Hofman J, Hafner M, Janta B. *Psychological Wellbeing and Work: Improving Service Provision and Outcomes*. London: Department of Work and Pensions, Department of Health, 2014.

68. Black C, Frost D. *Health at Work—An Independent Review of Sickness Absence*. Norwich: The Stationery Office, 2011.

69. Department for Work and Pensions (DWP). *Evaluation of the Statement of Fitness for Work (Fit Note): Quantitative Survey of Fit Notes. Research Report No 841*. London: DWP, 2013.

70. Shiels C, Gabbay M, Hillage J. Factors associated with prevalence and types of 'may be fit' advice on fit notes: a cross-sectional primary care analysis. *British Journal of General Practice* 2014; **64**: e137–e143.

71. Department for Work and Pensions. An evaluation of the Statement of Fitness for Work (fit note): quantitative survey of fit notes. Research Report 841. Available at: https://www.gov.uk/government/publications/evaluation-of-the-statement-of-fitness-for-work-fit-note-quantitative-survey-of-fit-notes-rr-841 (accessed 28 November 2018).

72. Gabbay M, Shiels C, Hillage J. Sickness certification for common mental disorders and GP return-to-work advice. *Primary Health Care Research & Development* 2016; **17**: 437–447.

73. Kausto J, Viikari-Juntura E, Virta LJ, Gould R, Koskinen A, Solovieva S. Effectiveness of new legislation on partial sickness benefit on work participation: a quasi-experiment in Finland. *BMJ Open* 2014; **4**: e006685.

74. Markussen S, Mykletun A, Røed K. The case for presenteeism—evidence from Norway's sickness insurance program. *Journal of Public Economics* 2012; **96**: 959–972.

75. Boardman J. Work and employment. In: Holloway F, Kaladindi S, Killaspy H, Roberts G. (eds) *Enabling Recovery*. 2nd ed. London: RCPsych Publications, 2015, pp. 308–323.

76. Perkins R, Farmer P, Litchfield P. *Realising Ambitions: Better Employment Support for People with a Mental Health Condition*. London: Department for Work and Pensions, 2009.

77. Taylor M. *Good Work: The Taylor Review of Modern Working Practices*. London: Department for Business, Energy & Industrial Strategy, 2017.

78. Benach J and Muntaner C. Precarious employment and health: developing a research agenda. *Journal of Epidemiology and Community Health* 2007; **61**: 276.

79. Murphy GC, Athanasou JA. The effect of unemployment on mental health. *Journal of Occupational and Organizational Psychology* 1999; **72**: 83–99.

80. Tinson A, Ayrton C, Barker K, Born TB, Aldridge H, Kenway P. *Monitoring Poverty and Social Exclusion 2016*. York: Joseph Rowntree Foundation, 2016.

81. **Hick R, Lanau A.** *In-work Poverty in the UK: Problem, Policy Analysis and Platform for Action.* Cardiff: Cardiff University, 2017.

82. **Evans-Lacko S, Henderson C, Thornicroft G.** Public knowledge, attitudes and behaviour regarding people with mental illness in England 2009–2012. *British Journal of Psychiatry* 2013; **202** (Suppl. 55): s51–s57.

83. **Shepherd G, Boardman J, Slade M.** *Making Recovery a Reality.* London: Sainsbury Centre for Mental Health, 2008.

84. **Boardman J, Currie A, Killaspy H, Mezey G.** *Social Inclusion and Mental Health.* London: RCPsych Publications, 2010.

Chapter 24

Conclusions

Dinesh Bhugra, Antonio Ventriglio,
João Castaldelli-Maia, and Layla McCay

It is apparent that the environment in which we are born in, live in, and work and play in has a major impact on our physical and mental health. Urban environment can impact on people's mental health and mental well-being, as well as physical health in a number of ways, and not all of these are entirely clear. It is apparent that biological vulnerabilities, which may be influenced by environmental factors, as well as social and psychological factors, will influence the mental health of individuals and the population as a whole. As this book has shown, some of these factors are clearly identifiable, whereas others are only beginning to emerge now. The relationship of the individual in the city and with the city can create conditions for better mental health. However, it can also contribute to mental ill health by taking away resilience and other protective factors such as social support. Unemployment, poverty, and overcrowding can strongly influence mental and physical health. Internal migration can further contribute to living in poor conditions with poorly paid jobs and job insecurity with low social support, which may make individuals more prone to mental ill health. Urban living for women and children undoubtedly carries differential risks. Epidemiological studies indicate that people living in cities have higher rates of psychiatric disorders but not of other disorders. This is not to say that rural living is idyllic, but there appear to be clear differences. It must be recognized that the physical environment of cities, such as pollution from vehicles, light pollution, and lack of clean and green spaces, may well further contribute to physical ill health, which may, in turn, contribute to poor mental health. As many of the authors in this volume have shown, green, active, pro-social, and safe spaces contribute to better mental health for people.

The reality is that in spite of best efforts researchers and clinicians can only do so much. The key to improving the mental health of the population lies in clinicians and physicians coming together with policymakers and urban planners.

In many cities—as shown in Vancouver, New York, and Tokyo—things are beginning to change, with cities taking clear responsibility in promoting and supporting good mental health as part of the overall health improvement. Thus, there are clear opportunities for urban planners and designers to improve population mental health through a number of strategies that help build resilience and foster protective factors for good mental health. As Layla McCay illustrated in Chapter 3, the World Health Organization defines public health as 'the art and science of preventing disease, prolonging life and promoting health through the organized efforts of society'. It is crucial that in a rapidly urbanizing world, urban mental health and urban public mental health take on the importance they deserve in order to prioritize the promotion of mental health and well-being for their citizens through better designs and better urban planning. Such an approach is critical at population, local, regional and national or federal, and at international levels.

We do not need to repeat the statistics regarding the number of people living in urban areas or the potential numbers developing mental illness and the resulting burden of disease. Thus, it is self-evident that investment is needed in developing cities that are dweller-friendly and help reduce mental illness and distress. The scale and potential impact of urban mental health problems is truly massive and challenging, but there is no doubt that a lot can be achieved if suitable partnerships are developed. Of course, cities by themselves are not responsible for the mental ill health of dwellers, as genetic, biological, psychological, social, and environmental factors can all interact at various levels and contribute to the development of mental disorders. As various contributors to this volume have argued persuasively, that just as the causes of mental health problems are multifactorial, so too are the solutions, which also require multidisciplinary approaches.

Life in the city, as with life elsewhere carries with it factors that exert both positive and negative influences on mental health. Cities also offer education and economic opportunities, and cultural enrichment, along with a wide variety of housing and transport options to suit different incomes and needs. Cities can also provide sexual and ethnic diversity, more health and social services, and more support services for people with drug and alcohol addictions, along with a range of opportunities that may be less accessible in the rural areas and can contribute to good mental health.

It is entirely possible that vulnerable individuals move to the anonymity of cities and perhaps cheaper accommodation. Disparities and segregation in cities may add to vulnerability, and overcrowding and lack of personal and individual space may further add to stress. Cities also tend to take away protective factors such as social support and move from joint families to nuclear families, creating further difficulties. As McCay argues persuasively in this volume, the complexity of mental disorder aetiology tends to give urban designers implicit permission to dismiss any mental health promotion responsibilities. People may come to the city with their own personal vulnerabilities but it is not beyond the realm of possibility that urban planning and design can mitigate and modify risk factors to create a setting that exerts a potential positive impact on people's mental health. Of course, urban planners cannot mitigate the risk of genetic factors or unemployment, but across several generations it must be possible to create an affordable, reliable, and safe public transport system, which helps people seeking jobs and able to commute, thereby increasing opportunities.

Green spaces, the ability to carry out physical activities and exercises, and opportunities for better social interaction and sense of safety in the city should be considered as paramount factors in improving the mental health of city dwellers. Therefore, the evidence for factors that contribute to mental ill health needs to be employed in urban settings, and all the design effort should focus on simple things like reducing commute duration and stressfulness; increasing leisure, social, and sleep time; increasing physical activity; and increasing connectivity and public gathering spaces that are accessible and safe. Furthermore, walkways and bikeways to enable safe, convenient, efficient, and cost-effective transit around the city, along with safe cycle lanes and pedestrianized zones, will improve physical and mental health. There is no doubt that, depending upon the size of the city and the size of the population, each city may have to develop individual solutions, but it is important to learn from examples of good practice and yet ensure local ownership meeting local needs.

Index

Tables, figures, and boxes are indicated by an italic *t*, *f*, and *b* following the page number.

individual responses, potential 306
internal migration 66
  refugees 75, 76, 78
  sex 250, 252
  Tokyo 284, 286, 291–4, 295, 297
  urban design 35–6, 42–4
  urbanization 84, 86
  urban mental health strategies 316
social isolation 305–6, 317*t*
  crime 310
  gender and sexual minorities 261
  happiness, self-reported 179
  internal migration 61
  psychogenic city 126
  research approaches 157
  suicide 240, 242, 243
  Tokyo 283–4
  unemployment 339
  urban design 35–6, 42
social media
  adolescents 194
  internal migration 65, 67
  sex 249, 250, 253, 255
  urbanization 86
social phobia 228
social psychology 152, 156, 164
social services
  supported employment 345
  urban mental health strategies 316
social stress
  common mental disorders 231
  psychoses 134*t*, 138–9, 156, 157
social support, fragmentation of 5
sociodemographic characteristics, psychogenic
  city 133*t*, 137
socio-economic status 34–5
  adolescent mental health 195
  globalization and urbanization 53
  inequalities 59
  New York 280
  psychogenic city 129
  urbanization 85
  see also low income; poverty
sociology 6–7, 16–31, 154, 155, 164
  Chicago School 6, 16–18, 19, 122
  neo-Marxism 18–20
Somalia 76, 77, 78
somatic neurosis 228
somatization, immigrants 54
somatoform disorders 227, 228–9, 235
South Africa 260
  see also Johannesburg
South Korea 158, 241–2, 243–4, 339
space
  and power 22–8
  see also private spaces; public spaces
Spain 128
  see also Madrid

Sri Lanka 242
stigma
  city living, US 179
  dementia 295
  gender and sexual minorities 259, 261
  Indian women with mental disorders 325,
    327, 330, 333, 335
  marginalization 104–5
  migrants 62, 68, 159
  sexually transmitted infections 103
  sex workers 254
  Thrive NYC 280
  Tokyo, mental ill health in 284, 296
  unemployment 339, 341, 347
  urban design 35
stimulation, excessive 308–9, 317*t*
Stockholm 55
street children 53
stress 190–1, 308–9, 317*t*, 355–6
  acculturative 62
  adolescents 189, 191, 192, 193, 196, 198
  air pollution 89
  common mental disorders 226, 227, 228–9,
    230, 231–2, 235
  commuting 41, 175, 314
  economic *see* poverty
  gender and sexual minorities 259–60, 261
  globalization 51
  goal-striving 88
  green spaces 38, 39
  marginalization 97
  migrants 60–5, 68, 69, 170
  neuroscience 117, 141, 143, 239
  physical activity 40
  post-traumatic stress disorder 74, 293
  psychogenic city 122, 134*t*, 136, 138–9,
    141, 143
  psychoses 155–61, 163
  research challenges 170, 174, 178, 180
  rural–urban migration 173
  sex workers 254
  shinrin yoku (forest bathing) 288
  social *see* social stress
  Tokyo 284, 288, 289, 290, 293, 294, 296
  urban design 38, 39, 40, 41, 90
  urbanization 51, 85, 87–8, 324
  work-related 232
stress reduction theory 38
substance abuse 34, 232, 304–5, 317*t*
  association versus causation 304–5
  children, in Mexico City 221, 223
  community responses, potential 305
  concentrated mental illness risk factors 304
  and crime 310
  diagnostic issues 51
  employment 343
  gender and sexual minorities 259, 260,
    263, 265